Female Sexual Pain Disorders

We dedicate this book to those people who are most important in our lives: our patients, past, present, and future, who have and continue to suffer from sexual pain; our mentors, Stanley Marinoff, Irv Binik, and Robert J. Krane, who both taught and inspired us to follow in their paths and continue on our own; and most especially our families; our spouses Gail Goldstein, Michael Roberts and Sue Goldstein, children Lena, Mimi, Julia, Connor, Bryan, Lauren, and Andrew, and our parents with appreciation for their love, support and faith in us.

Female Sexual Pain Disorders

EDITED BY

Andrew T. Goldstein, MD
Department of Obstetrics and Gynecology
George Washington University School of Medicine and Health Sciences
Washington, DC, USA

Caroline F. Pukall, PhD
Department of Psychology
Queen's University
Kingston, Ontario, Canada

Irwin Goldstein, MD
Sexual Medicine, Alvarado Hospital
Department of Surgery, University of California at San Diego
San Diego, CA, USA

FOREWORD BY

Yitzchak M. Binik, PhD

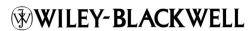

WILEY-BLACKWELL
A John Wiley & Sons, Ltd., Publication

Contents

Contents

List of Contributors

Premlatha Amalraj
The Women's Health Institute
New Brunswick, NJ, USA

Alison Amsterdam
Mount Sinai Medical Center
New York, NY, USA

Stanley J. Antolak, Jr.
Center for Urologic and Pelvic Pain
Lake Elmo, MN, USA

Gloria A. Bachmann
The Women's Health Institute
New Brunswick, NJ, USA

Lorraine Benuto
Department of Psychology
University of Nevada
Las Vegas, NV, USA

Sophie Bergeron
Department of Sexology
Université du Québec à Montréal
Montréal, Québec, Canada

Vanda Bianco
Outpatient Department of Vulvar Disease
V. Buzzi Hospital, Milan, Italy

Yitzchak M. Binik
Department of Psychology McGill University
Sex and Couple Therapy Service,
McGill University Health Centre
Montréal, Québec, Canada

Lori A. Boardman
University of Central Florida College of Medicine
Orlando, FL, USA

Jacob Bornstein
The Rappaport Faculty of Medicine
Hatechnion University
Nahariya, Israel

Stéphanie C. Boyer
Department of Psychology
Queen's University, Kingston, Ontario, Canada

Joe Brooks
The Arizona Vulva Clinic
Phoenix, AZ, USA

Lara J. Burrows
The Center for Vulvovaginal Disorders
Washington, DC, USA

Nadya M. Cinman
The Smith Institute for Urology
Long Island Jewish Medical Center
New York, NY, USA

Matthew F. Davies
Department of Obstetrics and Gynecology
Penn State University, College of Medicine
Hershey PA, USA

Gordon Davis
The University of Arizona School of Medicine
Phoenix, AZ, USA

Don Dizon
Brown Medical School and Women &
    Infants' Hospital of Rhode Island
Providence, RI, USA

Robyn L. Donaldson
Department of Psychology
University of Nevada, Las Vegas, NV, USA

Douglas A. Drossman
UNC Center for Functional GI and Motility Disorders
University of North Carolina
Chapel Hill, NC, USA

Jennifer Droz
Advanced Laparoscopy
University of Rochester Medical Center
Rochester, NY, USA

Melissa A. Farmer
Department of Psychology
McGill University, Montréal, Québec, Canada

David C. Foster
University of Rochester School of Medicine and Dentistry
Rochester, NY, USA

Nancy D. Gaba
The George Washington University Medical Center
Washington, DC, USA

David Goldmeier
St Mary's Hospital, Imperial College Healthcare NHS Trust
London, UK

Gail R. Goldstein
Annapolis Dermatology Center
Annapolis, MD, USA

Andrew T. Goldstein
Department of Obstetrics and Gynecology
George Washington University School of
    Medicine and Health Sciences
Washington, DC, USA

Irwin Goldstein
Sexual Medicine
Alvarado Hospital, San Diego, CA, USA

Allan S. Gordon
Wasser Pain Management Center
University of Toronto, Toronto, Ontario, Canada

Alessandra Graziottin
Center of Gynecology and Medical Sexology
H. San Raffaele Resnati
Milan, Italy

Hope K. Haefner
Department of Obstetrics and Gynecology
University of Michigan Medical Center
Ann Arbor, MI, USA

Dee Hartmann
Dee Hartmann Physical Therapy for Women
Chicago, IL, USA

Richard D. Hayes
University of Melbourne
Melbourne, Australia

Fred M. Howard
Division of Obstetrics and Gynecology
University of Rochester School of
    Medicine and Dentistry
Rochester, NY, USA

Chad Huckabay
The Smith Institute for Urology
Long Island Jewish Medical Center
New York, NY, USA

Crista Johnson
Maricopa Integrated Health System
Southwest Interdisciplinary Research Center
    Arizona State University
Phoenix, AZ, USA

Sarah Kelly
The Women's Health Institute
New Brunswick, NJ, USA

Colleen M. Kennedy
University of Iowa
Iowa City, IA, USA

Michael L. Krychman
Hoag Hospital
Newport Beach, CA, USA

Angela S. Kueck
Division of Obstetrics and Gynecology
University of Michigan Medical Center
Ann Arbor MI, USA

Tina Landry
Department of Psychology
Université du Québec à Montréal
Montréal, Québec, Canada

Catherine M. Leclair
Oregon Health & Science University
Portland, OR, USA

Bianca Leclerc
Department of Psychology
Université du Québec à Montréal
Montréal, Québec, Canada

Ahinoam Lev-Sagie
Department of Obstetrics and Gynecology
Division of Immunology and Infectious Diseases
Weill Medical College of Cornell University
New York, NY, USA

Colin MacNeill
Department of Obstetrics and Gynecology
Penn State University, College of Medicine
Hershey, PA, USA

Phyllis Mate
National Vulvodynia Association
Silver Spring, MD, USA

Marta Meana
Department of Psychology
University of Nevada
Las Vegas, NV, USA

Alison Mears
Genitourinary and Sexual Medicine
St Mary's Hospital, Imperial College
    Healthcare NHS Trust
London, UK

Gaby Moawad
The George Washington University
Washington, DC, USA

Jeffrey S. Mogil
Department of Psychology
McGill University
Montréal, Québec, Canada

Robert M. Moldwin
The Smith Institute for Urology
Long Island Jewish Medical Center
New York, NY, USA

Filippo Murina
Outpatient Department of Vulvar Disease
V. Buzzi Hospital, Milan, Italy

Paul Nyirjesy
Drexel University College of Medicine
Philadelphia, PA, USA

Ann Partridge
Dana-Farber Cancer Institute
Boston, MA, USA

Philip W.H. Peng
Toronto Western Hospital &
    Wasser Pain Management Center
University of Toronto
Toronto, Ontario, Canada

Caroline F. Pukall
Department of Psychology
Queen's University
Kingston, Ontario, Canada

Gianluigi Radici
Outpatient Department of Vulvar Disease
V. Buzzi Hospital, Milan, Italy

Barbara D. Reed
Department of Family Medicine
University of Michigan Health System
Ann Arbor, MI, USA

Elke D. Reissing
School of Psychology
University of Ottawa
Ottawa, Ontario, Canada

John T. Repke
Department of Obstetrics and Gynecology
Penn State University, College of Medicine
Hershey, PA, USA

Jennifer M. Rhode
Department of Obstetrics and Gynecology
Wright-Patterson Medical Center
Dayton, OH, USA

Talli Y. Rosenbaum
Urogynecological Physiotherapy Private Practice

Caitlin Shaw
Pelvic Pain Research Unit
University of North Carolina
Chapel Hill, NC, USA

Mario Sideri
Preventive Gynecology Unit
European Institute of Oncology
Milan, Italy

Kelly B. Smith
Department of Psychology
Queen's University
Kingston, Ontario, Canada

Jack D. Sobel
Division of Infectious Diseases
Wayne State University School of Medicine
Detroit, MI, USA

Susan Kellogg Spadt
Drexel University College of Medicine
Philadelphia, PA, USA

Ami D. Sperber
Department of Gastroenterology
Soroka Medical Center, Faculty of Health Sciences
Ben-Gurion University of the Negev
Beer-Sheva, Israel

Amy Stein
Beyond Basics Physical Therapy
New York, NY, USA

Katherine S. Sutton
Department of Psychology
Queen's University, Kingston, Ontario, Canada

Rochele Torgerson
Mayo Clinic, Rochester, MN, USA

Christin Veasley
National Vulvodynia Association
Silver Spring, MD, USA

Kristene E. Whitmore
Pelvic and Sexual Health Institute
Drexel University College of Medicine
Philadelphia, PA, USA

Doron Zarfati
The Rappaport Faculty of Medicine
Hatechnion University
Nahariya, Israel

Denniz Zolnoun
University of North Carolina
Chapel Hill, NC, USA

Foreword

It is hard to find a topic in the field of human sexuality or pain where there are not already too many books. My typical reaction to a book proposal is that we do not need to rehash old ideas and data yet again; we need to produce some systematic new information or theories. When it comes to dyspareunia, I was dead wrong. As far as I can tell, there are no previously published (edited or authored) books on the topic of dyspareunia. This is an extraordinary and gaping hole in our scholarship and work. If you are not familiar with the impact of "sexual pain," read the chapters on the prevalence (Chapter 2) and relevance (Chapter 3) of dyspareunia and the physical and interpersonal suffering it causes (Chapters 5 and 31).

This volume is extraordinary in many other ways. Its comprehensive coverage of all aspects of dyspareunia research and therapy is unusual. It is not surprising that there are chapters on evaluation/assessment or on treatment options; this would be expected in most volumes of this type. It is also not surprising that there are three chapters on introital, vaginal, and deep dyspareunia. This reflects our current and somewhat limited understanding of how to classify the different dyspareunic syndromes.

It is surprisingly wonderful, however, to see the range of topics that the editors have included in their introductory, relevant aspects, and conclusion sections. As a former history student, I was overjoyed to see a chapter on the history of dyspareunia (Chapter 1). In the health sciences, we are constantly "reinventing" the wheel and forgetting what was previously learned. I was also very happy to see a chapter on the "Power of Patient Advocacy" (Chapter 38). The sad truth of this field is that we are not close to a cure and the importance of patient advocacy groups in providing support and information to the public and influencing those who control health care funding cannot be underestimated. Topics that have been ignored in the literature and clinical practice (e.g., postpartum dyspareunia, Chapter 34; cancer and dyspareunia, Chapter 33; genital

cutting, Chapter 36) receive attention in chapters written by experts. I was somewhat taken aback by a chapter entitled "Hidradenitis Supperurativa" (Chapter 10) because I had no clue what the term meant. I clearly have things to learn from this book even after working in this field for 20 years.

Not only is the coverage extraordinarily broad but so is the expertise. How many books have you seen that are co-edited by a psychologist, a urologist, and a gynecologist? I have been in a fair number of hospitals where these disciplines do not talk to one another let alone write books together.

Although each editor is already well known in this field, each brings a special type of experience and expertise to the preparation of this book. Andrew Goldstein is one the world's most perceptive clinician gynecologists when it comes to dyspareunia. Caroline Pukall has applied the methods of experimental psychology in innovative and striking ways to the study of genital pain. Irwin Goldstein has almost single-handedly shifted the focus of sexual medicine from a male-dominated perspective to a more egalitarian model. This multidisciplinary and multifaceted authorship encourages my hope that the new fields of sexual health/medicine will follow through on their stated goal of adopting a truly biopsychosocial perspective. In addition to the disciplines of the editors, there are chapters by epidemiologists, infectious disease specialists, physical therapists, lay patient advocates, neurologists, psychiatrists, and dermatologists. The message is clear: no one discipline has a monopoly on understanding dyspareunia.

Naturally, no book is without its faults, though I am hard pressed to find any serious ones in this volume. I could quibble with the medical treatment emphasis, which is not empirically based though I think this reflects current practice. I would have liked to see a chapter focussed on pain mechanisms, though this is dealt with in several chapters. I would have also liked to see a more life-span coverage of dyspareunia including separate chapters on dyspareunia in adolescence (Landry & Bergeron, in press) and postmenopausal dyspareunia (see Kao et al., in press).

Two chapters—"The Relevance of Dyspareunia" by Meana et al. and "The Future of Vulvodynia Research" by Foster—initially caught my attention because of their titles. I cannot remember the word "relevance" in many book titles. I also know that social and health scientists are abysmal at predicting the future of their own fields. Neither chapter, however, disappointed me; on the contrary, despite the fact that one was written by psychologists and the other by a gynecologist, they sounded remarkably alike. Both highlighted the need for improved classification/assessment and for the development of better outcome measures leading to more efficacious and empirically based multidisciplinary treatment. These chapters and the editors' preface all reflect the stridently biopsychosocial framework of this book. Hallelujah!

Basically, I am thankful to the editors who have put together virtually all of the world's expertise on dyspareunia into one volume. I will be proud to have this book on my shelf. There is little question in my mind that any clinician or researcher who is interested in dyspareunia will have to start here.

Yitzchak M. Binik, PhD

References

Kao A, Binik YM, Kapuscinski A, Khalifé S. (2008) Dyspareunia in postmenopausal women: a critical review. *Pain Research and Management* **13**, 243–54.

Landry T, Bergeron S. (in press) How young does vulvo-vaginal pain begin? Prevalence and characteristics of dyspareunia in adolescents. *The Journal of Sexual Medicine.*

Preface

It's all in your head … or is it? Historically, women have been told that the sexual pain they were experiencing was just that—in their heads. As soon as a woman complained to her health care provider about sexual pain, she was referred to a mental health professional, ignoring possible concomitant biologic concerns.

A total of 21% of women have sexual pain, but because it involves the genital region there is no one discipline devoted to the management and treatment of the pain. Providers have found it difficult to believe women's self-reports without objective testing. Today, we are studying the physiology of the brain with the ability to convert a descriptive field into one with outcomes assessment, including psychologic, neuronal, hormonal, and genetic testing. An animal model of genital pain for the purposes of researching pain assessment and management is now furthering our knowledge in the field. What was once considered purely psychologic can be paired with the biologic.

So how did the editors get involved in the study of pain? Andrew Goldstein started practice as a general gynecologist in 1998 with sufficient time with each patient to perform a review of systems including questions about the woman's sexual health: libido, pain, and orgasm. The number of women with sexual problems wanting help overwhelmed him. To gain further knowledge, Dr. Goldstein attended the Female Sexual Function Forum, the earlier name of the International Society for the Study of Women's Sexual Health (ISSWSH). There was little mention of sexual pain at that meeting. In 2001, while writing a chapter for the Johns Hopkins *Manual on Gynecology and Obstetrics*, Dr. Goldstein came across many references to vulvar pain written by a local practitioner, Stanley Marinoff, a leading vulvar pain specialist during the 1980s and 1990s. Dr. Goldstein spent time training with him and eventually took over his practice.

Dr. Pukall quickly realized that although sex was generally a forbidden subject, people had a lot of questions and misinformation about it. As a college and undergraduate student, she took every human sexuality course available, until one semester her interest in psychology and sexual health coalesced. In 1995, after taking courses in psychophysics, pain, and human sexuality simultaneously, young Dr. Pukall offered to work in Yitzchak Binik's laboratory. Her work as a research assistant with Sophie Bergeron gave Dr. Pukall an opportunity to observe participants undergoing the cotton swab test and to speak with them afterward to learn about their experiences. Dr. Pukall was left wondering why they had such severe pain despite their healthy looking vulvas. It was at this point that Dr. Pukall recognized her interest in studying this taboo topic, to prove that the pain from which these women suffered was not purely psychologic, and to be able to give something back to them.

In 1998, with the appearance of sildenafil, Irwin Goldstein started receiving phone calls from women seeking help for their sexual dysfunction. A percentage of these women presented with pain and were referred to their gynecologists, who generally sent them back. Initially, Dr. Goldstein thought pain was related to either blood flow or hormones, and found that some women were helped with hormone therapy. After attending the annual meetings of the Female Sexual Function Forum and then ISSWSH and listening to presentations by Yitzchak Binik, Sophie Bergeron, Andrew Goldstein, and Caroline Pukall, Dr. Goldstein realized how much he had to learn about sexual pain. He decided to begin wearing loupes when examining women, allowing for better visualization of the painful genital areas. Having seen thousands of women with sexual problems, he concluded that there is nothing worse than sexual pain.

This book has been written to help those women in pain, to assist health care professionals in treating women with sexual pain, and to promote research in the field, with the intention of ultimately helping women who are suffering. The reader should note that there is overlap within the chapters because there is overlap within this field, rather than distinct categories of symptoms or disorders. Any redundancy is intentional, with the purpose in mind that it will make that chapter more understandable and meaningful to the reader than having to find that information elsewhere. In this way, the book parallels the field as bio-psycho-social. It may be for this very reason that it has taken so long for a definitive text in sexual pain disorders to be written.

Woven throughout the book is the theme of effective management. What is effective management? Is it permanent—a cure—or a temporary treatment? For how long after treatment stops should the patient be symptom-free for the treatment to be considered effective? For many kinds of sexual pain, the only option is management that allows the woman to have decreased symptoms. In some cases, the only absolute cure may be surgery. This textbook presents the spectrum of treatments so that you, the practitioner, can choose the most appropriate and effective ones for your individual patients.

It is remarkable the alacrity with which this textbook has been produced. Andrew Goldstein and Caroline Pukall were perusing the books available at ISSWSH in February 2007, and discussed the need for a text solely on sexual pain disorders in women. They shared their idea with Irwin Goldstein who readily agreed regarding the necessity for evidence-based information in this field. Authors were invited in October 2007, the contents were completed in May 2008, and first publication coincided with the February 2009 annual ISSWSH meeting. Despite there being several societies at which sexual pain disorders are discussed, this is the first evidence-based textbook of female sexual pain disorders in publication. In respect to the multidisciplinary nature of the book, its editors, and its contributors, the editors have proudly gifted all proceeds from this textbook to the multidisciplinary organization, ISSWSH.

The friendships of the three editors and respect they have for one another have deepened during the course of assembling this book. The editors, 10 associate editors, and dozens of authors involved in this project share a passion for the field of sexual pain and compassion for their patients who are suffering.

Andrew T. Goldstein
Caroline F. Pukall
Irwin Goldstein

Acknowledgments

The editors wish to acknowledge the dedication and commitment of many colleagues without whom this project would have not been completed. In particular, we wish to thank the senior associate editor, Lara Burrows. We are indebted, as well, to all the associate editors of the book: Lori Brotto, Melissa Farmer, Gail Goldstein, Sue Goldstein, Arielle Metz, Leah Millheiser, Talli Rosenbaum, Kelly Smith, Katherine Sutton, and Denniz Zolnoun. We would also like to thank all the authors who took valuable time from their already busy lives to write chapters for this book, especially those who authored more than one chapter, demonstrating their dedication and commitment to the field.

In addition, we would like to thank Martin Sugden and Charlie Hamlyn of Wiley-Blackwell Publishing; Martin for having the foresight to see the need for this book, and Charlie for supporting us constantly. We would also like to express our appreciation to Brigitte Wilke who served as our development editor, seeing that authors' paperwork and deadlines were maintained, and providing guidance to us when necessary.

Last but not least, we all have people without whom each of us would not have been able to proceed with this project. Andrew Goldstein would like to acknowledge his office staff, Ruth Bradford, Tamika Hill, and Alice Hickling as well as his good friend and webmaster, Stan Felder. Caroline Pukall offers her thanks to her research assistants, Sasha Segal and Emma Dargie. Irwin Goldstein would like to give his appreciation to Sue Goldstein, Andrew Goldstein, and Caroline Pukall.

"I can no other answer make, but, thanks, and thanks."
—William Shakespeare.

CHAPTER 1
Historical Perspective of Vulvodynia

Premlatha Amalraj, Sarah Kelly, Gloria A. Bachmann
The Women's Health Institute, New Brunswick, NJ, USA

History of Vulvodynia

Vulvodynia, or chronic vulvar pain, is a syndrome that appears to have been recognized for centuries, but was not fully described until recently. It is thought that early Egyptian papyri, including the Kahun Gynecological Papyrus and the Ramesseum Papyrus, were the first texts to address gynecological issues including vulvar pain [1, 2]. The condition may have been described in ancient medical literature by Soranus of Ephesus, who referred to a condition similar to what we call vulvodynia today as "satyriasis in females" [3]. However, no documented, medically accurate descriptions of the condition appear in the medical literature until modern times.

History of the Term
Provoked Vestibulodynia

Initial discussions of vulvodynia focused on the main complaint of women presenting to their physicians: dyspareunia (i.e., pain during sexual intercourse), a term coined by Barnes in 1874 [4]. In the late nineteenth century, Thomas [5] and Skene [6] described a condition of hypersensitivity in the vulvar region. Thomas [5] described this condition as an "excessive sensibility of the nerves supplying the mucous membrane of some portion of the vulva, sometimes confined to the vestibule... [and] other times to one labium minus." He noted that a primary complaint of women with this condition was dyspareunia. Similarly, in 1889, Skene [6] and Kellogg [7] reported that sensitive areas around the vaginal opening could cause problems with sexual intercourse. Very little new information on

dyspareunia was reported for a period of four decades, and then in 1928 the condition reemerged in the literature. Kelly [8] expanded on the damaging effects of vulvar pain on sexual intercourse, describing it "as a fruitful source of dyspareunia."

Information regarding the specific part(s) of the vulvar area implicated in the pain appeared later in published reports. Dickinson [9] found that almost 75% of his dyspareunic patients had a physical reason for their pain, with many suffering from problems of the hymen, urethral meatus, and fourchette. Hunt [10] stated that the minor vestibular gland structures had no link to the pain, and this claim was supported by Dickinson's report [9]. Over time, assertions regarding the cause of this pain began to appear in the literature. O'Donnell [11] believed that the cause of the pain was chronic inflammation attributed to an incomplete rupture of the hymen. Further supporting the involvement of inflammation in dyspareunia were the reports of Pelisse and Hewitt [12], Davis et al. [13], and Woodruff and Parmley [14]. For example, Pelisse and Hewitt [12] found histopathological evidence of chronic and acute inflammation in the posterior vestibule of affected women. Names for this condition, reflecting the role of inflammation (-itis), began to emerge and included the following: focal vulvitis [15], vestibular adenitis [16], focal vestibulitis vulvae [17], and vulvar vestibulitis syndrome [18].

The term *vulvar vestibulitis syndrome* (VVS) is commonly used to describe a condition in which localized, provoked dyspareunia is the main presenting complaint. According to Friedrich [18], the diagnostic criteria for VVS are "severe pain on vestibular touch or attempted vaginal entry, tenderness to pressure localized within the vulvar vestibule, and physical findings confined to vestibular erythema of various degrees." Today, the relevance

Female Sexual Pain Disorders 1st edition. Edited by A. Goldstein, C. Pukall & I. Goldstein. © 2009 Blackwell Publishing, ISBN: 9781405183987.

of Friedrich's criterion is questioned and most clinicians make the diagnosis by the exclusion of other etiologies of pain. Additionally, one major problem with the terminology exists: "vestibulitis" implies inflammation. However, the finding of inflammatory indices in the vestibules of women with VVS is not a consistent finding in the literature. As such, the International Society for the Study of Vulvovaginal Disease (ISSVD) renamed VVS to provoked vestibulodynia (PVD) [19].

History of the Term
Generalized Vulvodynia
In 1975, the ISSVD described generalized vulvodynia (GVD; also known as "essential" or "dysesthetic" vulvodynia) as "burning vulva syndrome" at its world congress. Eight years later, the ISSVD adopted the first standard definition of GVD as chronic vulvar discomfort, characterized by the patient's complaint of burning and sometimes stinging, irritating, or raw sensations.

The Emergence of Two Major Vulvodynia Subtypes
The first empirical attempt to delineate subtypes of dyspareunia was described by Meana and colleagues in 1997 [20]. These investigators proposed that dyspareunia was a heterogeneous disorder including at least three different diagnostic groups, and they emphasized the importance of the pain component of this condition. As a result of this foundational work, conceptualizations began to shift from focusing on "pain during intercourse" to "vulvar pain" conditions in which dyspareunia could potentially be a symptom. This focus is reflected in the ISSVD's classification of vulvar pain. It describes vulvodynia as "vulvar discomfort, most often described as burning pain, occurring in the absence of relevant and visible findings or specific, clinically identifiable, neurological disorder" and lists dyspareunia as one possible expression of vulvodynia [19]. In addition, this classification system includes temporal pain characteristics and pain location as the main categories into which to classify vulvodynia subtypes.

Depending on pain characteristics, two main types of vulvodynia are recognized: PVD and GVD. PVD refers to provoked pain that is localized to the vaginal opening, whereas GVD refers to unprovoked, diffuse vulvar pain affecting the entire vulvar region. Sometimes the pain in GVD may radiate to the anal region, to the lower back or

thighs, or to other areas consistent with the distribution of the pudendal nerve. PVD appears to be more common in premenopausal women, while GVD is most often diagnosed in peri- and postmenopausal women [21]. The pain of GVD can be intermittent or constant, and although the pain is typically unprovoked, it worsens with provocation in many cases. Periods of unexplained relief and/or flare-ups may occur, and erythema may or may not be present. The ISSVD classification also applies to other forms of vulvar pain, such as clitorodynia, reflecting the fact that multiple subtypes of vulvodynia exist.

Vulvodynia Versus Chronic Vulvar Pain Due to an Existing Condition
In the past (and to a lesser extent today), chronic pain conditions—including vulvodynia—that existed in the absence of physical findings were considered suspicious. Often, women with vulvodynia were told that there was nothing "physically wrong" with their genitals, implying that psychosexual problems were the root of the pain. However, as the field of chronic pain evolved, it became known that identifiable physical findings simply did not exist in most cases of chronic pain. This knowledge has been applied to vulvodynia as well.

The term *vulvodynia* is reserved for those cases of chronic vulvar pain that occur in the absence of physical findings [19]. Only in the event that possible contributors to the pain are ruled out can the diagnosis of vulvodynia be made. Specifically, conditions of infectious, inflammatory, neoplastic, and immunologic origin, as well as evidence for any systemic illness, physical trauma to the vulva, dermatologic conditions, urinary tract syndromes, and neurological disorders should be ruled out prior to making a diagnosis of vulvodynia [19]. However, "chronic vulvar pain" can coexist with several conditions and should still be carefully managed and assessed.

Several conditions can contribute to chronic vulvar pain, including the following: (i) infections due to, for example, Bartholin's gland abscess, vulvovaginal candidiasis, herpes genitalis, herpes zoster, human papillomavirus, molluscum contagiosum, and trichomoniasis; (ii) neoplasms, such as vulvar intraepithelial neoplasia and invasive squamous cell carcinoma; (iii) immunological changes due to, for example, altered levels of interleukin-1, tumor necrosis factor and interferon-α; (iv) systemic illnesses, such as Bechet's disease, Crohn's disease, Sjogren's syndrome, and systemic lupus erythematosus; (v) hormonal changes, such as those leading to atrophic vaginitis; (vi) dermatological conditions (e.g., allergic and contact dermatitis, eczema, hidradenitis suppurativa, lichen planus, lichen sclerosus, and psoriasis); and (vii) neurological disorders, such as those resulting from pudendal nerve entrapment, injury, or previous surgery.

Are We There Yet?

There has been a tremendous effort to classify, diagnose, study, and treat vulvodynia over the past 15 years. Because of this movement and the active discussion to improve all aspects of vulvodynia assessment, treatment, and support, it is likely that the terms used and the subtypes will continue to be refined for many years to come.

References

1 Barns JWB. (1956) *Five Ramasseum Papyri.* University Press, Oxford.

2 Griffith FL. (1898) *Hieratic Papyri from Kahun and Gurob.* Bernard Quartich, London, pp. 5–11.

3 McElhiney J, Kelly S, Rosen R *et al.* (2006) Satyriasis: the antiquity term for vulvodynia? *The Journal of Sexual Medicine* **3**, 161–63.

4 Barnes RA. (1874) *Clinical History of the Medical and Surgical Diseases of Women.* Henry C. Lea, Philadelphia.

5 Thomas TG, Mundae PF. (1891) *A Practical Treatise on the Diseases of Women,* 6th ed. Lea Brothers & Co., Philadelphia.

6 Skene AJC. (1889) *Treatise on the Diseases of Women.* Appleton & Co., New York.

7 Kellogg JH. (1889). *Plain Facts for Old and Young: Embracing the Natural History and Hygiene of Organic Life.* IF Segner, Burlington, VT.

8 Kelly HA. (1928) *Medical Gynecology.* WB Saunders, Philadelphia.

9 Dickinson RL. (1949) *Human Sex Anatomy,* 2nd ed. Williams & Wilkins, Baltimore.

10 Hunt I. (1948) *Disease of the Vulva.* Mosby, St. Louis.

11 O'Donnell RP. (1959) Relative hypospadias potentiated by inadequate rupture of the hymen: a cause of chronic inflammation of the lower part of the female urinary tract. *Journal of International College of Surgeons* **32**, 374.

12 Pelisse M, Hewitt J. (1976) Erythamous vulvitis en plaques. In: *Proceedings of the Third Congress of the International Society for the Study of Vulvar Disease, Cocoyoc, Mexico.* International Society for the Study of Vulvar Disease, Milwaukee, pp. 35–37.

13 Davis J, Shapiro L, Baral J. (1983) Vuvitis circumscripta plasma cellularis. *Journal of the American Association of Dermatology* **8**, 413–16.

14 Woodruff JD, Parmley TH. (1983) Infection of the minor vestibular gland. *Obstetrics and Gynecology* **62**, 609–12.

15 Peckham BM, Maki DG, Patterson JJ, *et al.* (1986). Focal vulvitis: a characteristic syndrome and cause of dyspareunia. *American Journal of Obstetrics and Gynecology* **154**, 855–64.

16 Friedrich EG. (1983) Therapeutic studies on vulvar vestibulitis. *The Journal of Reproductive Medicine* **33**, 514–17.

17 Tovell HMM, Young AW. (1991) *Diseases of the Vulva in Clinical Practice.* Elsevier, New York.

18 Friedrich EG. (1987) Vulvar vestibulitis syndrome. *The Journal of Reproductive Medicine* **32**, 110–14.

19 Haefner HK. (2007) Report of the International Society for the Study of Vulvovaginal Disease Terminology and Classification of Vulvodynia. *Journal of Lower Genital Tract Disease* **11**, 48–49.

20 Meana M, Binik I, Khalifé S, *et al.* (1997) Dyspareunia: sexual dysfunction or pain syndrome? *The Journal of Nervous and Mental Disease* **185**, 561–69.

21 Harlow BL, Wise LA, Stewart EG. (2001) Prevalence and predictors of chronic lower genital tract discomfort. *American Journal of Obstetrics and Gynecology* **185**, 545–50.

CHAPTER 2

The Prevalence of Dyspareunia

Richard D. Hayes
University of Melbourne, Melbourne, Australia

Introduction

Dyspareunia has a substantial impact on women's health, relationships, and quality of life [1]. Reliable prevalence data are needed to understand the burden that dyspareunia places on women in the community and to enable comparisons across populations or over time. Prevalence studies can also allow a greater understanding of the risk factors associated with this condition and may aid in identifying subgroups of women who are most likely to be affected. This information can assist in effectively targeting public health strategies.

Reported prevalence estimates of dyspareunia vary considerably. In a recent systematic literature review, some dyspareunia prevalence estimates were as low as 0.4%, whereas others were as high as 61% [2]. Further reviews have also reported a broad range of estimates [3–7]. Some of this variation may be due to true differences between populations surveyed. However, there is a growing body of evidence to suggest that much of this variation is due to inconsistent use of case definitions, variation in study design and conduct, and different outcome measures used to assess dyspareunia [2–4, 8].

Definitions

There is ongoing debate in the scientific literature regarding what constitutes female sexual dysfunction (FSD) and dyspareunia [9, 10]. In fact, there are differences between the definitions of dyspareunia provided by professional

Female Sexual Pain Disorders 1st edition. Edited by A. Goldstein, C. Pukall & I. Goldstein. © 2009 Blackwell Publishing, ISBN: 9781405183987.

organizations [11–13]. These inconsistencies have the potential to affect prevalence estimates reported. For example, the American Psychiatric Association's DSM-IV [12] and the World Health Organization's ICD-10 [13] define dyspareunia as pain associated with sexual intercourse. In the last decade, Basson et al. have revised definitions of FSD [11]. They broaden the definition of dyspareunia to also include pain with attempted or completed vaginal entry. As a result of this broader definition, studies using Basson et al.'s more encompassing definition are likely to report relatively higher prevalence estimates.

Painful intercourse can be associated with a range of conditions such as endometriosis, interstitial cystitis (IC), and vaginismus [6, 14]. DSM-IV and ICD-10 stipulate that sexual pain resulting from "general medical conditions" or "local pathology" should not be classified as dyspareunia [12, 13]. In addition, diagnostic systems usually classify dyspareunia and vaginismus as separate, mutually exclusive sexual dysfunctions [11–13]. Some authors have debated whether this distinction is appropriate, pointing to the lack of evidence related to the clinical presentation of vaginismus and superficial dyspareunia [6, 14]. ICD-10 and DSM-IV also exclude sexual pain due to lubrication problems. Many studies, however, do not exclude women who suffer from these conditions when reporting the prevalence of dyspareunia [8, 15]. Consequently, these studies may overestimate the prevalence of dyspareunia.

Study Design and Conduct

There is increasing evidence that aspects of study design and conduct have a substantial impact on the prevalence of dyspareunia reported in published studies. A recent meta-analysis investigated associations between the prevalence of sexual difficulties reported in 55 published studies and the design features of those studies [2]. Data collection procedures, inclusion criteria, duration of sexual difficulty recorded, sample size, and response rate were all significantly associated with the reported prevalence of at least one type of sexual difficulty.

Reported prevalence estimates of sexual pain were lower in studies that conducted interviews in person compared with studies that used self-administered questionnaires. It is possible that interviewing in person is a more accurate way of gathering data on dyspareunia. Alternatively, when women are interviewed in person, embarrassment and social desirability may bias responses.

Studies in which the duration of sexual pain recorded was longer (3–6 months or more) also reported lower prevalence estimates [2]. These associations between prevalence and study design were independent of likely predictors of true variation in prevalence such as study location, study year, and age range of participants. There is further evidence that dyspareunia can persist for varying durations [3, 16]. It is therefore plausible that investigations that only record longer-lasting difficulties will report lower prevalence estimates. In addition, some investigations recruit participants from clinical settings [17, 18], which may limit the generalizability of the results obtained. Women recruited in this way may be different from the general population in a range of ways that could affect their sexual function, such as being less healthy generally and belonging to a demographic that has better access to health care.

Instruments Used to Assess Dyspareunia

A wide variety of instruments have been used to assess dyspareunia. Studies that have employed simple questions are common in the literature [16, 19] and include well-cited and influential studies such as that by Laumann et al. [15]. These simple questions often ask respondents to report if they have experienced sexual pain for a month or more during the previous year [16, 19]. By contrast, a range of validated multi-item instruments have been developed [20, 21] and are being increasingly used in prevalence studies [8, 18].

Predominantly these multi-item instruments use a recall of the previous month. Multi-item instruments offer the advantage of being capable of measuring the intensity and frequency of pain experienced rather than simply assessing whether pain is present or absent. This approach corresponds better with DSM-IV and Basson definitions of dyspareunia that stipulate that sexual pain must be persistent or recurrent. Studies that only include persistent or recurrent pain as opposed to any pain with intercourse are likely to report a lower prevalence estimate of dyspareunia. Recently, a side-by side comparison of instruments was conducted in the one sample of women. Initially, simple instruments commonly used to assess dyspareunia were compared. Changing the recall period from "one month or more in the previous year" to "the previous month" reduced the prevalence estimate from 23% to 11% [8]. When dyspareunia was assessed using a multi-item scale (also with a recall of the previous month) in the same group of women, the prevalence estimate produced was only 3% [8].

Sexually Related Distress

Sexual distress refers to negative and distressing feelings that a woman may experience about her level of sexual function. DSM-IV stipulates that a woman can only be diagnosed with dyspareunia if she is also distressed by her sexual pain [12]. Sexual distress has attracted increasing attention in the literature [22]. Validated measures of sexual distress have also been developed [23]. This has created an opportunity for researchers to measure both the low sexual function and sexually related personal distress components of dyspareunia. Despite this, many studies do not take sexual distress into account [15, 16, 19].

Approximately one-third of women with dyspareunia (aged 18–70) experience some degree of sexually related distress [1, 8]. A range of issues including psychological and relationship factors may influence whether a woman feels distressed about her own sexual functioning [24]. An investigation of women in the United States and Western Europe reported that the proportion of women who are sexually distressed declines with age, although the proportion of women with low sexual function increases [25]. That investigation focused on low desire. We currently do not know if this age-related decline in distress holds true for distress caused specifically by sexual pain. There is evidence from a number of investigations that the decision to include sexual distress in outcome measures used to assess dyspareunia can significantly reduce the prevalence estimate obtained [1, 8] and may also affect risk factors reported. There is currently debate as to whether sexual distress should continue to be part of the official definition of dyspareunia [9]. The final outcome of this debate is likely to have a substantial impact on prevalence estimates of dyspareunia reported in future studies.

What Can Prevalence Studies Tell Us About Sexual Pain?

Novel approaches have extracted useful information from the heterogeneous literature in this area. One approach has been to investigate the prevalence of dyspareunia relative to other types of FSD. Within the one study, population characteristics and study design are likely to have a similar impact on all types of FSD investigated. For example, studies that report a relatively higher prevalence of dyspareunia often report a correspondingly higher prevalence of other types of FSD as well [19]. Consequently, the relationships between the different types of FSD are likely to be more consistent across studies than the absolute prevalence. This approach has shown that desire difficulty is the most common difficulty experienced and sexual pain is the least common [3]. However, on average, sexual pain still accounts for 26% of the sexual difficulties experienced by women. A further analysis compared the prevalence of dyspareunia across studies that used case definitions of different durations. Among women experiencing sexual pain, less than 20% of cases had lasted for a relatively short period of time (one month to less than several months), more than 50% of cases were of intermediate duration (several months to less than 6 months) and close to one-third of cases were more chronic, persisting for 6 months or more [3].

A meta-analysis of prevalence studies found that studies that included younger women and studies conducted in European countries (compared to a range of other countries, including the United States) reported lower prevalence estimates of dyspareunia [2]. Interestingly, these results had been statistically adjusted for differences in design features of those studies including the data collection procedure, the duration of sexual pain, recall, inclusion criteria, sampling method, use of validated outcome measures, the year the study was conducted, sample size, and response rate [2].

These results are consistent with data indicating that higher numbers of older women experience poor sexual function generally [26]. However, a number of studies have reported that dyspareunia declines with age [15, 19, 26]. This apparent decline in dyspareunia may simply be a consequence of older women engaging less often in sexual activities and fewer older women remaining sexually active [27]. There may also be changes in the type of sexual activities women engage in with age. A systematic shift from penetrative sex to other sexual activities would also cause an apparent reduction in the prevalence of dyspareunia among these women. These women may also be missed by assessment methods that focus exclusively on sexual intercourse.

Recommendations and Conclusions

Clinicians should be aware that there is diversity in the duration of time over which sexual pain may persist. In addition, the epidemiological data suggests that simply enquiring about the presence or absence of sexual pain may result in a different response compared to asking about persistent or recurrent sexual pain. Not all women will be distressed by sexual pain, indicating that some women will not be motivated to report it.

The literature on the prevalence of dyspareunia is extremely heterogeneous. There are substantial discrepancies in the way studies are designed and conducted. From the data presented in this chapter, it is apparent that inconsistencies in study design and outcome measures have a substantial effect on reported prevalence estimates. These inconsistencies make it difficult to combine data from studies on the prevalence or etiology of dyspareunia and undermine our ability to make comparisons between populations. In accordance with current definitions, researchers investigating the prevalence of dyspareunia may choose to exclude women experiencing various medical conditions. However, it would assist comparisons across studies if authors also reported the original unaltered prevalence estimates of sexual pain.

Novel approaches to extracting information from the current literature can only ever provide limited, general information. What is needed is consistency in research practice across investigations. In particular, this area of research would benefit from the consistent use of the same outcome measure in all studies. The absence of a standard, generally accepted instrument for determining the presence of dyspareunia represents a major limitation in current research. This issue has been raised previously [28, 29]. Changes in our understanding of dyspareunia are likely to result in new instruments being developed to assess this disorder. New instruments could be added to surveys along side a standard instrument with this standard instrument facilitating comparisons between studies, across populations and over time.

References

1 Oberg K, Fugl-Meyer KS. (2005) On Swedish women's distressing sexual dysfunctions: some concomitant conditions and life satisfaction. *The Journal of Sexual Medicine* **2**, 169–80.

2 Hayes RD, Bennett CM, Dennerstein L, *et al.* (2008) Are aspects of study design associated with the reported prevalence of female sexual difficulties? *Fertility and Sterility* **90**, 497–505.

3 Hayes RD, Bennett CM, Fairley CK, *et al.* (2006) What can prevalence studies tell us about female sexual difficulty and dysfunction? *The Journal of Sexual Medicine* **3**, 589–95.

4 Dunn KM, Jordan K, Croft PR, *et al.* (2002) Systematic review of sexual problems: epidemiology and methodology. *Journal of Sex and Marital Therapy* **28**, 399–422.

5 Lewis RW, Fugl-Meyer KS, Bosch R, *et al.* (2004) Epidemiology/risk factors of sexual dysfunction. *The Journal of Sexual Medicine* **1**, 35–39.

6 Schultz WW, Basson R, Binik Y, *et al.* (2005) Women's sexual pain and its management. *The Journal of Sexual Medicine* **2**, 301–16.

7 DeRogatis LR, Burnett AL. (2008) The epidemiology of sexual dysfunctions. *The Journal of Sexual Medicine* **5**, 289–300.

8 Hayes RD, Dennerstein L, Bennett CM, *et al.* (2008) What is the "true" prevalence of female sexual dysfunctions and does the way we assess these conditions have an impact? *The Journal of Sexual Medicine* **5**, 777–87.

9 Segraves R, Balon R, Clayton A. (2007) Proposal for changes in diagnostic criteria for sexual dysfunctions. *The Journal of Sexual Medicine* **4**, 567–80.

10 Sand M, Fisher WA. (2007) Women's endorsement of models of female sexual response: the nurses sexuality study. *The Journal of Sexual Medicine* **4**, 708–19.

11 Basson R, Leiblum S, Brotto L, *et al.* (2003) Definitions of women's sexual dysfunction reconsidered: advocating expansion and revision. *Journal of Psychosomatic Obstetrics and Gynecology* **24**, 221–29.

12 *APA Diagnostic and Statistical Manual of Mental Disorders*, 4th ed. (2000) American Psychiatric Association, Washington DC.

13 World Health Organization. (2000) *Manual of the International Statistical Classification of Diseases and Related Health Problems, 10th Revision* (ICD-10).

14 De Kruiff ME, Ter Kuile MM, Weijenborg PTM, *et al.* (2000) Vaginismus and dyspareunia: is there a difference in clinical presentation? *Journal of Psychosomatic Obstetrics and Gynecology* **21**, 149–55.

15 Laumann E, Paik A, Rosen R. (1999) Sexual dysfunction in the United States, prevalence and predictors. *Journal of the American Medical Association* **281**, 537–44.

16 Mercer CH, Fenton KA, Johnson AM, *et al.* (2003) Sexual function problems and help-seeking behaviour in Britain: national probability sample survey. *British Medical Journal* **327**, 426–27.

17 Amsterdam A, Carter J, Krychman M. (2006) Prevalence of psychiatric illness in women in an oncology sexual health population: a retrospective pilot study. *The Journal of Sexual Medicine* **3**, 292–95.

18 Nobre PJ, Pinto-Gouveia J, Gomes FA. (2006) Prevalence and comorbidity of sexual dysfunctions in a Portuguese clinical sample. *Journal of Sex and Marital Therapy* **32**, 173–82.

19 Richters J, Grulich AE, de Visser RO, *et al.* (2003) Sex in Australia: sexual difficulties in a representative sample of adults. *Australian and New Zealand Journal of Public Health* **27**, 164–70.

20 Quirk FH, Heiman JR, Rosen RC, *et al.* (2002) Development of a sexual function questionnaire for clinical trials of female sexual dysfunction. *Journal of Women's Health and Gender-Based Medicine* **11**, 277–89.

21 Rosen R, Brown C, Heiman J, *et al.* (2000) The female sexual function index (FSFI): a multidimensional, self-report instrument for the assessment of female sexual function. *Journal of Sex and Marital Therapy* **26**, 191–208.

22 Bancroft J, Loftus J, Long JS. (2003) Distress about sex: a national survey of women in heterosexual relationships. *Archives of Sexual Behaviour* **32**, 193–208.

23 Derogatis L, Rosen R, Leiblum S, *et al.* (2002) The Female Sexual Distress Scale (FSDS): initial validation of a standardized scale for assessment of sexually related personal distress in women. *Journal of Sex and Marital Therapy* **28**, 317–30.

24 Hayes RD, Dennerstein L, Bennett CM, *et al.* (2008) Risk factors for female sexual dysfunction in the general population: exploring factors associated with low sexual function and sexual distress. *The Journal of Sexual Medicine* **5**, 1681–93.

25 Hayes RD, Dennerstein L, Bennett CM, *et al.* (2007) Relationship between hypoactive sexual desire disorder and aging. *Fertility and Sterility* **87**, 107–12.

26 Hayes R, Dennerstein L. (2005) The impact of aging on sexual function and sexual dysfunction in women: a review of population-based studies. *The Journal of Sexual Medicine* **2**, 317–30.

27 Barlow D, Cardozo L, Francis R, *et al.* (1997) Urogenital ageing and its effect on sexual health in older British women. *British Journal of Obstetrics and Gynaecology* **104**, 87–91.

28 Hayes RD. (2008) Assessing female sexual dysfunction in epidemiological studies: why is it necessary to measure both low sexual function and sexually-related distress? *Sexual Health* **5**, 215–18.

29 DeRogatis L, Burnett AL. (2007) Key methodological issues in sexual medicine research. *The Journal of Sexual Medicine* **4**, 527–37.

CHAPTER 3

The Relevance of Dyspareunia

Marta Meana, Lorraine Benuto, Robyn L. Donaldson

University of Nevada, Las Vegas, NV, USA

Introduction

Fifteen years ago, sexual pain disorders appeared to have been cast into the dustbin of undifferentiated psychosomatic conditions. Little research attention was devoted to their description, etiology, or treatment. Since then, much research and clinical activity has recognized dyspareunia as a serious impairment imposing a significant burden. Its study has raised important research, diagnostic, and treatment questions with the potential to inform other pain syndromes and sexual dysfunctions. This chapter will focus on the relevance of dyspareunia to individuals, society, and the research and clinical enterprise.

Individual and Societal Burden

Research suggests that dyspareunia exacts a high individual and societal cost. In addition to comorbid sexual difficulties [1–2], affected women also suffer from negative affect [2–4] and relationship concerns [5–7]. Dyspareunia is often experienced as one of the most disturbing symptoms of genital pain disorders.

In one study of interstitial cystitis (IC), a condition marked by intense bladder pain, painful intercourse and relationship strain were ranked as the most disturbing consequences of the condition [8]. Another study that compared women with dyspareunia to women with chronic pelvic pain (CPP) found that both groups reported similar impairments as a purported function of their pain [9].

Female Sexual Pain Disorders 1st edition. Edited by A. Goldstein, C. Pukall & I. Goldstein. © 2009 Blackwell Publishing, ISBN: 9781405183987.

Chronic pain disorders have long been associated with high healthcare expenditures, lower work productivity, and many other societal costs [10]. There are currently no reliable estimates of healthcare expenditures associated with dyspareunia. As an acute, recurrent pain disorder typically provoked by sexual intercourse, dyspareunia is unlikely to exact as high a cost as lower back pain or migraine. However, healthcare costs associated with dyspareunia may be high. First, it is highly comorbid with other treatment-resistant pain-related conditions with high associated costs such as IC [11], irritable bowel syndrome [12], pelvic inflammatory disease [13], CPP [14], and endometriosis [15]. Second, the heterogeneity of its etiology [16] indicates that appropriate treatments may not be immediately identifiable. Third, its interference with quality of life likely creates a charged emotional context which, coupled with the elusiveness of effective treatment, makes dyspareunia an ideal candidate for doctor-shopping, uncoordinated multiple treatment attempts, and low adherence to strategies that fail to demonstrate immediate effects. For instance, in one online study of 428 women with vulvar pain, close to half reported consulting 4–9 physicians [5]. Only 40% trusted their current physician to manage the pain, and 57% reported their pain had stayed the same or worsened since initiating treatment. The estimate of medical care expenses incurred ranged from under $500 to over $75,000.

An additional cost of dyspareunia stems from its potential impact on relationships. Although Davis and Reissing [17] note that a number of studies fail to show relationship maladjustment in couples coping with dyspareunia, it is difficult to imagine that it would not affect the relationship dynamic. Extant studies of couple adjustment may fail to capture those couples who may not have survived the problems engendered by pain. In Gordon et al.'s vulvar pain study [5], 76% of respondents reported fearing that the pain would ruin their relationships. Although objective causes of relationship dissolution are difficult to ascertain, problems with sexual intimacy are often listed as one of most common reasons [18]. Infidelity has also been associated with divorce and linked to sexual dissatisfaction [19].

Challenging Definitions

The study of dyspareunia has engaged the field in a fruitful debate about current conceptualizations of sexual dysfunction. It has also stimulated the realization that female and male sexual responses may diverge sufficiently to merit a gender-differentiated approach. The empirical investigation of pain characteristics coupled with the lack of validation for old notions of dyspareunia as a somatic manifestation of psychic conflict has led researchers to question whether dyspareunia is better characterized as a pain disorder rather than as a sexual dysfunction [16, 20]. The focus on its interference (with sexual intercourse) rather than on its presenting symptom (pain) has not led to advances in etiological theory or in treatment. In contrast, pain properties appear to directly indicate potential etiologies and treatment approaches.

The research shift from the sexual aspects of dyspareunia to its pain culminated in Binik's appeal to eliminate the sexual pain disorders from the sexual dysfunction section of the DSM and have them subsumed under the pain disorders section [21]. This suggestion has its detractors, but the dilemma of classifying dyspareunia has forced the issue of nosological accuracy in sexual dysfunction and has made us consider the sociocultural forces that shape its development. This momentum has been concurrent with broader initiatives to reconceptualize female sexual dysfunction [22–23] in an attempt to untether ideas of sexual normalcy for women from those for men. One such argument posits that dyspareunia is the only true female sexual dysfunction [24] given that, unlike differing levels of arousal and desire, pain is unacceptable at any level. These theoretical and empirical forays make us examine presuppositions and correct damaging social constructions of pathology related to individuals' sexual well-being.

Defying Old Dualisms

Dyspareunia has also shone a spotlight on the futility of attempts to tease apart the psychological aspects from the physical aspects regarding sexuality. Sexual response is simultaneously a psychological and physiological process that defies attempts to situate problems in one domain or another, despite the DSM's insistence on the identification of pure psychogenicity.

Dyspareunia is almost always a function of both factors. Furthermore, it introduces an acutely social dimension. The pain does not just occur in the presence of others; it is technically provoked by others (the sexual partner), creating a complex configuration of potential etiological factors that makes the search for a single causal pathway almost futile. Even when there is some certainty about an originating factor, the experience of pain during intercourse is likely to have engendered physical (e.g., nerve dysfunction), sexual (e.g., desire/arousal problems), emotional (e.g., anxiety/hypervigilance), and relational (e.g., guilt/anger) dynamics that threaten to perpetuate the pain long past the resolution of the original problem.

For example, many women with dyspareunia report a history of vaginal infections (e.g., candidiasis), or seem convinced that such an infection was a significant contributor to the development of their pain [5, 25–26]. The findings linking active infection and dyspareunia in real time, however, are mixed [2, 27]. Perhaps women with dyspareunia are overestimating infection frequency in an attempt to make sense of their current condition. However, they may be accurate reporters. These infections and/or their treatment may have instated nociceptor sensitization that persists in the absence of active infection. The infection may have been the first-order etiological factor, the sensitization becomes a second-order one, and the emotional/relational strain of persistent pain may create other dynamics that become as instrumental in the pain experience as any of their etiological predecessors. There is little room for simplistic dualisms in this picture.

Multidisciplinary Treatment

A concerted appeal to bring the expertise of various relevant disciplines to bear on the assessment and treatment of dyspareunia in an integrated fashion has been apparent.

Considering the myriad predisposing and perpetuating factors likely involved in its development and maintenance, we can no longer leave its assessment and treatment to one discipline [28]. Ideally, most cases of dyspareunia should involve a physician, a psychologist/sex therapist, and a physical therapist. Although many women report they have consulted with some or all of these specialties in a serial fashion, the effort should be coordinated and each treatment component should be reasonably informed by the findings of the others.

This type of interdisciplinary collaboration is suited for most sexual dysfunctions and has already proven to be clinically and cost-effective in the treatment of other chronic pain disorders [10]. However, it poses two main challenges. First, different healthcare providers should suspend biases for one potential treatment avenue over another. For example, data indicates that surgery for provoked vestibulodynia (PVD) is successful, yet reluctance to consider this option persists [29–30]. However, data also indicate that surgery without concomitant sex therapy is unlikely to be effective [29].

Second, issues related to patient cost and structural difficulties in assembling treatment teams exist. However, the monetary cost of serial treatments with little individual efficacy is likely high, not to mention the burden of continued pain and distress. It behooves the healthcare system to invest in the organization of treatment teams that will deliver coordinated care for better long-term clinical outcomes and cost-effectiveness.

Outcome Issues

The multidimensionality of dyspareunia has also raised the issue of determining which outcome measures should be considered indicators of treatment success. Whereas one can easily define treatment success when pain reduction (as measured via a clinical examination) coincides with increased frequency of sexual intercourse, this definition is less clear when there is a misalignment between this measure of pain reduction and the woman's self-report.

In Bergeron et al.'s [31] treatment outcome study for PVD, surgery evidenced the greatest gains in pain reduction, measured clinically, in comparison to group cognitive-behavioral therapy (GCBT) and biofeedback. However, the three treatments did not differ from one another with regard to sexual function or self-reported intercourse pain.

The discrepancy between quantitative sensory measurement and naturalistic pain self-report points us toward the need for a more holistic conceptualization of treatment success. If dyspareunia is often characterized by fear, hypervigilance, and avoidance, it is probable that reductions in clinically measured pain consequent to an intervention may not have a close correspondence to the experience of pain in the naturalistic context of sexual intercourse. Intercourse may have become paired with pain through a classical conditioning paradigm. Additionally, sex may evoke other emotional and relational issues that do not arise in the context of pain measurement in a gynecology clinic. Ultimately, treatment outcome needs to center on the woman's sexual experience.

Developing New Assessment and Treatment Technologies

One of the most exciting aspects of recent research on dyspareunia has been the development of new assessment and treatment technologies. Researchers have started to focus on quantitative pain and sensory measurement. The administration of the *McGill Pain Questionnaire* [32] to women with dyspareunia revealed that the pain was significant in its intensity and that different subtypes were characterized by distinctive descriptors [16]. This was followed by attempts to locate and measure the intensity of vestibular pain in a more systematic fashion by way of the vestibular pain index, a composite of pain ratings in response to cotton-swab stimulation of six different sites in the vulvar vestibule [31]. Notably, Pukall and colleagues made a significant leap forward with the design of the vulvalgesiometer, a hand-held instrument that standardized the measurement of pressure-pain thresholds [33]. There are also instruments now available to measure vaginal sensitivity to temperature, vibration, and distention [34–35].

In terms of treatment, biofeedback and physical therapy have made significant contributions specifically in relation to pelvic floor tonicity. The old standard of undifferentiated vaginal dilatation in the absence of information about the individual woman's tonicity status has been replaced by customized protocols that may include pelvic floor manipulations (including dilatation), home exercises, sEMG biofeedback, electrical stimulation, and perineal ultrasound [36]. GCBT for dyspareunia has also been manualized by Bergeron et al. [31] and shown to be as effective as surgery in the treatment of PVD at long-term follow-up [29].

The development of new technologies or the novel application of techniques used with other pain disorders is a testament to the vibrancy of the current research effort on the sexual pain disorders. It augers well for (i) our understanding of basic physiological mechanisms of pain; (ii) the operationalization of symptoms; and (iii) the diversification of treatment options in the management of this complex and multifaceted disorder.

Conclusion

The recent prominence of the sexual pain disorders in the collective clinical and research consciousness has been long overdue. The study of dyspareunia indicates areas of burden but also offers opportunities. It promises to continue challenging outdated notions of sexual health and pathology and to contribute to the refinement and development of enhanced assessment and treatment approaches. Many of these advances are likely to prove useful in the management of many sexual difficulties, whether they rise to the level of dysfunction or not.

References

1 Farmer MA, Meston CM. (2007) Predictors of genital pain in young women. *Archives of Sexual Behavior* **36**, 831–43.
2 Meana M, Binik YM, Khalifé S, *et al.* (1997) Biopsychosocial profile of women with dyspareunia. *Obstetrics and Gynecology* **90**, 583–89.
3 Danielsson I, Eisemann M, Sjoberg I, *et al.* (2001) Vulvar vestibulitis: a multifactorial condition. *British Journal of Obstetrics and Gynaecology* **22**, 456–61.
4 Gates EA, Galask RP. (2001) Psychological and sexual functioning in women with vulvar vestibulitis. *Journal of Psychosomatic Obstetrics and Gynecology* **22**, 221–28.
5 Gordon AS, Panahian-Jand M, McComb F, *et al.* (2003) Characteristics of women with vulvar pain disorders: responses to a web-based survey. *Journal of Sex and Marital Therapy* **29**, 45–58.
6 Graziottin A, Brotto LA. (2004) Vulvar vestibulitis syndrome: a clinical approach. *Journal of Sex and Marital Therapy* **30**, 125–39.
7 NylanderLundqvist E, Bergdahl J. (2003) Vulvar vestibulitis: evidence of depression and state anxiety in patients and partners. *Acta Dermato-Venereologica* **83**, 369–73.
8 Azevedo K, Nguyen A, Rowhani-Rahbar A, *et al.* (2005) Pain impacts sexual functioning among interstitial cystitis patients. *Sexuality and Disability* **23**, 189–208.
9 Grace V, Zondervan K. (2006) Chronic pelvic pain in women in New Zealand: comparative well-being, comorbidity, and impact on work and other activities. *Health Care for Women International* **27**, 585–99.
10 Turk DC, Burwinkle TM. (2005) Clinical outcomes, cost-effectiveness and the role of psychology in treatments for chronic pain sufferers. *Professional Psychology: Research and Practice* **36**, 602–10.
11 Wu EQ, Birnbaum H, Mareva M, *et al.* (2006) Interstitial cystitis: cost, treatment and comorbidities in an employed population. *Pharmacoeconomics* **24**, 55–65.
12 Nyrop KA, Palsson OS, Levy RL, *et al.* (2007) Costs of health care for irritable bowel syndrome, chronic constipation, functional diarrhea and functional abdominal pain. *Alimentary Pharmacology and Therapeutics* **26**, 237–48.
13 Rein DB, Kassler WJ, Irwin KL, *et al.* (2000) Direct medical cost of pelvic inflammatory disease and its sequelae: decreasing, but still substantial. *Obstetrics and Gynecology* **95**, 397–402.
14 Mathias SD, Kupperman M, Liberman RF, *et al.* (1996) Chronic pelvic pain: prevalence, health-related quality of life, and economic correlates. *Obstetrics and Gynecology* **87**, 321–27.
15 Mirkin D, Murphy-Barron C, Iwasaki, K. (2007) Actuarial analysis of private payer administrative claims data for women with endometriosis. *Journal of Managed Care Pharmacy* **13**, 262–72.
16 Meana M, Binik YM, Khalifé S, *et al.* (1997) Dyspareunia: sexual dysfunction or pain syndrome? *Journal of Nervous and Mental Disease* **185**, 561–69.
17 Davis HJ, Reissing ED. (2007) Relationship adjustment and dyadic interaction in couples with sexual pain disorders: a critical review of the literature. *Sexual and Relationship Therapy* **22**, 245–54.
18 Amato PR, Previti D. (2003) People's reasons for divorcing: gender, social class, the life course, and adjustment. *Journal of Family Issues* **24**, 602–26.
19 Hall JH, Finchman FD. (2006) Relationship dissolution following infidelity. In: Fine MA, Harvey JH (eds.) *Handbook of Divorce and Relationship Dissolution.* Lawrence Erlbaum Associates, Inc, Philadelphia, pp. 153–68.
20 Binik YM, Meana M, Berkley K, *et al.* (1999) The sexual pain disorders: is the pain sexual or the sex painful? *Annual Review of Sex Research* **10**, 210–35.

21 Binik YM. (2005) Should dyspareunia be retained as a sexual dysfunction in DSM-V? A painful classification decision. *Archives of Sexual Behavior* **34**, 11–21.

22 Basson R, Berman J, Burnett A, *et al.* (2000) Report of the international consensus development conference on female sexual dysfunction: definitions and classifications. *Journal of Urology* **163**, 888–93.

23 Tiefer L. (2001) A new view of women's sexual problems: why new? why now? *Journal of Sex Research* **38**, 89–96.

24 Tiefer L. (2005) Dyspareunia is the only valid sexual dysfunction and certainly the only important one. *Archives of Sexual Behavior* **34**, 49–51.

25 Meana M, Binik YM, Khalifé S, *et al.* (1999) Psychosocial correlates of pain attributions in women with dyspareunia. *Psychosomatics* **40**, 497–502.

26 Edgardh K, Abdelnoor M. (2007) Vulvar vestibulitis and risk factors: a population-based case-control study in Oslo. *Acta Dermato-Venereologica* **87**, 350–54.

27 Rylander E, Berglund AL, Krassny C, *et al.* (2004) Vulvovaginal candida in a young sexually active population: prevalence and association with orogenital sex and frequent pain at intercourse. *Sexually Transmitted Infections* **80**, 54–57.

28 Binik YM, Bergeron S, Khalifé S. (2007) Dyspareunia and vaginismus: so-called sexual pain. In: Leiblum SR (ed.) *Principles and Practice of Sex Therapy*, 4th ed. Guildford Press, New York, pp. 124–56.

29 Bergeron S, Khalifé S, Glazer HI, *et al.* (2008) Surgical and behavioral treatments for vestibulodynia. *Obstetrics and Gynecology* **111**, 159–66.

30 Goldstein AT, Klingman D, Christopher K, *et al.* (2006) Surgical treatment of vulvar vestibulitis syndrome: outcome assessment derived from a postoperative questionnaire. *The Journal of Sexual Medicine* **3**, 923–31.

31 Bergeron S, Binik YM, Khalifé S, *et al.* (2001) A randomized comparison of groups cognitive-behavioral therapy, surface electromyographic biofeedback, and vestibulectomy in the treatment of dyspareunia resulting from vulvar vestibulitis. *Pain* **91**, 297–306.

32 Melzack R, Katz J. (2001) The McGill Pain Questionnaire: appraisal and current status. In: Turk DC, Melzack R (eds.) *Handbook of Pain Assessment*, 2nd ed. Guilford Press, New York, pp. 35–52.

33 Pukall CF, Young RA, Roberts MJ, *et al.* (2007) The vulvalgesiometer as a device to measure genital pressure-pain threshold. *Physiological Measurement* **28**, 1543–50.

34 Vardi Y, Gedalia U, Gruenwald I. (2006) Neurologic testing: quantified sensory testing. In: Goldstein I, Meston CM, Davis SR *et al.* (eds.) *Women's Sexual Function and Dysfunction: Study, Diagnosis, and Treatment.* Taylor & Francis, New York, pp. 399–403.

35 Bohm-Starke N, Hilliges M, Brodda-Jansen G, *et al.* (2001) Psychophysical evidence of nociceptor sensitization in vulvar vestibulitis syndrome. *Pain* **94**, 177–83.

36 Rosenbaum TY. (2007) Physical therapy management and treatment of sexual pain disorders. In: Leiblum SR (ed.) *Principles and Practice of Sex Therapy*, 4th ed. Guilford Press, New York, pp. 157–77.

CHAPTER 4

Medical History, Physical Examination, and Laboratory Tests for the Evaluation of Dyspareunia

Andrew T. Goldstein

George Washington University School of Medicine and Health Sciences, Washington, DC, USA

Introduction

Despite the high prevalence of sexual pain (i.e., dyspareunia), few comprehensive guidelines exist regarding its evaluation. This chapter provides an overview of the components of the medical history, physical examination, and laboratory tests that can help clinicians determine the diagnosis and cause of sexual pain.

Medical History

A patient's narrative of his/her illness provides essential information to determine the correct diagnosis of the presenting complaint. However, a woman's experience of dyspareunia is usually more complicated than other medical conditions. In addition to her pain, an affected woman may experience embarrassment, shame, guilt, loss of self-esteem, frustration, depression, and anxiety. Therefore, it is important for a clinician to use communication skills that enhance openness, comfort, trust, and confidence.

In general, a woman with sexual pain will see several clinicians in an effort to evaluate and treat her condition [1]. As a result, women may feel patronized, marginalized, and ostracized from these previous encounters, which can add to the burden of their illness. It is essential for the clinician to address these feelings in order to establish a constructive and trusting relationship with patients who experience sexual pain.

Furthermore, a clinician should refrain from being either too formal or too casual when obtaining the medical history. Providers should avoid being careless with words as patients may search for meaning in everything they say. A clinician should not display extreme reactions such as surprise, grimaces, or laughter while the patient gives her narrative. Privacy and assurances of confidentiality are essential when conducting the interview. Some patients may want a spouse, sexual partner, relative, or friend present during the interview or examination. While this may allow the patient to feel more comfortable, it also may inhibit the patient from disclosing pertinent aspects of her medical, social, relationship, or sexual history.

While it is important to ask direct questions to obtain specific information such as medication usage, it is equally essential to ask open-ended questions that allow a patient to describe her experience of the condition [2]. This process can be facilitated by encouraging the patient to give as much detailed information as possible and avoiding the temptation to frequently interrupt the patient's narrative. Throughout the whole process, displaying empathy, understanding, and acceptance is essential. Repeating the information back to the patient to confirm the accuracy of her history is also an important component.

While each clinician must establish his/her own routine, the author has found it especially helpful to provide a new patient the first 10 minutes of the interview to give her narrative of the experience of her condition. Before she starts, she is asked to try to be as specific as possible and to

Female Sexual Pain Disorders 1st edition. Edited by A. Goldstein,
C. Pukall & I. Goldstein. © 2009 Blackwell Publishing,
ISBN: 9781405183987.

try to follow a sequential timeline of her disease process. She is allowed to talk virtually uninterrupted for this time. Frequently, a patient will cry, and there may be moments of silence, but this can be cathartic for her and conveys the message that she will not be rushed, ignored, or devalued in the doctor–patient relationship. If there is not enough time to focus on a specific complaint during a single visit, the patient should be reassured of the importance of her problem and scheduled for a follow-up appointment to address that issue alone.

After taking the patient's history, it may be necessary to clarify her expectations. She may have several different complaints, so it will be important to determine which of these she feels is her chief complaint. For example, she may complain of generalized vulvar pain and burning, pain during intercourse, decreased libido, and difficulty achieving orgasm. While it is possible that one intervention can solve all of these problems, it is likely that a sequence of treatments will be needed.

After both an accurate history of present illness and chief complaint have been established, additional information should be gathered that may help the clinician narrow the differential diagnosis. Past medical, social, sexual, surgical, and medication history often provides essential information. Several tools may aid in gathering this information. The International Society for the Study of Vulvovaginal Disease has developed an extensive questionnaire that patients can fill out prior to their first appointment. This questionnaire is available online at www.ISSVD.org.

A list of questions that this author has found to be extremely valuable in the diagnosis of sexual pain disorders can be found in Table 4.1. Validated questionnaires can also be used to aid in the diagnosis of some sexual pain disorders, including irritable bowel syndrome [3], endometriosis [4], and interstitial cystitis [5]. The development of a validated instrument for vulvar pain or female sexual pain is currently ongoing. Until these instruments become available, the Female Sexual Function Index (www.fsfi-questionnaire.com), which has been validated in women with chronic pelvic pain [6], can be used.

Medication History

Many medications can cause dyspareunia. Therefore, it is essential to develop a timeline of medication use and com-

pare it to the timeline of the patient's sexual pain history. Because more than 90% of women take prescription medication [7], a discussion of the most commonly prescribed medications and their association with dyspareunia is warranted. In addition, it is important to note that patients frequently do not disclose use of herbal supplements to clinicians; thus, it is important to ask about herbs, vitamins, and alternative therapies during the medication history.

Antibiotics are the most common prescription medication that women use. While antibiotics do not directly cause sexual pain, long-term exposure does predispose women to chronic yeast infections, which may be a causative agent of the pain. Hormonal contraceptives (e.g., oral contraceptives, transdermal patch, vaginal ring) are the second most common prescription medication used by reproductive-aged women. The use of oral contraceptives is highly associated with vestibulodynia (formerly termed *vestibulitis*), the most common cause of dyspareunia in premenopausal women. In one case-control study, women who used oral contraceptives were 9.3 times more likely to develop vestibulodynia than controls [8]. In addition, women who used low-dose ethinyl estradiol oral contraceptives were more likely to develop vestibulodynia [9]. It has also been suggested that oral contraceptives may cause vestibulodynia by decreasing free circulating testosterone which may be harmful to the epithelium of the vulvar vestibule (see Chapter 28).

Lastly, approximately 20% of reproductive-aged women use prescription medications for anxiety and depression. Psychotropic medications are more frequently implicated as a cause of hypoactive sexual desire disorder (HSDD) and female sexual arousal disorder (FSAD), than sexual pain [10]. However, both HSDD and FSAD can contribute to dyspareunia due to their effects on vaginal lubrication.

It is also important to recognize that some aspects of a patient's medical history may be inaccurate. For instance, a woman's self-diagnosis of a vulvovaginal yeast infection is wrong about half the time [11]. In addition, studies surprisingly show that physician-aided diagnosis of candidiasis is frequently incorrect unless microscopy and culture are used [12]. While specific data are lacking, the author frequently finds that some women have a very difficult time localizing their sexual pain. They may incorrectly identify the location of their dyspareunia; localizing it to

Table 4.1 Useful questions when obtaining a sexual pain history.

Do you have a history of:	Suggestive of what condition
Physical, sexual, and emotional abuse or anxiety?	PFD, vaginismus
Low back or hip pain?	PFD, leiom
Urinary urgency, frequency, hesitancy, or incomplete emptying?	PFD, IC, leiom
Chronic constipation or rectal fissures.	PFD
Oral contraceptive pill use (especially OCPs with 20 µ of ethinyl estradiol, or the progestins norgestimate or drospirenone) preceding or during the onset of symptoms?	HMPVD
Ovarian suppression by Lupron, Depo-Provera?	HMPVD, AV
Decreased libido or decreased vaginal lubrication prior to the onset of dyspareunia?	HMPVD, AV
Peri-menopausal or menopausal symptoms such as hot flashes and night sweats?	HMPVD, AV
Contact allergies or skin sensitive to chemicals?	SPVD, LSC
Recurrent (culture positive) yeast infections?	SPVD, RC
Persistent yellowish vaginal discharge?	DIV, LP, trich, STI, semen allergy
Persistent white vaginal discharge?	RC
Severe burning or an allergic reaction to a topical medication on the vulva or in the vagina?	SPVD, LSC
Burning after intercourse?	PPVD, SPVD, HMPVD, LP, LS, semen allergy
Pain since first attempt at intercourse without any pain-free sex?	PPVD
Pain with first tampon use?	PPVD
Increased sensitivity of the umbilicus?	PPVD
Postcoital spotting or bleeding?	VGF, LS, LP, DIV
Vulvar itching?	RC, LS, LP, DIV, LSC, VIN, plasma cell vulvitis
Night-time scratching?	LS, LSC, RC
Diarrhea?	IBS
Midcycle spotting or pain?	Endo
Pain is worse in sexual positions with deep thrusting?	Endo, IBS, adenomyosis, ov, leiom
Vulvar ulcerations, tears, fissures?	RC, LS, LP, AV, LSC
Painful periods?	Endo, leiom
Chronic pelvic pain?	Endo, leiom, ov, PFD, PID, STI
Feeling of an obstruction in the vagina?	Recto, PFD, vaginismus, leiom,
Pain beginning after childbirth?	AV, VGF, PFD, HMPVD
Dribbling after urination?	Urethral diverticulum, PFD
Changes in coloration or architecture of the labia or vulva?	LS, LP, female genital cutting
Decreased clitoral sensation?	LS
Frequent bicycle riding?	PN
Aggressive abdominal muscle strengthening or Pilates?	PFD
Pain mainly at the clitoris?	Postherpetic neuralgia, PN
Since the pain during intercourse began, has there been completely pain-free intercourse? If yes:	PFD, RC
Do you have oral lesions or bleeding gums?	LP, mucous membrane pemphigoid
History of high-risk human papilloma virus or cervical dysplasia?	VIN

KEY: PFD = pelvic floor dysfunction; IC = interstitial cystitis; HMPVD = hormonally mediated provoked vestibulodynia; PPVD = primary provoked vestibulodynia; SPVD = secondary provoked vestibulodynia; PN = pudendal neuralgia; LS = lichen sclerosus; LP = lichen planus; AV = atrophic vaginitis; DIV = desquamative inflammatory vaginitis; PID = pelvic inflammatory disease; IBS = irritable bowel syndrome; VGF = vulvar granuloma fissuratum; leiom = leiomyoma; endo = endometriosis; RC = recurrent candidiasis; ov = ovarian mass; VIN = vulvar intraepithelial neoplasia; LSC = lichen simplex chronicus; STI = sexually transmitted infection.

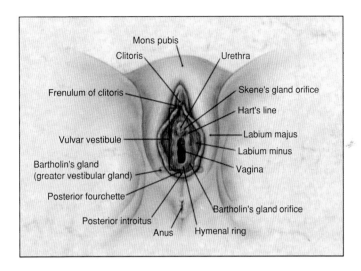

Figure 4.1 Vulvar anatomy.

Physical Exam

All women with dyspareunia should undergo a thorough physical examination. While this exam focuses primarily on the urogenital system, additional organ systems may need to be assessed depending on information gathered during the medical history. The goal of the physical examination is to gather data to determine the etiology of the sexual pain. This requires a meticulous and methodical exam. In addition, if the examiner can identify the correct location and by manual examination reproduce a woman's pain, she feels validated as this shows her that her sexual pain is primarily physical. In addition, it inspires confidence that the practitioner will be able to treat her pain.

It is useful if the patient watches the physical examination to establish a common nomenclature for the parts of the urogenital system (Figure 4.1). The author utilizes a video colposcope linked to a LCD monitor to aid in this didactic exercise. In addition, the video colposcope can magnify important structures, and digital photographs can then be printed. These photos can be used to monitor treatment progress and can be given to patients to help guide treatment when they are at home. It is important to obtain consent before taking any digital images [13].

Chapter 7 of this book is entirely devoted to the colposcopic examination of the vulva, commonly referred to as vulvoscopy, in women with sexual pain. If a video colposcope is unavailable, a patient can hold a hand mirror in order to visualize all aspects of the exam. Important findings that can be observed on the visual examination of the vulva include infection, trauma, and dermatitis. Specifically, the observer should note any inflammation, induration, excoriation, fissures, ulceration, lichenification, hypopigmentation, hyperpigmentation, scarring, or architectural changes, which may be evidence for dermatologic disease of the vulva (Figure 4.2). These diseases are discussed in greater detail in Chapter 9. While erythema is a nonspecific finding, intense redness at the ostia of the Bartholin and Skene glands is suggestive of vestibulodynia (Figure 4.3). Vestibulodynia is thoroughly discussed in Chapter 12.

A sensory exam of the vulva is performed using a moistened cotton swab to determine if there are areas that exhibit an abnormal pain response. Women with sexual pain can exhibit allodynia (i.e., the perception of pain upon provocation by a normally nonpainful stimulus such as being touched with a cotton swab) or hyperpathia (i.e., pain provoked by very light touch). This exam should be performed systematically to ensure that all areas of the anogenital region are tested. Initially, the medial thigh, buttocks, and mons pubis are palpated. These areas are typically not painful and this allows the patient to get comfortable with this exam.

The labia majora, clitoral prepuce, perineum, and intralabial sulci should then be palpated. Pain in these areas would suggest a process that is affecting the whole

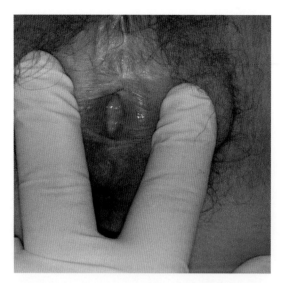

Figure 4.2 Lichenification, hypopigmentation, and architectural changes of lichen sclerosus.

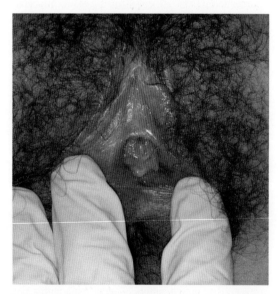

Figure 4.3 Erythema of PVD.

anogenital region including vulvar dermatoses, vulvovaginal infections, or neuropathic processes such as pudendal neuralgia. The labia minora are then gently palpated. First, the medial labia minora are gently touched lateral to Hart's line, which is the lateral boundary of the vulvar vestibule. The cotton swab is then used to gently palpate the vestibule at five locations: at the ostia of the Skene glands (lat-

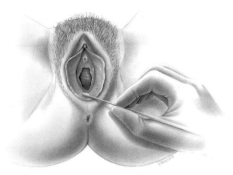

Figure 4.4 Cotton swab test.

eral to the urethra), at the ostia of the Bartholin glands (4 and 8 o'clock on the vestibule), and at 6 o'clock at the fossa navicularis (Figure 4.4). Patients with vestibulodynia will frequently experience allodynia with the cotton swab palpation confined to the tissue of the vulvar vestibule but have normal sensation lateral to this boundary. Chapter 8 discusses the differential diagnosis in a woman with vestibulodynia.

A speculum exam of the vagina is the next step in the physical examination of a woman with dyspareunia. In general, a pediatric-sized Graves speculum should be used and all efforts should be used to insert the speculum through the hymeneal ring without touching the vulvar vestibule.

Initially, the vagina should be examined for evidence of abnormal vaginal discharge. A cotton swab should be used to collect some discharge for pH testing, wet mount, and potassium hydroxide (KOH) prep. In addition, a culture should be obtained and sent for speciation and sensitivity. Important findings while visualizing the vagina include atrophy, erythema, erosions, ulcerations, abnormal discharge, or synechiae. These abnormalities are discussed in much greater detail in the following chapters: Chapter 11 examines sexually transmitted infections; Chapter 15 addresses other infectious causes of vulvovaginitis; and Chapter 16 outlines the evaluation and treatment of sterile vaginitis (atrophic vaginitis and desquamative inflammatory vaginitis).

A manual exam is then performed with one finger instead of the usual two fingers. The examiner's index finger is inserted through the hymen without touching the vestibule. The urethra and bladder trigone are gently palpated. Intrinsic tenderness of the urethra may be suggestive of a urethral diverticulum or interstitial cystitis, while tenderness of the bladder may be suggestive of either interstitial cystitis (Chapter 14) or endometriosis (Chapter 19). The levator ani muscles are then palpated for hypertonicity, tenderness, weakness, and trigger points, which can be evidence of pelvic floor muscle dysfunction (also known as levator ani syndrome or vaginismus).

Because pelvic floor dysfunction (PFD) is such an important and common cause of dyspareunia, three chapters are devoted its discussion: Chapter 6 focuses on the evaluation of the pelvic floor muscles; Chapter 13 examines the treatment strategies for PFD; and Chapter 35 examines additional aspects of the evaluation and treatment of vaginismus.

The ischial spine is then located and the pudendal nerve is palpated as it enters Alcock's canal. Tenderness of the pudendal nerve is suggestive of pudendal neuralgia or pudendal nerve entrapment discussed in Chapter 17. Next, a bimanual examination is performed to assess the uterus and adnexa (ovaries and fallopian tubes). Abnormalities in the size, shape, or contour may be indicative of a leiomyoma, further discussed in Chapter 29. A diffusely enlarged, "boggy" and tender uterus may be signs of adenomyosis (Chapter 19). Enlargement of the adnexa may represent an ovarian mass, which is reviewed in detail in Chapter 29. Tenderness of the adnexa can often be a sign of a sexually transmitted infection (Chapter 11), pelvic inflammatory disease (Chapter 20), or endometriosis. A recto-vaginal examination is then performed to assess the rectovaginal septum and the posterior cul-de-sac. Thickening or nodularity of the septum, nodularity of the uterosacral ligaments, or obliteration of the posterior cul-de-sac can be suggestive of endometriosis (Chapter 19). Traumatic neuromas can also be a source of significant pain in women who have had prior vaginal surgery, including repair of lacerations or episiotomies incurred during childbirth (discussed in Chapter 34).

Testing

Wet Mount and Cultures

As discussed above, vaginal discharge should be examined by wet prep, pH, and KOH testing. Specifically, vaginal discharge should be obtained on two cotton swabs from the upper third of the vagina, and the pH of the discharge should be tested. One swab is used to make a slide with saline and the other swab is combined with KOH. The wet mount should be examined with a microscope on both low- and high-power magnification. The saline slide is examined for normal squamous epithelial cells, increased white blood cells (WBC) (more than one WBC per epithelial cell), pathogens such as yeast cells (species other than candida albicans can be found on microscopy) and trichomonas, parabasal cells, clue cells, and normal flora such as lactobacilli. As microscopic examination frequently misses candidiasis and trichomoniasis, a culture obtained at the time of vaginal inspection should be sent for speciation and sensitivity. In addition, if there is significant leukorrhea, a swab should be obtained for an immunochromatographic assay for trichomonas (Genzyme Corporation, Cambridge, MA).

Histology

A vulvar or vaginal biopsy should be obtained if there are specific findings on colposcopic exam of the vulva suggestive of a dermatoses, intraepithelial neoplasia, or neoplasia. It is unlikely, however, that the biopsy will prove useful if the physical findings are just nonspecific erythema. The biopsy should be obtained at the edge of any ulcerations or erosions if present using a 5 mm punch biopsy. All biopsies should be closed with one or two stitches of absorbable suture such as 4-0 Vicryl-rapide (Ethicon, Inc., Somerville, NJ).

The author recommends that all vulvovaginal biopsies should be sent with a description of the physical findings to pathologists who, when possible, specialize in dermatologic disorders. When vulvovaginal ulcerations are present, a second biopsy may be obtained and sent in Michel's transport media for direct immunofluorescence to rule out the immunobullous diseases such as mucous membrane pemphigoid [14]. This should only be done when the more common sources of ulceration, such as genital herpes, have been ruled out.

Serum Testing

Because hormonal abnormalities are common causes of sexual pain, blood should be obtained for serum estradiol, total testosterone, free testosterone, albumin, sex hormone binding globulin (SHBG), follicle stimulating hormone, and prolactin. A decreased serum estradiol is frequently found in women with vestibulodynia or atrophic vaginitis. Elevated SHBG and decreased free testosterone and estradiol are frequently found in women with vestibulodynia caused by hormonal contraceptives. An elevated prolactin level can cause anovulation which leads to atrophic vaginitis. Herpes serology should be obtained in women with symptoms of generalized vulvar burning or tingling, or in those with pain concentrated in the clitoris (clitorodynia).

Serum testing is not necessary in all cases of sexual pain, but may help when the etiology of the pain is not obvious. For example, serum estradiol does not need to be drawn if a woman is postmenopausal and has signs of atrophic vaginitis, or if the patient is on hormonal contraceptives. In the latter case, she would be expected to have low serum levels of free testosterone and estradiol and higher SHBG.

Additional Testing

Referrals for additional tests should be based on findings during the history and physical examination. Radiographic or ultrasonographic imaging may be appropriate to evaluate the uterus, ovaries, pelvis, or lower spine. Diagnostic laparoscopy may be necessary if there is significant evidence of endometriosis or utero-ovarian pathology that does not respond to initial conservative management. Colonoscopy, barium enema, and/or a CT scan with contrast may be used to rule out pathology of the lower gastrointestinal tract if deep thrusting dyspareunia is present along with dyschezia, hematochezia, or symptoms consistent with inflammatory bowel disease. Cystoscopy may be used to aid in the diagnosis of interstitial cystitis. An electromyelogram may be used to assess the tone and strength of the levator ani muscles when there is evidence of pelvic floor dysfunction.

Conclusions

A combination of a thorough medical history, physical examination, and appropriate testing should give a clinician enough evidence to establish either a specific diagnosis or a differential diagnosis of the etiology of a woman's sexual pain. In addition, the process of obtaining this history and physical examination establishes a rapport between the clinician and patient, which is essential in the treatment of sexual pain disorders.

References

1 Harlow BL, Stewart EG. (2003) A population-based assessment of chronic unexplained vulvar pain: have we underestimated the prevalence of vulvodynia? *Journal of the American Medical Women's Association* **58**, 82–88.

2 Seidel HM, Ball JW, Dains JE, *et al.* (eds.) (1991) *Mosby's Guide to Physical Examination.* Mosby-Year Book, Inc, St. Louis.

3 Wiklund IK, Fullerton S, Hawkey CJ, *et al.* (2003) An irritable bowel syndrome-specific symptom questionnaire: development and validation. *Scandinavian Journal of Gastroenterology* **38**, 947–954.

4 Fedele L, Bianchi S, Carmignani L, *et al.* (2007) Evaluation of a new questionnaire for the presurgical diagnosis of bladder endometriosis. *Human Reproduction* **22**, 2698–2701.

5 Brewer ME, White WM, Klein FA, *et al.* (2007) Validity of pelvic pain, urgency, and frequency questionnaire in patients with interstitial cystitis/painful bladder syndrome. *Urology* **70**, 646–49.

6 Verit FF, Verit A. (2007) Validation of the female sexual function index in women with chronic pelvic pain. *The Journal of Sexual Medicine* **4**, 1635–41.

7 Glover DD, Rybeck BF, Tracy TS. (2004) Medication use in a rural gynecologic population: prescription, over-the-counter, and herbal medicines. *American Journal of Obstetrics and Gynecology* **190**, 351–57.

8 Bouchard C, Brisson J, Fortier M, *et al.* (2002) Use of oral contraceptive pills and vulvar vestibulitis: a case-control study. *American Journal of Epidemiology* **156**, 254–61.

9 Greenstein A, Ben-Aroya Z, Fass O, *et al.* (2007) Vulvar vestibulitis syndrome and estrogen dose of oral contraceptive pills. *The Journal of Sexual Medicine* **4**, 1679–83.

10 Clayton AH, Campbell BJ, Favit A, *et al.* (2007) Symptoms of sexual dysfunction in patients treated for major depressive disorder: a meta-analysis comparing selegiline transdermal system and placebo using a patient-rated scale. *Journal of Clinical Psychiatry* **68**, 1860–66.

11 Ferris DG, Nyirjesy P, Sobel JD, *et al.* (2002) Over-the-counter antifungal drug misuse associated with patient-diagnosed vulvovaginal candidiasis. *Obstetrics and Gynecology* **99**, 419–25.

12 Ledger WJ, Monif GRG. (2004) A growing concern: inability to diagnose vulvovaginal infections correctly. *Obstetrics and Gynecology* **103**, 782–84.

13 Berle I. (2008) Clinical photography and patient rights: the need for orthopraxy. *Journal of Medical Ethics* **34**, 89–92.

14 Raghu AR, Nirmala NR, Sreekumaran N. (2002) Direct immunofluorescence in oral lichen planus and oral lichenoid reactions. *Quintessence International* **33**, 234–39.

CHAPTER 5

Psychological Evaluation and Measurement of Dyspareunia

Caroline F. Pukall,[1] *Marta Meana,*[2] *Katherine S. Sutton*[1]

[1]Queen's University, Kingston, Ontario, Canada
[2]University of Nevada, Las Vegas, NV, USA

Introduction

Despite the high prevalence of dyspareunia, few comprehensive guidelines exist regarding its evaluation. This chapter provides an overview of the clinical interview, standardized measures, and psychophysical methods used to assess this condition.

The Clinical Interview

The clinical interview is uniquely equipped to cover multiple areas affected by dyspareunia and to elicit descriptions important to treatment planning. Although there is no standardized interview for the assessment of sexual pain disorders, the empirical literature has charted a clear path to relevant areas. Obtaining a psychosexual history is recommended [1]; it can provide invaluable information about predisposing factors such as family of origin and cultural schemas about sexuality, formative sexual experiences, and any history of sexual abuse/trauma. Of more proximal relevance is the assessment of pain properties, mediators, and interference, comorbid disorders, and self-reported effectiveness of past treatment attempts.

Pain Properties

The clinical interview starts with patients' general descriptions of their difficulties and reasons for seeking treatment. This open-ended characterization is important as it can communicate much about the patient's cognitive and

Female Sexual Pain Disorders 1st edition. Edited by A. Goldstein,
C. Pukall & I. Goldstein. © 2009 Blackwell Publishing,
ISBN: 9781405183987.

emotional disposition toward the problem prior to treatment suggestion or intervention. It is followed by more specific questions about the properties of the pain. Of diagnostic importance are the lifetime onset of the pain, onset within an intercourse episode, duration of the pain, and its specific location (it is helpful to provide patients with a diagram/model of the genital and pelvic region), qualitative descriptions, and severity [2]. Open-ended characterizations of the pain should also be followed up with the administration of a pain descriptor list. Finally, the severity of pain can be elicited via visual analog or numerical rating scales.

Pain Mediators

Pain is a complex subjective experience that can be impacted by a variety of factors ranging from the mechanics of stimulation to emotional states [3]. Identifying factors that mediate pain is essential to diagnostic assessment and treatment interventions. It is important to elicit details regarding conditions that patients have identified as affecting their pain experience. For example, what tends to exacerbate or improve the pain? Some potential mediators include length of foreplay, intercourse positions, use of lubrication aids, level of desire/arousal, timing, fatigue, stress, mood, feelings toward the sexual partner, and overall relationship quality. Any one or combination of these factors may affect the pain experience and provide clues to its successful management.

Pain Interference and Comorbid Problems

Pain can also have a significant impact on other aspects of patients' lives and interfere with their sexual function, psychological well-being, and relationships. The comorbidity of other sexual dysfunctions, mood disturbances, and relationship difficulties are relatively well documented, although it can be difficult to separate cause and consequence. Regardless, comorbid disorders and/or problems require therapeutic attention and are thus important targets for assessment.

Women who experience pain with intercourse tend to report higher levels of difficulties with desire, arousal, and orgasm [4]. It is important to ask women about all aspects of their sexual function and satisfaction and to administer sexual function measures that allow for comparison to norms. Women with dyspareunia also report higher levels of mood disturbances, negative affect, somatization [4, 5], and a hypervigilant and catastrophizing cognitive style [6, 7]. Inquiring about patients' theories regarding their coital pain also can be fruitful, as these have been related to distress and relationship adjustment [8].

Relationship Adjustment

A disorder that interferes with sex is likely also to affect relationship dynamics. In turn, the quality of the relationship probably influences the experience of dyspareunia. It is thus ideal to involve the partner in the assessment process. Research on dyadic adjustment in the context of dyspareunia is scarce, but studies have shown an association between pain intensity and marital adjustment, partner solicitousness, and partner hostility [9, 10].

General relationship adjustment inquiries can be aided by self-administered measures. However, it is also crucial to ask specific questions about how the couple navigates the difficulties posed by intercourse pain. Examples of such questions are: How does each person react to difficult or aborted attempts at intercourse? What does the partner think the cause of the problem might be? What are fears about the possible impact of dyspareunia on the viability of their relationship? How does each person personalize the difficulty as a reflection of their desirability? What would happen if the pain went away? Comorbid sexual dysfunction in the partner is also important to assess as it can have a significant impact on the development of treatment strategies.

Previous Treatment Attempts

Finally, it is recommended that the patient be asked about the types and outcomes of treatments she may have already engaged in, if any. It is important to respect these reports and preferences, but the clinician should keep in mind that not all treatments are delivered in the same fashion by all providers and that not all patients adhere to treatment regimens as recommended. Obtaining as many details as possible about prior treatment attempts can be useful in the determination of future steps.

Self-Administered Measures

Self-administered measures of pain, sexual function, and psychological and relationship adjustment complement the interview and are essential to implementing and monitoring treatment efficacy.

Pain

Dyspareunic pain has been measured primarily in terms of its intensity and qualitative description. Intensity is probably best captured via visual analog or numerical rating scales anchored at "no pain" and "extreme pain," or variants thereof. These scales can be administered such that women rate the intensity of their pain retrospectively, or they can be part of a pain diary completed after every intercourse attempt. Descriptors of pain have been predictive of dyspareunia type [2] and thus constitute an important assessment tool.

The most widely used and validated pain measure with dyspareunic women is the McGill–Melzack Pain Questionnaire (MPQ) [11]. It consists of a list of pain descriptors about sensory, affective, and evaluative factors, while also providing an overall pain rating index. Because psychological reactions to pain can have as much of an impact on one's life as the sensory aspect, it is useful to determine the level of distress incurred by attempted or penetrative intercourse especially in the formulation of cognitive treatment strategies. The Pain Catastrophizing Scale (PCS) [12] can be invaluable because it taps into emotions and cognitions that accompany the pain experience.

Sexual Function

Sexual function questionnaires can shed light on comorbid sexual dysfunctions and can be used to monitor treatment progress on multiple levels. There is no single standardized questionnaire designed exclusively for the assessment of sexual pain, but there are several appropriate sexual function and satisfaction measures.

Measures applicable to both men and women include the Golombok–Rust Inventory of Sexual Satisfaction (GRISS) [13], a 56-item (28 on the male version and 28 on the female version) measure of sexual function and relationship quality in heterosexual relationships. It yields scores on several subscales (e.g., orgasmic difficulties) and provides a global score of overall sexual quality of the relationship and the couple's sexual function. The Changes in Sexual Functioning Questionnaire (CSFQ) [14, 15] can be clinician-administered as a structured interview or self-administered as a gender-specific questionnaire. It measures five dimensions of sexual functioning: sexual pleasure, sexual desire/frequency, sexual desire/interest, arousal, and orgasm.

Measures specifically designed for women include the Female Sexual Function Index (FSFI) [16], a 19-item measure of female sexual function yielding a total score, as well as scores on desire, arousal, lubrication, orgasm, satisfaction, and pain. It has shown good discriminant validity in the assessment of chronic vulvar pain [17]. The Sexual Function Questionnaire (SFQ) [18] is a 34-item instrument developed to measure multiple aspects of sexual function and relationship quality. The McCoy Female Sexuality Questionnaire (MFSQ) [19] is a 19-item measure that assesses recent levels of sexual interest and response. The Sexual Satisfaction Scale for Women (SSS-W) [20] is a 30-item scale assessing five domains: contentment, communication, compatibility, relational concern, and personal concern. Finally, because distress is an important mediator of the pain experience, the 12-item Female Sexual Distress Scale (FSDS) [21] can be used to estimate levels of distress over sexual difficulties.

Psychological Function

If depression or anxiety is suspected, the Beck Depression Inventory II (BDI-II) [22] and the Beck Anxiety Inventory (BAI) [23] are psychometrically sound and brief. They each consist of 21 items rated on 4-point scales. For a global profile of psychological function, the 344-item Personality Assessment Inventory (PAI) [24] has superior psychometric properties and has been validated with chronic pain populations [25]. The administration of any measure of psychological symptomatology should be prefaced with a clear explanation of its function (i.e., the investigation of pain mediators/contributors). Iatrogenic harm can be inflicted if the patient perceives the clinician as believing her pain is "not real."

Relationship Adjustment

The Dyadic Adjustment Scale (DAS) [26] consists of 32 items assessing dyadic consensus, satisfaction, cohesion, and affective expression. Total scores have been shown to discriminate between distressed and nondistressed couples and to identify at-risk marriages. It is easy to administer and provides information about the relational context within which the sexual pain disorder exists. An alternative is the older Locke–Wallace Marital Adjustment Test (LWMAT) [27] which remains valid for married couples despite its age [28].

Quantifiable Measures of Dyspareunic Pain

In addition to self-report measures, hands-on techniques that quantify pain sensitivity via the use of quantitative sensory testing (QST) can be used to explore potential mechanisms involved in dyspareunia and the real-time pain responses of patients. QST has been most often applied to provoked vestibulodynia (PVD), although it is gaining in popularity for use in other dyspareunic conditions.

Pressure–Pain Measurement

Although not a QST method per se, the cotton swab test [29] can be a measure of pain sensitivity when combined with the recording of pain ratings. This test is the standard gynecological test for diagnosing PVD, and it consists of palpating vulvar sites with a cotton swab. It can be performed in a variety of ways; however, the order of the vestibular palpations should be randomized to control for sensitization [30]. PVD patients have reported significantly higher mean pain ratings at the vulvar vestibule than pain-free controls [7], demonstrating the utility of this test in distinguishing between PVD patients and control women.

While the cotton swab test is useful in clinical practice, it is prone to measurement error and may not be ideal for experimental purposes [30]. The most problematic aspect of this test is the consistency of pressure application. Individuals may apply different amounts of pressure and vary in terms of pressure application over time, leading to difficulty in comparing pain ratings. However, a new device, the vulvalgesiometer, exerts standardized pressures to measure pressure–pain thresholds [31, 32].

A set of five vulvalgesiometers exerts a range of 26 predetermined pressures from 3 to 950 g [32]. Each vulvalgesiometer is a handheld device containing springs with different compression rates. At the end of each device is a disposable cotton swab, the only part that comes into contact with the test area. Although the diagnostic ability of the vulvalgesiometers has yet to be determined, they have been used to measure vestibular pressure–pain thresholds in several studies [33]. The vulvalgesiometers replicate the sharp/burning sensation reported by women with PVD when describing their pain during intercourse [32]. Thresholds measured via the vulvalgesiometers and other spring-based pressure–pain devices discriminate between women with and without PVD [32, 34].

Methods to assess vaginal pressure–pain sensitivity may be useful in vaginal dyspareunia conditions. The vaginal algometer [35] assesses pressure–pain threshold on the lateral walls of the vagina via a thimblelike probe on the clinician's index finger. When it is inserted into the vagina, the algometer is positioned over the pudendal nerve and the pressure level is increased by 2 newtons per second until the patient reports pain. It is well tolerated by healthy women, and thresholds are not influenced by parity or menstrual phase [35]. It is also capable of discriminating between women with and without chronic pelvic pain (CPP) [36].

Measurement of Other Forms of Stimulation

Genital sensitivity to other forms of stimulation (e.g., temperature, vibration) can also be measured. The Medoc Thermal Genital Sensory Analyzer includes the only probe designed for use on the genitals and inside the vagina [37]. Its temperature range is 0–50°C, different sized probes are available, and several threshold programs can be used. Studies indicate that the heat–pain threshold discriminates between women with and without PVD [38], but not between women with and without interstitial cystitis (IC) [39]. In addition, the Medoc Vibratory Sensory Analyzer is a vibratory probe designed for use in the vagina and over the clitoris. It has a fixed vibration frequency at 100 Hz and amplitude range of 0–130 μm. Studies indicate that the measurement of vibration thresholds is reliable and valid [37]; however, it does not discriminate between women with and without PVD [38].

Sensitivity to vaginal distension at the introitus or deeper can be measured with a small rubber balloon, connected by a plastic tube to a pressure gauge, inserted to the desired vaginal depth. Bohm-Starke et al. [38] dilated the vaginal introitus of women with and without PVD until pain was reported. Women with PVD experienced pain at a lower distension level than the control group.

Sensitivity to bladder distention has been used in the IC literature to discriminate between affected and nonaffected women. Saline is typically infused into the bladder at a rate of 50 cc/min via a transurethral catheter until the pain can no longer be tolerated. Results of studies indicate that women with IC report their first desire to void and pain tolerance level at lower volumes than nonaffected women, and they also report higher pain intensity ratings than do control women at comparable distension levels [39].

While the measurement of thresholds is empirically useful, it may not be practical for clinical settings, because it is time-consuming, the equipment is costly, training may be required, and information gleaned from threshold measurement does not necessarily aid in the diagnosis of dyspareunia.

Discussion

Measuring pain and associated factors in multiple ways is optimal for a comprehensive understanding of the patient's experience and for efficacious treatment planning. It is important, however, to keep in mind that decreasing dyspareunic pain does not necessarily lead to a restoration of sexual function, as has been shown in a randomized trial involving women with PVD [40]. Only an interdisciplinary treatment approach to dyspareunia can target both restoration of sexual function and pain reduction. In addition, pre- and posttreatment quantification of genital sensitivity while recording pain intensity can lead to advances in the optimization of treatment success and a deeper understanding of the pathophysiology of dyspareunia.

References

1 Maurice WL. (1999) *Sexual Medicine in Primary Care.* Mosby, St. Louis.

2 Meana M, Binik YM, Khalifé S, *et al.* (1997a) Dyspareunia: sexual dysfunction or pain syndrome? *Journal of Nervous and Mental Disease* 185, 561–69.

3 Price DD. (1999) *Psychological Mechanisms of Pain and Analgesia.* IASP Press, Seattle.

4 Meana M, Binik YM, Khalifé S, *et al.* (1997b) Biopsychosocial profile of women with dyspareunia: searching for etiological hypotheses. *Obstetrics and Gynecology* **90**, 583–89.

5 Danielsson I, Eisemann M, Sjoberg I, *et al.* (2001) Vulvar vestibulitis: a multifactorial condition. *British Journal of Obstetrics and Gynaecology* **22**, 456–61.

6 Payne KA, Binik YM, Amsel R, *et al.* (2005) When sex hurts, anxiety and fear orient toward pain. *European Journal of Pain* **9**, 427–36.

7 Pukall CF, Binik YM, Khalifé S, *et al.* (2002) Vestibular tactile and pain thresholds in women with vulvar vestibulitis syndrome. *Pain* **96**, 163–75.

8 Meana M, Binik YM, Khalifé S, *et al.* (1999) Psychosocial correlates of pain attributions in women with dyspareunia. *Psychosomatics* **40**, 497–502.

9 Meana M, Binik YM, Khalifé S, *et al.* (1998) Affect and marital adjustment in women's ratings of dyspareunic pain. *Canadian Journal of Psychiatry* **43**, 381–85.

10 Desrosiers M, Bergeron S, Meana M, *et al.* (2008) Psychosexual characteristics of vestibulodynia couples: partner solicitousness and hostility are associated with pain. *The Journal of Sexual Medicine* **5**, 418–27.

11 Melzack R, Katz J. (2001) The McGill Pain Questionnaire: appraisal and current status. In: Turk DC, Melzack R (eds.) *Handbook of Pain Assessment*, 2nd ed. Guilford Press, New York, pp. 35–52.

12 Sullivan MJL, Bishop SR, Pivik J. (1995) The pain catastrophizing scale: development and validation. *Psychological Assessment* **7**, 524–32.

13 Rust J, Golombok S. (1986) The GRISS: a psychometric instrument for the assessment of sexual dysfunction. *Archives of Sexual Behavior* **15**, 157–65.

14 Clayton AH, McGarvey EL, Clavet GJ. (1997) The Changes in Sexual Functioning Questionnaire (CSFQ): Development, reliability, and validity. *Psychopharmacology Bulletin* **33**, 731–45.

15 Keller A, McGarvey EL, Clayton AH. (2006) Reliability and construct validity of the Changes in Sexual Functioning Questionnaire Short-Form (CSFQ-14). *Journal of Sex and Marital Therapy* **32**, 43–52.

16 Rosen R, Brown C, Heiman J, *et al.* (2000) The Female Sexual Function Index (FSFI): a multidimensional self-report instrument for the assessment of female sexual function. *Journal of Sex and Marital Therapy* **26**, 191–208.

17 Masheb RM, Lozano-Blanco C, Kohorn EI, *et al.* (2004) Assessing sexual function and dyspareunia with the Female Sexual Function Index (FSFI) in women with vulvodynia. *Journal of Sex and Marital Therapy* **30**, 315–24.

18 Quirk FH, Heiman JR, Rosen RC, *et al.* (2002) Development of a sexual function questionnaire for clinical trials of female sexual dysfunction. *Journal of Women's Health and Gender-Based Medicine* **11**, 277–89.

19 McCoy NL, Matyas JR. (1998) McCoy Female Sexuality Questionnaire. In: Davis CM, Yarber WL, Bauserman R, *et al.* (eds.) *Handbook of Sexuality Related Measures.* Sage Publications, Thousand Oaks, CA, pp. 249–51.

20 Meston CM, Trapnell P. (2005) Development and validation of a five-factor sexual satisfaction and distress scale for women: the Sexual Satisfaction Scale for women. *The Journal of Sexual Medicine* **2**, 66–81.

21 Derogatis LR, Rosen R, Leiblum S, *et al.* (2002) The Female Sexual Distress Scale (FSDS): initial validation of a standardized scale for assessment of sexually related personal distress in women. *Journal of Sex and Marital Therapy* **28**, 317–30.

22 Beck AT, Steer RA, Brown GK. (1996) *Beck Depression Inventory Manual*, 2nd ed. Psychological Corporation, San Antonio.

23 Beck AT, Steer RA. (1990) *Beck Anxiety Inventory.* Psychological Corporation, San Antonio.

24 Morey LC. (2007) *Personality Assessment Inventory: Professional Manual*, 2nd ed. Psychological Assessment Resources, Odessa.

25 Bradley LA, Haile JM, Jarkowski TM. (1992) Assessment of psychological status using interviews and self-report instruments. In: Turk DC, Melzack R (eds.) *Handbook of Pain Assessment*, 2nd ed. Guilford Press, New York, pp. 193–213.

26 Spanier GB. (1976) Measuring dyadic adjustment: new scales for assessing the quality of marriage and similar dyads. *Journal of Marriage and Family* **38**, 15–28.

27 Locke HJ & Wallace KM. (1959) Short marital adjustment and prediction tests: their reliability and validity. *Marriage and Family Living* **21**, 251–55.

28 Freeston MH, Plechaty M. (1997) Reconsideration of the Locke–Wallace Marital Adjustment Test: is it still relevant for the 1990's? *Psychological Reports* **81**, 419–34.

29 Friedrich EG, Jr. (1987) Vulvar vestibulitis syndrome. *The Journal of Reproductive Medicine* **32**, 110–114.

30 Pukall CF, Payne KA, Binik YM, *et al.* (2003) Pain measurement in vulvodynia. *Journal of Sex and Marital Therapy* **29**, 111–20.

31 Pukall CF, Binik YM, Khalifé S. (2004) A new instrument for pain assessment in vulvar vestibulitis syndrome. *Journal of Sex and Marital Therapy* **30**, 69–78.

32 Pukall CF, Young RA, Roberts MJ, *et al.* (2007) The vulvalgesiometer as a device to measure genital pressure-pain threshold. *Physiological Measurement* **28**, 1543–50.

33 Pukall CF, Kandyba K, Amsel R, *et al.* (2007) Effectiveness of hypnosis for the treatment of vulvar vestibulitis syndrome: a

CHAPTER 5

preliminary investigation. *The Journal of Sexual Medicine* **4**, 417–25.

34 Lowenstein L, Vardi Y, Deutsch M, *et al.* (2004) Vulvar vestibulitis severity: assessment by sensory and pain testing modalities. *Pain* **107**, 47–53.

35 Curnow JSH, Barron L, Morrison G, *et al.* (1996) Vulval algesiometer. *Medical and Biological Engineering and Computing* **34**, 266–69.

36 Tu FF, Fitzgerald CM, Kuiken T, *et al.* (2007) Comparative measurement of pelvic floor pain sensitivity in chronic pelvic pain. *Obstetrics and Gynecology* **110**, 1244–48.

37 Vardi Y, Gedalia U, Gruenwald I. (2006) Neurologic testing: quantified sensory testing. In: Goldstein I, Meston CM, Davis SR, *et al.* (eds.). *Women's Sexual*

Function and Dysfunction: Study, Diagnosis, and Treatment. Taylor & Francis, New York, pp. 399–403.

38 Bohm-Starke N, Hilliges M, Brodda-Jansen G, *et al.* (2001) Psychophysical evidence of nociceptor sensitization in vulvar vestibulitis syndrome. *Pain* **94**, 177–83.

39 Ness TJ, Powell-Boone T, Cannon R, *et al.* (2005) Psychophysical evidence of hypersensitivity in subjects with interstitial cystitis. *The Journal of Urology* **173**, 1983–87.

40 Bergeron S, Binik YM, Khalifé S, *et al.* (2001) A randomized comparison of group cognitive-behavioral therapy, surface electromyographic biofeedback, and vestibulectomy in the treatment of dyspareunia resulting from vulvar vestibulitis. *Pain* **91**, 297–306.

CHAPTER 6

Physical Therapy Evaluation of Dyspareunia

Talli Y. Rosenbaum
Urogynecological Physiotherapy Private Practice

Introduction

Dyspareunia refers to pain associated with intercourse and is classically viewed as the result of either a medical or psychological cause. Therefore, practitioners who treat dyspareunia have traditionally been physicians with expertise in the urogenital organs (gynecologists, urologists) or mental health professionals with expertise in sexuality (psychologists, sex therapists). However, when the presenting symptom is pain, physical therapists (PTs), who are well versed in evaluating and treating pain disorders, should be a part of the treatment team. Moreover, while the etiology of dyspareunia was once considered *either* physical *or* psychological [1] the contemporary approach recognizes that psychosexual, relational, physiological, and contextual factors combine to create and/or perpetuate painful sex [2]. This approach validates the presence of pain even in the absence of a clear medical pathology, such as infection or skin disease.

The goal of a physical therapy intervention is to identify the source of dyspareunia and provide treatment that reduces pain and improves sexual function [3]. Common tools employed by PTs in performing a comprehensive evaluation include obtaining an accurate history; assessing posture; observing gait and movement patterns; evaluating muscle strength, tone, and endurance; and assessing joint and soft tissue mobility. PTs who have specialized training in the evaluation and treatment of pelvic floor disorders are skilled at assessing the musculoskeletal components involved in genital and pelvic pain.

Pelvic Anatomy

A detailed understanding of the anatomic structures that comprise the pelvis is essential in determining the musculoskeletal components of dyspareunia. The bony pelvis is comprised of three bones on each side—the ilium, ischium and pubis bones, which together form the ox coxae. Also referred to as the innominate bone, they are joined anteriorly at the symphysis pubis and posteriorly to the sacrum and coccyx. The endopelvic portion of the pelvis surrounds the pelvic organs, which include the bladder, urethra, uterus, and rectum, as well as the perineum, which supports the viscera and gives structure to the urethra, vagina, and anus. The abdominal peritoneum extends inferiorly, covering the uterus, bladder, and rectum. Dynamically, the pelvis allows transfer of weight bearing forces between the trunk and lower limbs, provides protection of the pelvic organs, attachments for muscle, fascia, and ligaments in and around the midsection, and directs propulsive forces during parturition. Mobility and function are influenced by the muscles and soft tissues that attach to the pelvis, hips, and spine. In addition, the pelvic viscera and their fascial attachments within the pelvis (broad ligament, uracus, pubovesical ligament, vesicovaginal fascia) provide support to the bladder and urethra. The uterosacral, broad, and round ligaments support the uterus.

The pelvic floor is divided into layers. The deepest layer comprises the pelvic viscera and its supportive

Female Sexual Pain Disorders 1st edition. Edited by A. Goldstein,
C. Pukall & I. Goldstein. © 2009 Blackwell Publishing,
ISBN: 9781405183987.

endopelvic fascia. These fascial structures are composed of loose connective tissue, smooth muscle, elastic fibers, blood vessels, and nerves, more closely resembling a mesentery than skeletal ligaments. The endopelvic fascia serves to suspend the pelvic viscera to the pelvic side walls. The middle layer comprises the levator ani muscles, which include the pubococcygeous and iliococcygeus which support the viscera and allows for the urethral, vaginal, and anal opening. The puborectalis muscles act together with the external anal and urethral sphincters to contract the sphincters and prevent urinary or fecal leakage. Superficial to this layer is the urogenital diaphragm which crosses the anterior pelvic outlet, connecting the perineal body to the ischiopubic rami and securing the distal urethra. Most superficial are the bulbocavernosus, ischiocavernosus, and superficial transverse perineal muscles of the anterior urogenital triangle and the anal sphincter of the posterior anal triangle. As a whole, the pelvic floor muscles function to support the pelvic organs, to assist in both fecal and urinary continence, to provide support for the rectum and inhibition to the bladder, and to assist in pelvic–spinal stability. In addition, the pelvic floor is involved in enhancing sexual pleasure for both partners [4].

Pelvic floor muscle dysfunction generally refers to disorders of laxity (hypotonus) or overactivity (hypertonus). Hypotonus disorders, due to hormonal factors, mechanical damage, or weakness are generally associated with urinary and fecal incontinence, as well as pelvic organ prolapse. They have also been implicated in contributing to pelvic pain and dyspareunia. However, it is generally believed that pelvic floor hypertonus is the primary pelvic floor dysfunction causing sexual pain disorders.

Medical History

As this book demonstrates, there are many pain disorders in which a physical therapist may be involved in treatment including pudendal neuralgia, fibromyalgia, low back pain, endometriosis, bowel disorders, interstitial cystitis, generalized or localized vulvodynia, postpartum dyspareunia, postmenopausal dyspareunia, and vaginismus. Therefore, a physical therapy evaluation must begin with a detailed medical, gynecological, and sexual history (described in depth in Chapter 4). A thorough history focuses on the location, timing, and nature of the pain. Additionally, the PT should ask about urinary symptoms

(frequency, urgency, stress or urge incontinence, hesitancy) and changes in bowel function (frequency, consistency of stool, urgency, constipation, bloating, flatulence, or fecal incontinence). A PT should inquire about prior musculoskeletal problems or injuries including back pain, hip pain, scoliosis, and ruptured or herniated vertebral discs. Lastly, obstetrical, surgical, and accident/trauma history should be discussed.

In some cases, patients may present for treatment of a primary pain condition such as generalized vulvodynia, chronic pelvic pain, fibromyalgia, or interstitial cystitis, in which dyspareunia is just one component of a constellation of symptoms affecting overall quality of life. In other cases, the presenting complaint may refer directly to sexual function, such as the inability to have sexual intercourse. For example, a patient may have always had localized vestibulodynia which prevented her from using tampons, but her inability to have intercourse is the current trigger for seeking treatment. Understanding the context of the patient's presentation and her current sexual relationship is important in the assessment, as one of the major aims of obtaining an accurate history is to determine the goals for both the patient and her partner and consider suggesting concurrent relationship counseling or sex therapy.

The Physical Exam

General Observation and Posture
The physical evaluation of a patient actually begins when she initially walks through the door. Relevant data that can be gained from this first observation includes an assessment of body language, posture, and gait. For example, a PT should look for evidence of anxiety which is associated with upper respiratory breathing patterns, which in turn can lead to decreased pelvic joint mobility and shortening of the muscles of the hips and pelvis [5].

The physical exam begins by asking the patient to stand, preferably in her bra and underwear, and observing her from posterior, anterior, and lateral positions. Gross postural abnormalities, such as scoliosis, may be noted which may contribute to postural or breathing abnormalities. Spinal, sacral, and pelvic alignment are checked and examples of noteworthy observations include increased lumbar lordosis, asymmetrical pelvic alignment, and a flattened thoracic spine. Abnormal musculoskeletal presentations may include pelvic obliquities, decreased spinal mobility, sacroiliac dysfunction, and pubic symphysis misalignment. These findings have been associated with vulvodynia and pelvic floor dysfunction [6].

Musculoskeletal Exam

The musculoskeletal exam consists of assessing the bones, muscles, joints, and connective tissue. The mobility, length, and strength of the trunk, pelvis, and extremities should be assessed. The cervical, thoracic, and lumbar spine, sacrum, coccyx, and pubic symphysis are examined in standing, supine, and prone positions. The position and mobility of the anterior and superior iliac spines are examined to determine if there is torsion or rotation of the ilia on the sacrum. The bony pelvis, coccyx, and pubic symphysis are palpated to assess mobility. Pelvic joint hypermobility may be indicative of joint laxity and, coupled with weak core musculature, may require stabilization exercises. Muscles are tested for length, strength, tone, and presence of trigger points. It is important to examine the musculature of the pelvis and hips including the piriformis, iliopsoas semimembranosus, semitendinosus and biceps femoris, quadriceps, transverse abdominus, and rectus abdominus muscles. These muscles are palpated to reveal tenderness, trigger points, hypertonus, decreased mobility, and abnormal sensory perception. Lastly, the visceral organs, including the digestive and urogenital organs, are gently palpated. This palpation may reveal organ hypermobility or hypomobility, local tenderness, or what is referred to in osteopathy as "positional torsion," which is treated with gentle manipulation techniques [7].

Pelvic and Genital Examination

It is essential that the PT reduce a patient's anxiety throughout the genital and pelvic exam. The PT should talk to the patient throughout the entire exam, maintain eye contact, and take frequent breaks if necessary. This allows the patient to feel in control during the exam and prevents her from disassociating during the exam. Dissociation is a phenomenon generally associated with sexual abuse or trauma and may be triggered by a strong emotional reaction such as feeling trapped, exposed, terrified, ashamed, or helpless. Dissociation can involve a range of presentations from altered awareness or attention to flashbacks and out-of-body experiences. As prevalence rates of child sexual abuse have been reported to be as high as 27%

[8], the PT must be aware of the possibility of dissociation during an exam that involves genital touch. However, even women who have not experienced a history of sexual trauma report anxiety with pelvic exams [9].

At the beginning of the pelvic and genital exam, general observations can be very useful. For example, is the patient able to separate her legs? Does she relax her head on the pillow, or is she constantly lifting her head? (This is significant because activation of the rectus abdominus muscles which occurs with head lifting will influence the pelvic floor muscle presentation [10]). Bringing the legs together, lifting the buttocks, and/or contracting the pelvic floor or gluteal muscles are common reactions often associated with the diagnosis of vaginismus.

The genitalia, perineum, and anus are examined to identify erythema, induration, scar tissue, or edema. The perineum is examined, noting its length and the presence of scars or fissures. Dryness or atrophy of the mucosa is noted as well as atrophy of the labia. Thorough observation may reveal a vulvar dermatosis such as lichen sclerosus or lichen planus that may contribute to dyspareunia. The clitoris and urethral meatus are examined in order to detect clitoral phimosis or urethral prolapse. Tender areas are palpated and the cotton swab test is performed as described in Chapter 5. The patient is asked to rate the pain on a numeric scale, which is helpful in providing objective evidence of pain reduction. When the cotton swab test clearly is a source of distress to the patient, it is the author's opinion that this part of the exam may be omitted if she has previously undergone this test with the referring physician. The patient is asked to perform pelvic floor contraction and relaxation while the PT observes the perineum for evidence of excursion. The patient is asked to cough or strain to determine if there is a paradoxical contraction of the pelvic floor, perineal bulging, or prolapse.

Before the internal examination, the PT asks the patient's permission to allow penetration through the introitus. One finger is introduced through the hymenal ring without touching the vestibule. Often it is necessary to wait until the patient's muscles relax enough to permit entry. The integrity of the introitus is noted, and the hymen is examined, palpating for thickness, elasticity, or septi. This is achieved by gently inserting a second finger with both fingers inserted only as far as the distal interphalangeal joints and separating the two fingers in a V shape. Internal examination includes transvaginal, digital palpation of the viscera, bones, and soft tissue structures. Internal

examination includes palpation for tenderness and mobility of the urethra, bladder, cervix, uterus and rectum.
Evidence of pelvic organ prolapse or descent may be noted
at this time. Bony landmarks including the coccyx, ischial
spine, and pubic rami are assessed for tenderness, asymmetry, or misalignment. The pudendal nerve in Alcock's
canal, just inferior to the arcus tendonus, can be palpated
and may reproduce neuropathic symptoms.

Pelvic Floor Examination

Assessment of the pelvic floor focuses on the function, balance, mobility, and integrity of the muscular, fascial, and
connective tissue components. Superficial internal palpation allows examination of the bulbospongiosus and is-
chiocavernous muscles, and slightly deeper palpation allows examination of the puborectalis, pubococcygeous,
and iliococcygeus muscles. The pelvic floor muscles, the
obturator internus, and the piriformis, are palpated to
determine their ability to contract and relax. In addition,
these muscles are evaluated for hypertonicity and trigger
points. Pelvic floor muscle strength testing is then performed by subjectively assessing the force of contraction
felt around the palpating finger, the presence of a perceiv-
able lift of the palpating finger, the number of contractions
performed, and the duration of the contractions [11]. In
assessing pelvic floor muscle tone, important markers include the patient's ability to isolate muscles, the patient's
muscle length, muscle tension, muscle stiffness, presence
of trigger points, and pelvic floor synergy or dysenergia
[12].

The Contribution of the Pelvic Floor Musculature to Dyspareunia

Pelvic floor muscle hypertonus has been demonstrated to
contribute to interstitial cystitis [13], provoked vestibulodynia [14], and generalized vulvodynia [15]. Various ter-
minologies have been used to describe hypertonus disorders of the pelvic floor including pelvic floor dysfunction,
levator ani syndrome, pelvic floor tension myalgia, vaginismus, anismus, coccyodynia, sphincter dysenergia, pelvic
floor spasm, and a shortened pelvic floor [16]. While
the mechanism of pelvic floor dysfunction is not completely understood, studies have demonstrated that pelvic
floor muscle hyperactivity is a part of an overall response
to heightened anxiety [17]. Genital pain may also trigger pelvic floor dysenergia. This phenomenon, characterized by paradoxical contraction of the pelvic floor muscles

when attempting to release them, is associated with constipation, incomplete bladder emptying, and penetration
difficulties [18].

While pain is a trigger for hypertonus, it should also be
noted that hypertonic muscles can also cause pain. Blood
vessels are compressed in hypertonic muscles thereby limiting blood flow and oxygenation, which in turn leads to a
build-up of lactic acidosis in the hypertonic muscles. Hypertonic muscles may also cause compression of nerves to
cause neuropathic pain such as pudendal neuralgia.

Electromyographic Assessment of the Pelvic Floor

Pelvic floor surface electromyography (sEMG) biofeedback is commonly used by physical therapists in the assessment and treatment of pelvic floor hypertonus related
to vulvar pain syndromes [19] and vaginismus [20]. Glazer
and his colleagues were the first to compare pelvic floor
sEMG findings in vulvodynia patients versus normal controls. The results indicated that women with vulvodynia
had increased pelvic floor tone and decreased pelvic floor
muscle stability [21]. Glazer reported that pelvic floor exercises assisted by a home biofeedback trainer resulted in
at least 50% effectiveness in reducing the pain of vulvodynia [22]. Subsequent studies produced similar findings.

The electomyographic assessment is generally performed once the patient is able to allow insertion of a
vaginal sensor probe. The practitioner and patient are then
able to view the muscle function on a computer screen.
The "Glazer protocol" tests baseline muscle tone at rest,
muscle strength, and contraction time with 1- and 10-sec
contractions, as well as return time and muscle stability.
Important variables in the Glazer protocol include signal
amplitude, standard deviation, recruitment, power latencies, coefficients of variance, power density, and spectral
frequency analysis. In clinical practice, baseline muscle
tone, strength, and stability are of most practical significance.

Summary of the Evaluation

The conclusion of the physical exam marks a critical junc-
ture for the patient. Because it is likely she has already
been to many practitioners, she will be interested in the
therapist's impressions and how physical therapy can help
to resolve her dyspareunia. The results of the physical

therapy evaluation should be summarized for the patient, and together the PT and patient should discuss the goals of the therapy and the plan of treatment. Physical therapy treatment techniques are discussed in Chapter 13.

Conclusion

Physical therapists play a unique role in the evaluation and treatment of women with dyspareunia. A PT must perform a through evaluation prior to initiating a treatment regimen that is individualized based on the patient's specific medical history and musculoskeletal dysfunction.

References

1 American Psychiatric Association. (2000) *Diagnostic and Statistical Manual of Mental Disorders.* 4th ed., text revision. American Psychiatric Publishing, Washington, DC.

2 Weijmar Schultz W, Basson R, Binik Y, *et al.* (2005) Women's sexual pain and its management. *The Journal of Sexual Medicine* **2**, 301–16.

3 Rosenbaum T. (2005) Physiotherapy treatment of sexual pain disorders. *Journal of Sex and Marital Therapy* **31**, 329–40.

4 Shafik A. (2000) The role of the levator ani muscle in evacuation, sexual performance, and pelvic floor disorders. *International Journal of Urogynecology* **11**, 361–76.

5 Haugstad GK, Haugstad TS, Kirste UM, *et al.* (2006) Posture, movement patterns, and body awareness in women with chronic pelvic pain. *Psychosomatic Research* **61**, 637–44.

6 Morrison P. (2007) Common physical therapy evaluation findings in women with chronic vulvar pain: a preliminary study. Presented at the *International Society for the Study of Vulvovaginal Disease XIX World Congress Meeting*, Alaska.

7 Barral JP, Mercier P. (2005) *Visceral Manipulation.* Eastland Press, Seattle.

8 Finklehor D, Hotaling G, Lewis IA, *et al.* (1990) Sexual abuse in a national survey of adult men and women: prevalence, characteristics, and risk factors. *Child Abuse and Neglect* **14**, 19–28.

9 Robohm JS, Buttenheim M. (1996) The gynecological care experience of adult survivors of childhood sexual abuse: a preliminary investigation. *Women and Health* **24**, 59–75.

10 Sapsford RR, Hodges PW, Richardson CA, *et al.* (2001) Co-activation of the abdominal and pelvic floor muscles during voluntary exercises. *Neurological Urodynamics* **20**, 31–42.

11 Laycock J. (1994) Pelvic muscle exercises: physiotherapy for the pelvic floor. *Urological Nursing* **14**, 136–40.

12 Rosenbaum T. (2008) The role of pelvic floor physical therapy in the treatment of pelvic and genital pain related sexual dysfunction. *The Journal of Sexual Medicine* **5**, 513–23.

13 Peters KM, Carrico DJ, Kalinowski SE, *et al.* (2007) Prevalence of pelvic floor dysfunction in patients with interstitial cystitis. *Urology* **70**, 16–18.

14 Reissing ED, Brown C, Lord MJ, *et al.* (2005) Pelvic floor muscle functioning in women with vulvar vestibulitis syndrome. *Journal of Psychosomatic Obstetrics and Gynecology* **26**, 107–13.

15 Glazer HI, Jantos M, Hartmann EH, *et al.* (1998) Electromyographic comparisons of the pelvic floor in women with dysesthetic vulvodynia and asymptomatic women. *The Journal of Reproductive Medicine* **43**, 959–62.

16 Fitzgerald MP, Kotarinos R. (2003) Rehabilitation of the short pelvic floor. I: Treatment of the patient with the short pelvic floor. *International Urogynecology Journal* **4**, 261–68.

17 Van der Velde J, Everaerd W. (2001) The relationship between involuntary pelvic floor muscle activity, muscle awareness and experienced threat in women with and without vaginismus. *Behavior Research and Therapy* **39**, 395–408.

18 Graziottin A, Bottanelli M, Bertolasi L. (2004) Vaginismus: a clinical and neurophysiological study. *Urodinamica* **14**, 117–21.

19 Glazer H, Rodke G, Swencionis C, *et al.* (1995) Treatment of vulvar vestibulitis syndrome with electromyographic biofeedback of pelvic floor musculature. *The Journal of Reproductive Medicine* **40**, 283–90.

20 Reissing ED, Binik YM, Khalifé S, *et al.* (2004) Vaginal spasm, pain, and behavior: an empirical investigation of the diagnosis of vaginismus. *Archives of Sexual Behavior* **33**, 5–17.

21 Glazer HI, Jantos M, Hartmann EH, *et al.* (1998) Electromyographic comparisons of the pelvic floor in women with dysesthetic vulvodynia and asymptomatic women. *The Journal of Reproductive Medicine* **43**, 959–62.

22 Glazer H, Rodke G, Swencionis C, *et al.* (1995) Treatment of vulvar vestibulitis syndrome with electromyographic biofeedback of pelvic floor musculature. *The Journal of Reproductive Medicine* **40**, 283–90.

CHAPTER 7

The Role of Vulvoscopy in the Evaluation of Dyspareunia

Mario Sideri,[1] *Filippo Murina,*[2] *Vanda Bianco,*[2]
Gianluigi Radici[2]

[1] European Institute of Oncology, Milan, Italy
[2] V. Buzzi Hospital, Milan, Italy

Introduction

Vulvoscopy, the colposcopic examination of the vulva, is an essential part of an examination of a woman who presents with dyspareunia. A colposcope is a low-power microscope with an integrated light source that was initially developed to examine dysplastic and neoplastic lesions of the vagina and cervix. However, in the 1970s it was reported that the colposcope could also be used to improve visualization of the structures of the vulva. It was observed that colposcopy of the vulva (i.e., vulvoscopy) gave the examiner enhanced visualization of the labia majora, labia minora, interlabial sulci, vestibule, glans clitoris, prepuce, frenulum, hymen, minor vestibular glands, perineum, and anus.

Vulvoscopy enhances the ability to detect subtle colors changes associated with inflammatory or neoplastic diseases of the vulva. Increased redness can be visualized when there are stromal changes due to inflammation, an immune response, or from neovascularization that occurs in association with neoplasia. In addition, there can be decreased vascularization, or fibrotic changes in the stroma, both of which appear pallid when viewed with a vulvoscope. Lastly, increased keratinization (lichenification) will appear as dense white areas of vulvar tissue.

Vulvoscopy can also help reveal scarring and architectural changes of the vulva. Chronic inflammatory disorders of the vulva, such as lichen sclerosus and lichen planus, frequently cause structural changes such as resorption of the labia minora, vulvar granuloma fissuratorum (chronic tearing of the posterior fourchette), and phimosis of the clitoris. These changes, which can be subtle, are best visualized with a vulvoscope.

In addition, inflammatory or dysplastic disorders of the vulva can cause fissures, ulcerations, erosions, and plaques. Magnification achieved with the vulvoscope gives the examiner the ability to characterize these lesions with much greater detail. For example, the vulvoscopist can determine if a lesion is a raised plaque or just a flat macule. In addition, the margins of the lesion can be characterized (e.g., are the lesions distinct or are the observed changes more diffuse?). The vulvoscope can also help make the distinction between different conditions with very similar findings, for example, a papilloma and a condyloma (discussed below).

Vulvoscopy microscopes can be combined with photography, which permits the pathologic lesion to be photographed and to be followed over time to assess treatment benefit. Another obvious benefit of vulvoscopy photography is the educational value for the patient.

According to most gynecologic literature, vulvoscopy should be performed after applying acetic acid to the vulva [1]. The use of acetic acid was extrapolated from its use in colposcopy of the cervix. When acetic acid is applied to the cervix, it induces changes in the protein structure of the cells of the epithelium causing them to

Female Sexual Pain Disorders 1st edition. Edited by A. Goldstein,
C. Pukall & I. Goldstein. © 2009 Blackwell Publishing,
ISBN: 9781405183987.

appear opaque. These changes are more readily apparent in dysplastic tissue because these regions have an increased nuclear density and concentration of proteins. The changes are known as acetowhite changes. In addition, the application of acetic acid helps in the detection of abnormal vasculature frequently seen in cervical dysplasia. However, as the epithelium of the vulva is histologically different from the epithelium of the cervix, acetowhite changes on the vulva are more common and less specific for dysplasia/neoplasia than on the cervix [1]. In addition, the application of acetic acid to the vulva of a woman with dyspareunia (who is already experiencing allodynia) frequently causes severe pain and distress. Recent articles that have reviewed this topic have thus questioned the benefit of acetic acid in vulvoscopy and have not recommended its use [1].

In the 1960s the use of the toluidine blue test (TBT) was first reported to aid in the colposcopic detection of cervical dysplasia and neoplasia [2]. As with acetic acid, the TBT was quickly adopted by vulvoscopists to help detect vulvar intraepithlial neoplasia (VIN) [1]. However, in 1985, Micheletti and colleagues reported a study of 93 women who had vulvoscopic-directed biopsies after the TBT. The false positive rate in this study was 26.9% and the false negative rate was 37.5%. The authors concluded that these rates were too high to justify the continued use of the TBT when performing vulvoscopy [3].

Normal Finding on Vulvoscopy

The vulva is a very complex organ that can make visualization difficult. There are folds, sulci, and ostia of several different glands. The tissue is derived from the ectoderm, mesoderm, and endoderm and contains mucous membrane, modified mucous membrane, and hair-bearing, keratinized skin.

During the vulvoscopic examination of the vulva, a wide variation of normal vulvar tissue should be recognized. The skin of the labia majora may be pigmented, and smooth, 1–2 mm large, white or yellow papules may be present especially in upper and inner parts of the labia majora as well as in the labia minora. These tiny elevations are referred to as Fordyce spots and represent normal sebaceous glands, which in this area open directly to the surface, while in hair-bearing areas they open to the hair follicles.

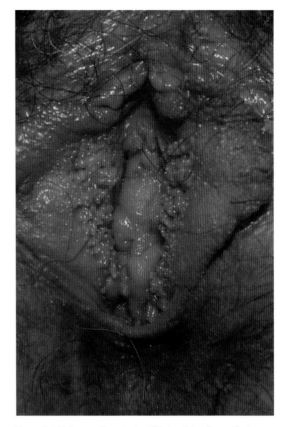

Figure 7.1 Vulvar papillomatosis widely involving the vestibule, a common nonpathological condition. Its bilateral and symmetrical array helps differentiate this normal vulvar feature from vestibular condyloma acuminate.

The mucosa of the labia minora and vestibule is generally pink and smooth; however, localized or widespread micropapillary or villiform patterns may sometimes be observed (Figure 7.1).

These occasionally coalesce to form tissue that can be misinterpreted as condyloma due to the human papillomavirus (HPV) virus. These papillae can be distinguished from HPV-induced lesions on the basis of their regular shape and distribution, uniform color, soft consistency, and lack of tendency to fuse. They are projections of connective tissue covered by a normal epithelium. In contrast, condylomas are pointed, soft, pink, or white finger-elongated excrescences (Figure 7.2). Prominently vascularised, they have fingerlike projections on the surface; their appearance differs according to the site affected.

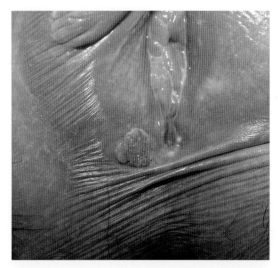

Figure 7.2 Condyloma acuminate. A single lesion is present on the vulvar vestibule.

On hair-bearing skin, they are flesh-colored and somewhat camouflaged; on hairless skin, they tend to be soft, papular, and strikingly white; on mucous membranes they are often fleshy, vascular, and filiform. While these vulvoscopic findings of the morphology of condylomata are quite specific, a vulvar biopsy can confirm the diagnosis and rule out VIN. In addition, polymerase chain reaction (PCR) can be performed on the biopsy to determine the strain(s) of HPV present.

Vulvoscopic Finding of Vulvodynia

The International Society for the Study of Vulvovaginal Disease (ISSVD) defines vulvodynia as vulvar discomfort occurring in the absence of relevant visible findings [4]. Allodynia and hyperalgesia are usually present, and are evidenced by discomfort from spontaneous and/or provoked pain. Dyspareunia is not always present, but most patients do have discomfort during sexual intercourse. Patients frequently complain of pain involving the introitus (vestibulodynia) or pain radiating to the labia majora, groin, and perineum (generalized vulvodynia). Most of the time, the only finding during the vulvoscopic examination of a women with vulvodynia is erythema of the vestibule, which is frequently most apparent at the ostia of the major and minor vestibular glands and Skene's glands.

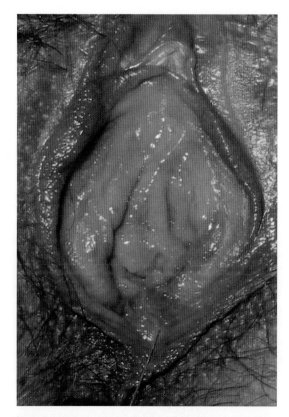

Figure 7.3 Vestibulodynia. The vulvoscopy shows no abnormality other than some degree of vestibular erythema.

Therefore, the vulvoscopist's main goal in a woman with suspected vulvodynia is to rule out specific diseases that can cause vulvar pain (Figure 7.3).

Vulvoscopic Finding of Ulcerative Conditions

Many different diseases can produce erosive, ulcerative, or desquamative lesions of the vulva. Vulvar aphthae, genital herpes, erosive lichen planus, Crohn's disease, Behcet's disease, pemphigus, and pemphigoid are conditions that should be considered in the differential diagnosis of ulcerative vulvar lesions. In addition, both benign and malignant neoplastic lesions can have an ulcerative appearance. Several ulcerative conditions of the vulva have concomitant oral lesions and are associated with other systemic or dermatologic manifestations (Table 7.1). The vulvoscopic

Table 7.1 Differential diagnosis of ulcerative conditions.

Disease	Nonvulvar sites	Histologic features	Characteristics
Lichen planus	Oral, skin	Submucosal infiltrate	Tissue immunofluorescence
Behçet	Oral, ocular	Vasculitis	Uveitis
Crohn's disease	Gastrointestinal tract	Noncaseating granulomas	Gastrointestinal symptoms
Herpes genitalis	—	Ballooning degeneration	Recurrences
Pemphigus	Oral	Acantholysis intraepid.	Intercellelular immunofluorescence
Pemphigoid	Oral, ocular, trunk	Acantholysis subepid.	Basement membrane immunofluorescence

findings seen in these diseases are discussed below. For a more thorough discussion of the etiology and treatment of these diseases, see Chapter 9.

Herpes Simplex Virus

Herpes simplex virus (HSV) (see Chapter 11) infection causes vesicular eruptions that result in shallow ulcers distributed in small patches (Figure 7.4). These ulcers may be single or multiple, and usually measure 1–2 mm in size. They are typically painful, nonindurated

lesions. HSV can appear on any part of the vulva, but most often affects the labia majora and minora, posterior fourchette, perineum, and the anus. The vesicles may coalesce and form large ulcerated areas, with irregular red borders and a pale yellow center.

Aphthous Ulcers

Vulvar aphthosis, a dermatological condition typically seen in young adolescent women, can present as ulcers with a yellow base and erythematous rim (Figure 7.5). They can be greater than 1 cm in size and are exquisitely tender. Generally, they are round, but irregular shapes (perhaps when two ulcers became confluent) may also be seen. Women with vulvar aphthosis frequently have oral aphthae, which are commonly known as canker sores. If a woman has recurrence of both oral and vulvar aphthae, she is given the diagnosis of complex aphthosis and she needs

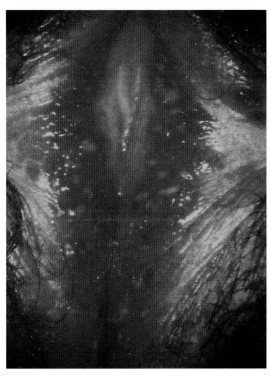

Figure 7.4 Multiple shallow ulcers of herpes simplex infection on the vulvar vestibule.

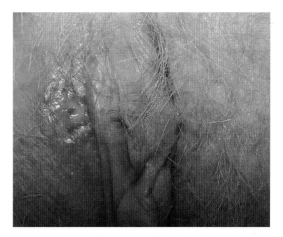

Figure 7.5 An acutely painful aphthous ulcer in a patient presenting with dyspareunia. This is a well-limited ulceration with a red border and a yellowish base, and negative virology, bacteriology, and histology.

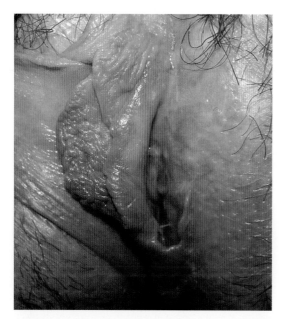

Figure 7.6 An ectopic manifestation of Crohn's disease presenting with painful vestibular ulceration.

a work-up to rule out Behcet's disease (see Chapter 9). Aphthosis is commonly confused with genital herpes as both have painful, recurrent ulcers. However, the lesions of genital herpes (see Chapter 11), after a brief blister stage, have the appearance of shallow erosions rather than the deeper ulcerations seen with aphthosis.

Crohn's Disease

Crohn's disease is a chronic, autoimmune, inflammatory bowel disease than can affect any part of the gastrointestinal tract from mouth to anus. Less commonly, Crohn's disease can affect the vulva. There are three different vulvar findings that may be found in women with Crohn's disease: fistulae, noncontinuous granulomatous metastates, and ulcers presenting as "knifelike cuts" (Figure 7.6). Typically, these lesions are unilateral and cause unilateral swelling of the labia majora.

Lichen Sclerosus

Lichen sclerosus (LS) is a chronic cutaneous disorder with a predilection for the vulva. The classic findings seen on vulvoscopy include epithelial thinning, loss of normal vulvar architecture, and porcelain-white papules and plaques.

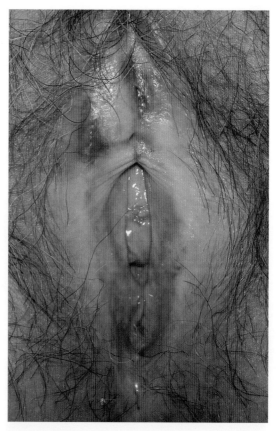

Figure 7.7 Lichen sclerosus. A well-demarcated area of whitening with vulvar fissuring, leading to severe dyspareunia.

Also common are areas of ecchymosis affecting the clitoral hood, clitoris, labia minora, and perineal body giving the appearance of a figure-eight or keyhole configuration (Figure 7.7). Phimosis of the clitoris and obliteration of the labia minora and periclitoral structures may be seen late in the course of disease (Figure 7.8).

There is typically no genital mucosal involvement, but the stenosis that may develop at the edge of mucocutaneous junctions can cause severe dyspareunia. The introitus may become so stenotic that the opening will barely admit one finger, even in parous women (Figure 7.9). As LS has a 3–5% malignant transformation potential, the vulvoscopist must be wary of any lesions that might be VIN or vulvar carcinoma (see below), and there should be a low threshold for performing a vulvar punch biopsy on any suspicious lesions.

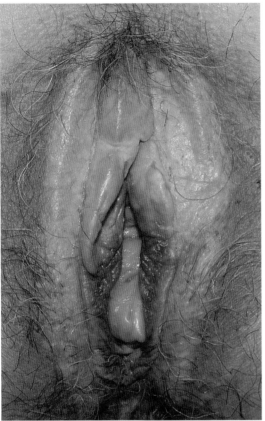

Figure 7.8 Lichen sclerosus with well-circumscribed white plaques.

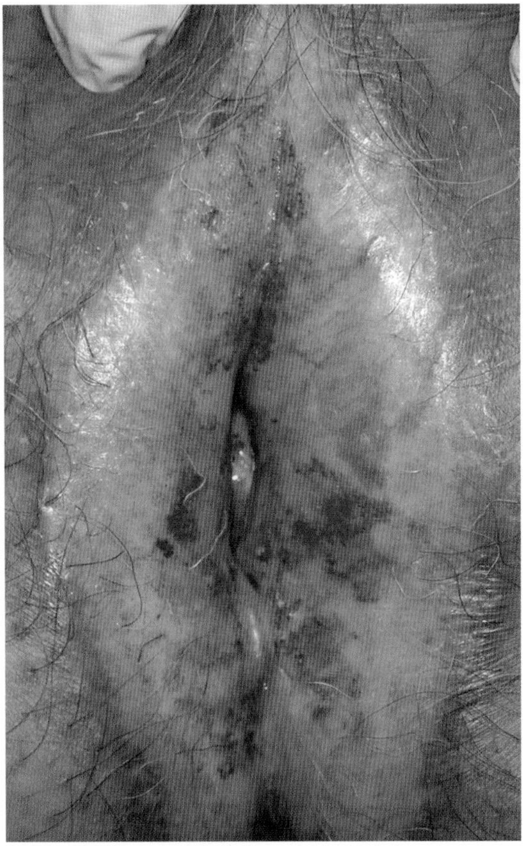

Figure 7.9 Advanced lichen sclerosus, with loss of all normal vulvar architecture and introital narrowing.

Lichen Planus

Lichen planus (LP) is an inflammatory, autoimmune, mucocutaneous disorder with multiple clinical variants that may involve both keratinized skin and mucosal surfaces. In addition to affecting keratinized skin of the trunk and extremities, LP often affects the oral and vulvovaginal mucosa. Vulvovaginal involvement can be associated with itching, burning, pain, dyspareunia, and destruction of the vulvar and vaginal architecture. The variant that typically affects the vulva and vagina is called erosive LP; this is the most painful form of the disease.

The main symptoms are vulvar burning, occurring spontaneously or after vulvar contact, and severe dyspareunia. Penetrative sexual intercourse often results in bleeding. The erosive LP may cause atrophy and stenosis of the vulva as a result of severe scarring. Unlike LS, erosive LP can extend into the vaginal mucosa. The vulvoscopic find-

ings include the following: the mucosa of the introitus is often denuded with a red, glazed appearance; there may be erythema of the vestibular mucosa with varying degrees of epithelial desquamation or frank erosions (Figure 7.10); a fern-like or lace-like pattern called Wickham's stria is frequently seen at the edge of erosions (Figure 7.11); and the borders or erosions may be slightly purple in color (a violacious border).

Lichen Simplex Chronicus

Lichen simplex chronicus (LSC) is the end-stage of a chronic itch-scratch cycle. The skin undergoes lichenification, which causes epithelial thickening and an increase in skin markings. On vulvoscopy, erosions, ulcers, broken hairs, pitting, and honey-colored serosanguineous crusting can be seen. Women with LSC often present with

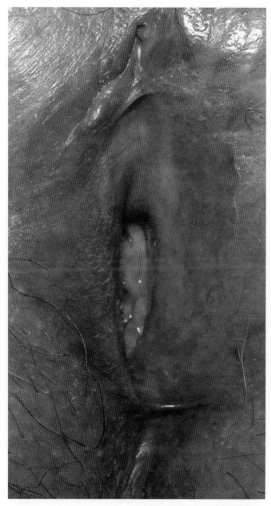

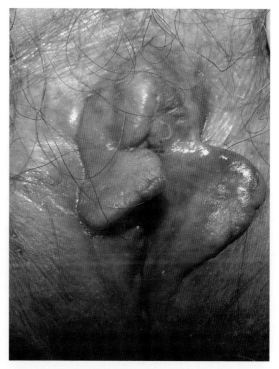

Figure 7.11 Erosive vulval lichen planus involving the labia minora and vestibule, with erosion of the vaginal anterior wall.

Figure 7.10 Erosive lichen planus. Erosive erythema of the vestibular mucosa. At the periphery, there is a narrow rim of white reticulation.

labia majora can appear edematous and excoriated. Small erosions and fissures are sometimes visible in the natural folds and satellite lesions are common (Figure 7.13).

Atrophic Vulvovaginitis

Women who are hypoestrogenic may experience vaginal dryness that causes a chafing sensation with intercourse. Patients are often able to identify that the vaginal dryness is due to lack of lubrication. In the early stages of atrophy, the capillary beds of the vestibule may have a diffuse, patchy red appearance. However, as the atrophy progresses, the capillary bed becomes sparse and the vulvar vestibule takes on a smooth, shiny appearance. Superficial fissuring of the posterior fourchette or intralabial sulci is not uncommon (Figure 7.14).

Vulvar Intraepithelial Neoplasia (VIN)

Many terms have previously been used to describe premalignant lesions of the vulva. This, together with the variable clinical presentation of these lesions, has led to much

pruritus, but pain may also be present due to excoriations from scratching or fissuring. Dyspareunia, if present, is usually a result of irritation from open lesions (Figure 7.12).

Chronic Vulvovaginal Candidiasis

Vulvar candidiasis is a common vulvovaginal infection that typically presents as pruritus, burning, and a thick, white vaginal discharge. However, vulvar pain, particularly dyspareunia, can be a major component of this syndrome, and may be the presenting symptom. The labia minora and vulvar vestibule may be erythematous. The

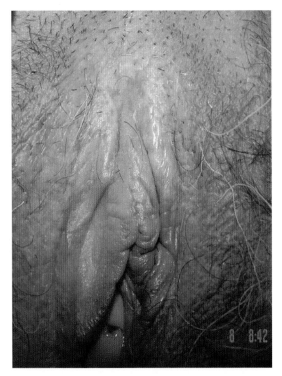

Figure 7.12 Vulvar lichen simplex. Diffuse thickening with a shiny surface criss-crossed by exaggerated skin markings.

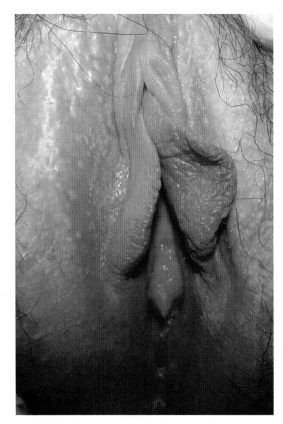

Figure 7.13 Chronic vulvovaginal candidiasis. The vulva is very erythematous and inflamed, involving the labia minora, the interlabial sulcus, and introitus.

confusion. However, the recent terminology proposed the by ISSVD has been helpful in clarifying the issues related to VIN [5]. It is recommended that the term *VIN 1* should no longer be used and high-grade lesions (VIN 2-3) should be divided into two groups: VIN usual type and VIN differentiated type. The usual type occurs in younger women and is related to HPV infection. The differentiated type is less common and seen primarily in older women; it often occurs in association with dermatoses such as LS.

VIN does not have a characteristic presentation. Some patients may have pruritus or burning, while others will notice an asymptomatic abnormality on the vulvar skin. VIN usual type commonly presents with a distinct lesion, typically on the posterior labia minora. The lesions may be raised or flat with a rough surface. The lesions may appear white or red or of mixed color (Figure 7.15). Patients with VIN differentiated type are often symptomatic. Vulvar lesions that do not respond to therapy or nonhealing ulcers/erosions should be biopsied in patients with chronic vulvar dermatoses (Figure 7.16).

Invasive Vulvar Cancer

Malignant diseases of the vulva comprise 4% (38%) of all primary genital tract malignancies [6]. Squamous cell carcinoma comprises 90% of all vulvar cancers diagnosed in women [7]. Symptoms include pruritus, pain, bleeding and/or the presence of a palpable lesion. A total of 70% of tumors arise on the labia. In 40% of cases, tumors can appear in the labia minora, and in 9–15%, the clitoris and perineum are affected [8]. More than half of the tumors (57–62%) are ulcerated; about one-third (27–40%) are papillary; and in the remaining cases (10%) they present as flat lesions [8] (Figures 7.17 and 7.18).

Vulvar Paget's Disease

According to the ISSVD, this condition is classified as a nonsquamous form of intraepithelial neoplasia of the

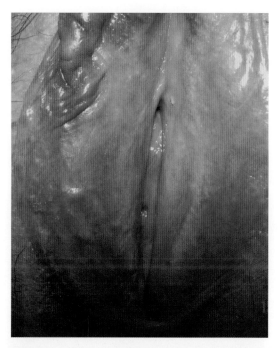

Figure 7.14 Atrophic vulvovaginitis. The mucosa appears pale, with little lubrication and the capillary bed is very evident.

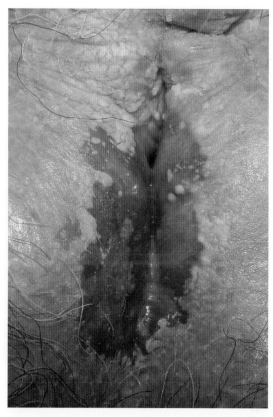

Figure 7.16 VIN 3. This patient presented with a thickened white area demarcated by a deep red lesion.

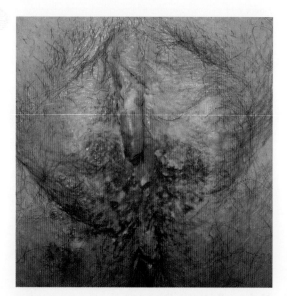

Figure 7.15 VIN 3. This patient presented with a diffuse involvement of the labia majora and minora, and the perianal area with red and white hypercheratotic lesions.

vulva [5]. A characteristic clinical finding is the so-called "weeping" Paget's disease that affects the moist parts of the vulva. In affected areas, hyperkeratotic tissue intersperse with rivulets of raw red tissue exist [9]. Multiple, erythematous, eczematous changes can be seen, well separated from the surrounding skin (Figure 7.19). They are scaly and resemble a geographical map. Sometimes, the patches are hyperkeratotic and white; occasionally however, they are papillary.

Conclusion

Vulvoscopy utilizes a microscope to enhance and facilitate the detailed examination of the vulva in women with dyspareunia and other conditions. Based on the comprehensive discussion of the pathology in this chapter,

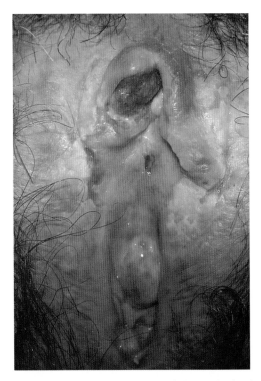

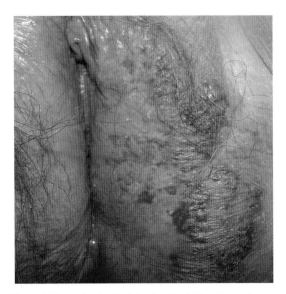

Figure 7.19 A red and white lesion involving labia majora and minora, with an asymmetrical extension beyond the right genitocrural fold, causing itching and dyspareunia. The vulvar biopsy revealed histological and immunohistochemical pattern of vulvar intraepithelial Paget's disease.

Figure 7.17 A vulvar ulcerated malignant lesion, causing burning and dyspareunia.

it appears logical that the appropriate clinical management of affected women involves use of the vulvoscopy during patient evaluation.

References

1 Micheletti L, Bogliatto F, Lynch PJ. (2008) Vulvoscopy: review of a diagnostic approach requiring clarification. *The Journal of Reproductive Medicine* **53**, 179–82.

2 Richart RM. (1963) A clinical staining technique for the in vivo delineation of dysplasia and carcinoma in situ. *American Journal of Obstetrics and Gynecology* **86**, 703–12.

3 Michelletti L, Borgno G., Barbero M, et al. (1986) Diagnosis of vulvar dystrophy. *Minerva Ginecologica* **38**, 1027–32.

4 Moyal-Barracco M, Lynch PJ. (2004) 2003 ISSVD terminology and classification of vulvodynia: a historical perspective. *The Journal of Reproductive Medicine* **49**, 772–77.

5 Sideri M, Jones RW, Wilkinson EJ, *et al.* (2005) Squamous vulvar intra-epithelial neoplasia. 2004 modified terminology, ISSVD Vulvar Oncology Subcommitee. *The Journal of Reproductive Medicine* **50**, 807–10.

6 Krupp PJ, Jr. (1992) Invasive tumours of vulva: clinical features, staging and management. In: Coppleson M (ed.)

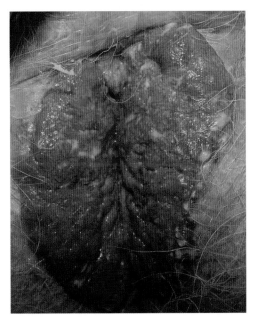

Figure 7.18 Vulvar carcinoma. A vegetans red vulvar lesion was the clinical feature of a patient with itching, burning, and dyspareunia.

Gynecological Oncology, 2nd ed. Churchill Livingstone, Edinburgh, pp. 479–92.

7 Japaze H, Dinh TV, Woodruf JD. (1982) Verrucous carcinoma of the vulva: study of 24 cases. *Obstetrics and Gynecology* **60**, 462–66.

8 Podratz KC, Symmonds RE, Taylor WF, *et al.* (1983) Carcinoma of the vulva: analysis of treatment and survival. *Obstetrics and Gynecology* **61**, 63–74.

9 Gunn RA, Gallager HS. (1980) Vulvar Paget's disease. *Cancer* **46**, 590–94.

8

CHAPTER 8
Provoked Vestibulodynia

Andrew T. Goldstein,[1] *Caroline F. Pukall*[2]
[1] George Washington University School of Medicine and Health Sciences, Washington, DC, USA
[2] Queen's University, Kingston, Ontario, Canada

Introduction

Vulvodynia refers to vulvar pain that occurs in the absence of physical findings or a specific disorder [1]. Vulvodynia is divided into two main categories based on the vulvar area affected by the pain. *Localized* vulvodynia refers to pain in one vulvar area (e.g., vestibule), and *generalized* vulvodynia refers to pain over the entire vulvar region. Each category is further divided according to the temporal pattern of the pain. Vulvar pain can be provoked (i.e., it occurs in response to stimulation of the affected area), unprovoked (i.e., it occurs independently of stimulation), or mixed. Provoked pain can occur during sexual, nonsexual, or both kinds of activities.

Perhaps the most common subtype of vulvodynia is provoked vestibulodynia (PVD), formerly termed *vulvar vestibulitis syndrome*. It has been estimated to affect 12% of premenopausal women in the general population [2]. PVD is characterized by a severe, burning/sharp pain that occurs in response to pressure localized to the vulvar vestibule [3]. Dyspareunia (i.e., painful intercourse) is the defining symptom of PVD and is often the patient's presenting complaint. Painful intercourse can be present from coitarche (i.e., the first intercourse attempt; primary PVD) or it may develop after a period of pain-free intercourse (i.e., secondary PVD).

Female Sexual Pain Disorders 1st edition. Edited by A. Goldstein,
C. Pukall & I. Goldstein. © 2009 Blackwell Publishing,
ISBN: 9781405183987.

Anatomy, Embryology, and Histology of the Vulvar Vestibule

The anatomic borders of the vulvar vestibule are Hart's line laterally, the hymen medially, the frenulum of the clitoris anteriorly, and the fourchette posteriorly [4] (Figure 8.1). These borders represent embryologically derived boundaries. The keratinized epithelium lateral to Hart's line is derived from ectoderm, whereas the stratified nonkeratinized squamous epithelium of the vestibule is derived from the primitive urogenital sinus. The hymen is the canalized outermost boundary of the vagina, which is derived from the Mullerian eminence [5]. Structures within the vulvar vestibule include the urethral orifice, ostia of the Skene's glands, ostia of the Bartholin's glands, and the minor vestibular glands [4]. The Bartholin's gland is the embryologic equivalent of the Cowper's gland in males, and the minor vestibular glands are embryologic analogues of the glands of Littre [6].

Etiology of PVD

The results of research examining the etiology of PVD are sometimes confusing and even contradictory. As the diagnosis of PVD is derived from signs and symptoms, not from a defined pathophysiology, it is likely that there are multiple etiologies for this disorder. As discussed above, the vulvar vestibule is embryologically derived from unique tissue. As such, it is possible that the epithelium of the vulvar vestibule responds differently to "environmental factors" than the outer vulva or the vagina. It is likely, therefore, that a wide range of factors or insults may negatively impact the vulvar vestibule mucosa and cause

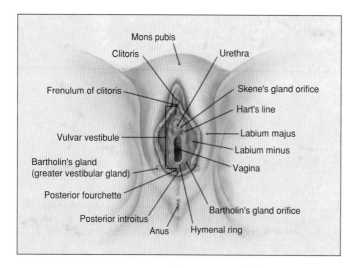

Figure 8.1 Vulvar anatomy.

PVD. These insults may include: hormonal changes, infections, an exaggerated immunologic or inflammatory response, hypoxic injury, congenital malformation, neuropathic injury, and trauma. A brief examination of the current research regarding the etiology of PVD is presented below.

Studies suggest that some cases of PVD are caused by a proliferation of C-afferent nociceptors in the vestibular mucosa [7]. It has been shown that there can be a tenfold increase in the density of these nerve endings in the vestibular mucosa of women with PVD [8]. Possible causes of this proliferation have also been examined, and support has been found for some specific triggers. For example, mast cells can induce this neuronal hyperplasia via nerve growth factor and heparanase, possibly in response to an allergen [8, 9] such as topical antifungal creams or seminal fluid [10, 11]. The role of mast cells in the pathogenesis of sexual pain disorders is discussed in detail in Chapter 27. In addition, certain genetic polymorphisms may predispose some affected women to an exaggerated inflammatory response leading to neuronal proliferation [12]. Additionally, because some women with primary PVD also have hyperpathia in the umbilicus (which is also embryologically derived from the primitive urogenital sinus), a congenital neuronal hyperplasia may be involved [13].

Further data implicate hormonal alterations as a potential cause of PVD. Specifically, it has been shown that the relative risk of developing PVD is 6.6 in women who have used oral contraceptive pills [14–17]. Supporting the role of hormones in increasing vestibular sensitivity are findings that oral contraceptive pills cause changes in hormonal receptors and an altered morphological pattern in the vestibular mucosa [15, 18, 19]. The exact mechanism by which hormonal alterations might cause PVD is not known, but it has been suggested that decreased free testosterone caused by elevated sex-hormone binding globulin in oral contraceptive users may be partially responsible.

As mentioned above, the tissue of the vulvar vestibule is embryologically analogous to the urogenital glands in males. These glands exhibit a high density of androgen receptors, which implies that adequate testosterone is essential for the maintenance of healthy tissue. It is possible therefore, that decreased free testosterone may be harmful to the vestibular epithelium. This theory is discussed in greater detail in Chapter 28.

PVD may also be related to pelvic floor muscle hypertonicity (i.e., increased muscle tension). Reissing et al. found that 90% of women with PVD had some form of pelvic floor dysfunction and suggested that it be considered a core characteristic of PVD [20]. The results of their study also suggest that the increase in muscle tension results from—and does not initially cause—the pain, as significant hypertonicity was present at the superficial, but not at the deep, muscle layers.

While the findings mentioned above implicate pathological alterations in the vestibule or pelvic floor muscles, studies also implicate nonlocal factors in the development and maintenance of PVD. For example, women with PVD report significantly more nonvulvar pain complaints (e.g., migraine) and are more sensitive to various kinds of stimulation (e.g., pressure, heat pain) in nonvulvar areas than nonaffected women [21]. These results imply that central, in addition to peripheral, factors play a role in PVD.

Consistent with this idea are findings from recent studies examining brain function and structure. Pukall et al. used functional magnetic resonance imaging (fMRI) to examine neural activation patterns in women with and without PVD during painful vestibular stimulation. Results indicated that women with PVD responded to such stimulation with an increased neural response as compared to nonaffected women [22]. In addition, [23] examined gray matter density in women with and without PVD and found increases in pain-related areas in affected women. These neural changes suggest that the symptoms of PVD may be mediated by abnormalities in the central nervous system.

Evaluation of PVD

Regardless of the cause(s) of PVD, a careful assessment is essential. An appropriate evaluation combines an in-depth medical history, history of present illness, a thorough physical exam, appropriate laboratory testing, and comprehensive psychosocial testing. The specific components of this evaluation are discussed in detail in Chapters 4 and 5.

Medical Treatment Options for PVD

Some vulvar specialists and treatment guidelines recommend a standard treatment algorithm for all women with PVD [24]. This treatment algorithm relies on vulvar care measures combined with standard treatment for neuropathic pain disorders. The assumption is that whatever the initial cause of PVD, there is a common endpoint of neuropathic pain. While these guidelines are useful for some patients, the authors of this chapter believe that a very thorough medical history, comprehensive laboratory testing, and a focused physical exam can frequently reveal subtle differences in patients with PVD that can be used

Table 8.1 Pelvic floor dysfunction as a cause of PVD.

History of
- Anxiety, panic attacks, compulsive behavior
- Low back or hip pain
- Urinary urgency, frequency, hesitancy, or incomplete emptying
- Chronic constipation or rectal fissures

Lab findings
- Surface electromyography showing elevated resting baseline above 2.0 microV

Physical exam findings
- Tenderness at 4, 6, and 8 o'clock on the vestibule
- Relatively nontender anterior vestibule
- Hypertonicity, tenderness, and trigger points when palpating the puboccygeus, transverse perinea, and (sometimes) the obturator internus muscles.

Treatment
- Pelvic floor physical therapy
- Cognitive behavior therapy focusing on stress and anxiety reduction (see Chapter 23)
- Hypnosis (see Chapter 23)
- Warm baths
- Muscle relaxants (cyclobenzaprine, metaxalone, diazepam, carisoprodol)
- Intralevator injections of botulinum toxin type A

to formulate a more individualized treatment regimen. These specific regimens are found in Tables 8.1–8.4 and are discussed below.

We acknowledge that many components of these treatment regimens are not derived from evidence-based literature. Unfortunately, there are very few well-designed treatment trials for PVD on which to base treatment. Therefore, we have relied on the clinical experience of specialists in sexual pain from a wide range of medical disciplines including gynecologists, dermatologist, urologists, physical therapists, and psychologists.

When pelvic floor hypertonicity is present (Table 8.1), the authors advocate a treatment approach that combines: pelvic floor physical therapy, electromyographic biofeedback, heat therapy, muscle relaxants (cyclobenzaprine, metaxalone, diazepam, carisoprodol), intralevator injections of botulinum toxin type A, cognitive behavior therapy focusing on stress and anxiety reduction, and hypnosis.

If evidence supports a hormonal etiology for PVD (Table 8.2), all hormonal contraceptives should be stopped

Table 8.2 Hormonal changes as a cause of PVD.

History of
- Oral contraceptive pill (OCP) use preceding the onset of symptoms, especially combined OCP with 20 μg of ethinyl estradiol, or the progestins norgestimate or drospirenone
- Ovarian suppression by Lupron or Depo-Provera
- Amenorrhea
- Gradual onset of symptoms
- Decreased libido or decreased vaginal lubrication prior to the onset of dyspareunia

Lab findings
- Serum estradiol < 30
- Calculated free testosterone < 0.4 ng/dL
- Sex hormone binding globulin > 50 nmol/L

Physical exam findings
- Diffuse tenderness of the vestibule
- Diffuse erythema or pallor of the vestibule
- Evidence of recurrent tearing at the posterior fourchette

Treatment
- Stop OCPs
- Estradiol 0.02% + testosterone 0.1% compounded in methylcellulose gel applied to the vestibule twice daily

Table 8.3 Acquired neuronal proliferation as a cause of PVD.

History of
- Contact allergies
- Recurrent yeast infections
- Repetitive use of topical antifungal creams
- Increased burning with the use of intravaginal medication

Lab findings
- Polymorphisms in genes encoding for IL-1RA, IL-1 beta, Mannose-binding lectin
- Increased density of C-afferent nociceptors in vestibular biopsy visualized using PGP 9.5 immunohistochemistry

Physical exam findings
- Tenderness at the ostia of the Bartholin and Skene's glands
- "Cherry red" spots at the ostia of the Bartholin and Skene's glands
- Concurrent pelvic floor dysfunction (frequently)
- Evidence of recurrent tearing at the posterior fourchette

Treatments
- Intralesional Interferon- alpha 12 injections on 1.5 million units
- Intralesional steroid injections (triamcinolone)
- Topical gabapentin 4% compounded in a acid mantel base twice daily
- Topical capsaicin 0.025% compounded in an acid mantel base daily for 6–12 weeks
- Topical lidocaine 5% prior to intercourse or nightly
- Oral tricyclic antidepressants (amitriptyline, nortriptyline, desipramine): start at 25 mg and increase to 100 mg as tolerated
- Oral antiepileptics (gabapentin, pregabulin, carbamazepine)
- Vulvar vestibulectomy with vaginal advancement if conservative treatments fail

and a compound of estradiol and testosterone should be applied to the vestibule twice daily. Patients should be made aware that they will not see significant improvement in their symptoms for approximately 3 months.

If there is evidence either acquired or congenital neuronal proliferation is the cause of the PVD (Tables 8.3 and 8.4), a more traditional treatment approach utilizing oral tricyclic antidepressants (amitriptyline, nortriptyline, desipramine starting at 25 mg and increased to 100 mg as tolerated), oral antiepileptics (gabapentin, pregabulin, carbamazepine), topical lidocaine 5% prior to intercourse or nightly, topical gabapentin (4% compounded in a acid mantel base applied to the vestibule twice daily), and topical capsaicin (0.025% compounded in a acid mantel base and applied daily for 6–12 weeks) can prove useful. If there is evidence that the PVD was caused by an exposure to an irritant or allergen, consider intralesional Interferon-alpha injections (a series of 12 injections of 1.5 million units or intralesional steroid injection (triamcinolone). Surgery (vulvar vestibulectomy with vaginal advancement) can be used if these conservative treatments fail. In addition, the author (AG) believes that surgery may be recommended as a first-line option for women with primary PVD.

Surgery for PVD

Woodruff first described surgery for PVD, calling it a modified perineoplasty [25]. This surgery is currently referred to as a vestibulectomy. Between 1981 and 2006, 32 published case series compromising a total of 1275 patients were reported [26]. These reports encompass several different surgical procedures, as modifications of the basic excision and reconstructive procedure have evolved. Despite these inconsistencies, 28 of the 32 papers demonstrate at least an 80% success rate for PVD [26].

A recent series of 104 women who underwent vestibulectomy demonstrated that 93% were satisfied with the procedure and would recommend the procedure to other women with similar symptoms [26]. Specific surgical techniques are discussed in Chapter 25. If performed by an experienced surgeon, complications from

Table 8.4 Congenital neuronal hyperplasia as a cause of PVD.

History of
- Pain since first tampon use
- Dyspareunia since coitarche (first attempt at intercourse)
- No episodes of completely pain-free intercourse
- Age of coitarche > 23

Lab findings
- Increased density of C-afferent nociceptors in vestibular biopsy visualized using PGP 9.5 immunohistochemistry

Physical exam findings
- Tenderness of the entire vestibule but greatest at the ostia of the Bartholin and Skene's glands
- "Cherry red" spots at the ostia of the Bartholin and Skene's glands
- Concurrent pelvic floor dysfunction is infrequent
- Relative umbilical hypersensitivity

Treatments
- Topical gabapentin 4% compounded in a acid mantel base twice daily
- Topical capsaicin 0.025% compounded in a acid mantel base daily for 6–12 weeks
- Topical lidocaine 5% prior to intercourse or nightly
- Oral tricyclic antidepressants (amitriptyline, nortriptyline, desipramine). Start at 25 mg nightly and increase by 10–25 mg weekly up to 100 mg
- Oral antiepileptics (gabapentin, pregabulin, carbamazepine)
- Vulvar vestibulectomy with vaginal advancement

vestibulectomy are infrequent and usually minor, but may include clinically relevant blood loss (<1%), wound infection or separation (1–3%), granulation tissue (1–3%), decreased orgasm (8%), increased pain (2–4%), Bartholin's cyst formation (1–3%), unfavorable cosmetic changes (4%), and decreased lubrication (20%) [26]. Vestibulectomy does not interfere with a woman's ability to have a vaginal delivery.

Multidisciplinary Approach to the Treatment of PVD

Most sexual pain specialists advocate a biopsychosocial approach for the treatment of PVD. Therefore, while this chapter has focused primarily on the medical or surgical treatments for PVD, the authors advocate enlisting the aid of psychologists, physical therapists, and other allied health care professionals (e.g. acupuncturists, hypnotherapists) in a multidisciplinary approach to the treatment of PVD. Specifically, Chapters 6 and 13 discuss the role of

physical therapists in the treatment of PVD, and Chapters 5 and 23 address the role of psychologists in the management of PVD.

Conclusion

PVD is the most common sexual pain disorder in premenopausal women. It is likely, however, that the constellation of signs and symptoms that we currently call "PVD" is, in fact, several different disease entities. As such, the authors believe that treatment should be individualized and based on relevant aspects of the patient's history of present illness, physical exam, laboratory tests, and psychosocial evaluation.

References

1 Moyal-Barracco M, Lynch PJ. (2004) 2003 ISSVD terminology and classification of vulvodynia: a historical perspective. *The Journal of Reproductive Medicine* **49**, 772–77.
2 Harlow BL, Wise LA, Stewart EG. (2001) Prevalence and predictors of chronic lower genital tract discomfort. *American Journal of Obstetrics and Gynecology* **185**, 545–50.
3 Bergeron S, Binik YM, Khalifé S, *et al.* (2001) Vulvar vestibulitis syndrome: reliability of diagnosis and evaluation of current diagnostic criteria. *Obstetrics and Gynecology* **98**, 45–51.
4 Edward J, Wilkinson IKS (eds.) (1995) *Atlas of Vulvar Disease.* Williams & Wilkins: Baltimore.
5 Ridley CM. (2002) Vulvar anatomy. In: Martin Black MM, Braude P, Vaughan S, Margesson L (eds.) *Obstetric and Gynecologic Dermatology*, Mosby, London, pp. 99–104.
6 Ginat Mirowsky LE. (2004) Genital anatomy. In: Edwards L (ed.) *Genital Dermatology Atlas*, Lippincott, Williams, & Wilkins, Philadelphia, pp.1–8.
7 Bohm-Starke N, Hilliges M, Falconer C, *et al.* (1998) Increased intraepithelial innervation in women with vulvar vestibulitis syndrome. *Gynecologic and Obstetric Investigation* **46**, 256–60.
8 Bornstein J, Goldschmid N, Sabo E. (2004) Hyperinnervation and mast cell activation may be used as histopathologic diagnostic criteria for vulvar vestibulitis. *Gynecologic and Obstetric Investigation* **58**, 171–78.
9 Bornstein J, Cohen Y, Zarfati D, *et al.* (2008) Involvement of heparanase in the pathogenesis of localized vulvodynia. *International Journal of Gynecological Pathology* **27**, 136–41.
10 Marinoff SC, Turner ML. (1991) Vulvar vestibulitis syndrome: an overview. *American Journal of Obstetrics and Gynecology* **165**, 1228–33.
11 Babula O, Bongiovanni AM, Ledger WJ, *et al.* (2004) Immunoglobulin E antibodies to seminal fluid in women with

vulvar vestibulitis syndrome: relation to onset and timing of symptoms. *American Journal of Obstetrics and Gynecology* **190**, 663–67.

12 Gerber S, Bongiovanni AM, Ledger WJ, *et al.* (2002) A deficiency in interferon-alpha production in women with vulvar vestibulitis. *American Journal of Obstetrics and Gynecology* **186**, 361–64.

13 Burrows LJ, Klingman D, Pukall CF, *et al.* (2008) Umbilical hypersensitivity in women with primary vestibulodynia. *The Journal of Reproductive Medicine* **53**, 413–416.

14 Bouchard C, Brisson J, Fortier M, *et al.* (2002) Use of oral contraceptive pills and vulvar vestibulitis: a case-control study. *American Journal of Epidemiology* **156**, 254–61.

15 Bohm-Starke N, Johannesson U, Hilliges M,*et al.* (2004) Decreased mechanical pain threshold in the vestibular mucosa of women using oral contraceptives: a contributing factor in vulvar vestibulitis? *The Journal of Reproductive Medicine* **49**, 888–92.

16 Berglund AL, Nigaard L, Rylander E. (2002) Vulvar pain, sexual behavior and genital infections in a young population: a pilot study. *Acta Obstetricia et Gynecologica Scandinavica* **81**, 738–42.

17 Greenstein A, Ben-Aroya Z, Fass O, *et al.* (2007) Vulvar vestibulitis syndrome and estrogen dose of oral contraceptive pills. *The Journal of Sexual Medicine* **4**, 1679–83.

18 Eva LJ, Maclean AB, Reid WMN, *et al.* (2003) Estrogen receptor expression in vulvar vestibulitis syndrome. *American Journal of Obstetrics and Gynecology* **189**, 458–61.

19 Johannesson U, Sahlin L, Masironi B, *et al.* (2008) Steroid receptor expression and morphology in provoked vestibulodynia. *American Journal of Obstetrics and Gynecology* **198**, 311–16.

20 Reissing ED, Brown C, Lord MJ, *et al.* (2005) Pelvic floor muscle functioning in women with vulvar vestibulitis syndrome. *The Journal of Psychosomatic Obstetrics and Gynaecology* **26**, 107–13.

21 Pukall CF, Binik YM, Khalifé S, *et al.* (2002) Vestibular tactile and pain thresholds in women with vulvar vestibulitis syndrome. *Pain* **96**, 163–75.

22 Pukall CF, Strigo IA, Binik YM, *et al.* (2005) Neural correlates of painful genital touch in women with vulvar vestibulitis syndrome. *Pain* **115**, 118–27.

23 Schweinhardt P, Kuchinad A, Pukall CF, *et al.* (in press) Increased grey matter density in young women with chronic vulvar pain. *Pain*

24 Haefner HK, Collins ME, Davis GD, *et al.* (2005) The vulvodynia guideline. *Journal of Lower Genital Tract Disease* **9**, 40–51.

25 Woodruff JD, Genadry R, Poliakoff S. (1981) Treatment of dyspareunia and vaginal outlet distortions by perineoplasty. *Obstetrics and Gynecology* **57**, 750–54.

26 Goldstein AT, Klingman D, Christopher K, *et al.* (2006) Surgical treatment of vulvar vestibulitis syndrome: Outcome assessment derived from a postoperative questionnaire. *The Journal of Sexual Medicine* **3**, 923–31.

CHAPTER 9

Vulvar Dermatoses as a Cause of Dyspareunia

Lara J. Burrows,[1] *Gail R. Goldstein,*[2] *Gaby Moawad,*[3]
Rochele Torgerson[4]

[1] The Center for Vulvovaginal Disorders, Washington, DC, USA
[2] Annapolis Dermatology Center, Annapolis, MD, USA
[3] The George Washington University, Washington, DC, USA
[4] Mayo Clinic, Rochester, MN, USA

Introduction

The vulva has received relatively little focus in the medical literature and has been referred to as "the forgotten pelvic organ" [1]. There are many ways in which the keratinized skin and mucocutaneous surfaces of the vulva differ from the skin on the rest of the body. It is the only area of the human body where epithelium from all three embryologic layers coalesce. In addition, the vulvovaginal tract encounters foreign proteins and antigens necessary for reproduction, and has evolved with a unique immunologic response [2]. Lastly, the subcutaneous tissue of the labia majora is looser, allowing for considerable edema to form.

Vulvar dermatoses may present in a variety of ways, ranging from asymptomatic to mildly bothersome to severely disabling. Vulvar dermatoses are often difficult to treat and severely impact a woman's quality of life. Vulvar dermatoses may present with dyspareunia. Symptoms may include sexual pain, nonsexual pain, itching, fissuring, and postcoital bleeding. Women may be embarrassed by the disfiguring vulvar changes that may occur and avoid sexual intimacy. Patients are frequently reticent to discuss their symptoms with a health care provider, and many clinicians feel challenged with respect to the management of vulvar disease. These factors may result

in women receiving suboptimal treatment, resulting in persistent symptoms and/or avoidance of sexual relationships altogether. The purpose of this chapter is to discuss the diagnosis and treatment of the vulvar dermatologic conditions that may be associated with dyspareunia.

Physical Examination

The vulva should be examined with a vulvoscope as it allows the clinician to see the disease process in greater detail, aiding in an accurate diagnosis (see Chapter 7). Digital photography is especially useful for documenting baseline findings, progress with treatment, and educating the patient. The vulvar examination should begin with the patient in the dorsal lithotomy position. Specifically, the vulva should be thoroughly examined for erythema, atrophy, induration, fissures, lichenification, ulceration, erosions, hypopigmentation, scarring, phimosis of the clitoris, narrowing of the introitus, and tenderness to palpation. A speculum exam should also be performed to look for ulcerations or synechiae in the vagina.

A vulvar biopsy is strongly recommended w' normalities are seen on vulvoscopy. A 4 biopsy should be performed under ' caine with epinephrine), and ' with one or two stitche' Vicryl-Rapide (Ethic is extremely useful in a

Female Sexual Pain Disorders 1st edition. Edited by A. Goldstein,
C. Pukall & I. Goldstein. © 2009 Blackwell Publishing,
ISBN: 9781405183987.

disorders that can present in similar ways. Working with an experienced dermatopathologist can help ensure the accuracy of biopsy results.

The Vulvar Dermatoses

The following dermatoses are commonly encountered when treating women with dyspareunia.

Lichen Sclerosus

Lichen sclerosus (LS) is a chronic, lymphocyte-mediated cutaneous disorder affecting approximately one in seventy women [3]. There is a bimodal peaked incidence in premenarchal girls and menopausal women with the average age of diagnosis being 51 years. Extragenital lesions may occur in 11% of female patients [4]. While the etiology has not been completely elucidated, LS is most likely an autoimmune disorder as it is associated with other autoimmune disorders including autoimmune thyroid disease, alopecia areata, vitiligo, pernicious anemia, and lichen planus [5–7]. In addition, there are high levels of circulating autoimmune antibodies in patients with LS. A genetic susceptibility to LS has been suggested because of reports of familial association. In addition, several studies have demonstrated increased prevalence in women with specific major histocompatability complex (HLA-complex) subgroups such as HLA-DQ7 [8]. Women with LS have a 4–5% risk of developing vulvar carcinoma [5]. LS has been found in greater than 60% of cases of squamous carcinoma of the vulva [9].

Clinically, while some patients are asymptomatic, most give a history of pruritis or pain [3]. One study that focused on the impact of lichen sclerosus on a woman's sexual satisfaction showed that women with LS were less likely to be sexually active (vaginal intercourse, oral intercourse, and masturbation) than control groups. Furthermore, 79% of women with LS reported chronic vulvar pain [10]. In another study by Dalziel, 76% of women with LS had dyspareunia and more than half of those women were completely apareunic because of LS [11].

Physical examination reveals white atrophic plaques ("cigarette paper"), depigmentation, ecchymoses, resorp-tion of the labia, narrowing of the introitus, and distor-tion of the vulvar architecture (Figure 9.1). Lichen scle-rosus may involve the labia minora and inner portion of labia majora, interlabial sulcus, clitoris, vestibule,

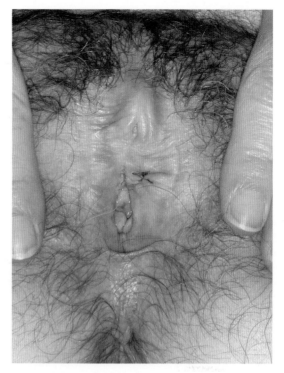

Figure 9.1 Lichen sclerosus.

perineum, and the perianal region, but almost never involves the vaginal mucosa. Scarring of the clitoral prepuce may cause "phimosis" of the glans clitoris, which in turn, can lead to formation of a smegmatic psuedocyst abscess between the prepuce and clitoris [12].

A biopsy specimen should be obtained to confirm the diagnosis because the histopathologic changes of LS are distinctive. Characteristic pathologic findings include hyperkeratosis of the epidermis, epidermal atrophy with loss of rete ridges, homogenization of the collagen in the upper dermis, and a lichenoid (bandlike) inflammatory infiltrate in the dermis (Figure 9.2). It is essential to obtain the biopsy prior to starting treatment because the pathognomonic changes described above can resolve with the application of corticosteroids [13].

The gold standard treatment for LS is an ultrapotent topical corticosteroid ointment, such as clobetasol propionate ointment, applied daily until all active disease has resolved [8]. More recently, tacrolimus and pimecrolimus, topical calcineurin inhibitors, have been described for the treatment of LS [14–16]. The potential advantage of these

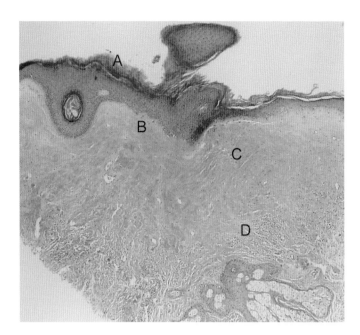

Figure 9.2 Histology of lichen sclerosus. (a) Hyperkeratosis of the epidermis. (b) Epidermal atrophy with loss of rete ridges. (c) Homogenization of the collagen in the upper dermis. (d) Lichenoid infiltrate in the dermis.

newer medications is they do not inhibit collagen synthesis so they do not cause dermal atrophy. Areas of ulceration or lichenification that do not resolve after adequate treatment must be biopsied to rule out vulvar intraepithelial neoplasia or carcinoma. After all active disease has resolved, patients may taper the frequency of treatment to twice per week. Patients should be counseled that LS is a chronic disease and that treatment only when symptomatic is not sufficient because there can be active disease without symptoms. Lastly, it should be noted that topical testosterone was historically used to treat LS, but controlled trials in the 1990s showed that this is an ineffective treatment [17].

In the past, surgery for lichen sclerosus was reserved for patients in whom there was associated high-grade vulvar intraepithelial neoplasia or carcinoma [18]. Surgery to correct architectural changes such as narrowing of the introitus or clitoral phimosis was contraindicated because of a process known as the koebner phenomenon. Koebnerization in LS is a pathological process in which normal skin becomes sclerotic after it is injured or traumatized [19]. However, koebnerization in women with LS can now be effectively prevented with ultrapotent corticosteroids. Perineoplasty has been shown to improve dyspareunia in 90% of women who had introital stenosis because of LS

[4]. In addition, surgery to correct clitoral phimosis has been shown to improve clitoral sensation and increase orgasms in women with LS [12].

Lichen Planus

Lichen planus (LP) is an intensely inflammatory, autoimmune, mucocutaneous disorder that may involve both keratinized skin and mucosal surfaces. In addition to affecting keratinized skin of the trunk and extremities, LP often affects the oral and vulvovaginal mucosae [20]. Vulvovaginal involvement can be associated with dyspareunia, itching, burning, pain, and destruction of the vulvar and vaginal architecture [21]. Approximately 1 in 400 women have vulvovaginal LP [22]. However, the true incidence of LP is difficult to assess because patients may present to a wide variety of specialists including dentists, dermatologists, gynecologists, and gastroenterologists [22]. The age of peak prevalence ranges from ages 30 to 60 years [23].

Erosive LP is characterized by glassy, brightly erythematous erosions associated with white striae (Wickham's striae). The disease may involve the labia minora and vestibule while sparing the outer vulva, or may be associated with loss of the labia minora, and narrowing of the introitus (Figure 9.3). Vaginal involvement has been

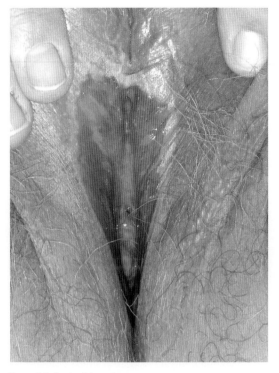

Figure 9.3 Erosive lichen planus

reported in up to 70% of patients with erosive LP [24]. On physical examination, the vulvar skin and vaginal mucosa are friable, and bleed easily upon insertion of a speculum. Patients frequently have copious yellow discharge composed of lymphocytes and parabasal cells [20]. In severe cases, intravaginal synechiae may form, causing partial or complete obliteration of the vaginal lumen [21].

Histologically, erosive LP is characterized by hyperkeratosis in areas of keratinized skin, irregular acanthosis with a sawtooth appearance of rete ridges, a prominent granular layer, and basal cell liquefaction. Apoptotic eosinophilic basal and prickle cells (colloid bodies) are sometimes present, as is a band-like dermal infiltrate composed primarily of T cells [25]. To help distinguish erosive LP from immunobullous diseases (mucous membrane pemphigoid, pemphigus vulgaris, and linear IgA bullous disease), a biopsy taken from normal tissue at the edge of an erosion should be sent for direct immunofluorescence studies [26].

In general, even though LP is more difficult to treat than LS, most authors recommend the same initial treat-

ments: ultrapotent corticosteroid ointments or topical macrolide immunosuppressants. Systemic immunosuppressive therapy may be necessary for patients who fail these therapies or with extensive disease affecting multiple areas of the body [20]. Vaginal LP may be treated with intravaginal hydrocortisone suppositories (commonly used formulations are those used to treat hemorrhoids). Other treatment options include inserting a Pyrex vaginal dilator coated with a potent corticosteroid ointment into the vagina [27]. This treatment helps to prevent or improve vaginal synechiea.

Topical calcineurin inhibitors have also been described for the treatment of vaginal LP [28, 29]. When applied with a vaginal applicator, serum levels of the calcineurin inhibitors may become high enough to achieve the side effect of systemic immunosuppression. However, when applied intravaginally with a finger, or with a suppository, serum levels are negligible. Patients must be counseled that LP is a chronic disease that likely increases the risk of developing vulvar or vaginal squamous cell carcinoma. Lifelong treatment and monitoring is required [21].

Irritant and Allergic Contact Dermatitis

Contact dermatitis is an inflammation of the skin due to an external agent acting as an irritant or allergen (Figure 9.4). An irritant is any substance that causes inflammation, erythema, and induration upon exposure to the skin or mucous membranes, whereas an allergen is any substance that stimulates a type IV delayed hypersensitivity reaction in previously sensitized individuals [30].

The incidence of vulvar contact dermatitis in the general population is unknown. However, the reported prevalence in a vulvar clinic in the United Kingdom was 20–30%, and in an Australian vulvar clinic, the prevalence was 15% [31, 32]. It is generally accepted among specialists in vulvar disease, however, that as women increasingly apply products to the vulva, the incidence of contact dermatitis is increasing. Common products containing chemicals that may cause contact dermatitis include soaps, menstrual pads, panty liners, toilet paper, diapers, laundry detergents, fabric softeners, feminine sprays, cosmetics, spermicides, shaving cream, depilatory agents, pessaries, and condoms. Additionally, topical medications that frequently cause contact dermatitis, include benzocaine, hormonal creams, corticosteroids, topical antifungals,

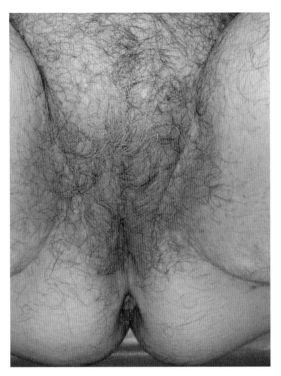

Figure 9.4 Irritant dermatitis.

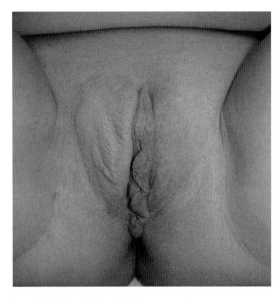

Figure 9.5 Lichen simplex chronicus.

and antibiotics, especially when topical medications are dissolved in the solvent propylene glycol [30].

Women with contact dermatitis present with burning, itching, dyspareunia, and fissuring around the introitus [31]. Physical examination findings may range from mild erythema to weeping lesions. Histologically, findings are nonspecific. One may see spongiosis, acanthosis, parakeratosis, and a dermal inflammatory infiltrate. The lax tissues of the vulva predispose to marked dermal edema. Continued exposure to the irritant and chronic rubbing or scratching may eventually lead to lichen simplex chronicus.

The diagnosis of contact dermatitis of the vulva is made by taking a detailed history and careful physical examination. One should not hesitate to perform a biopsy and rule out coexisting conditions. The differential diagnosis includes candidiasis, psoriasis, sebhorreic dermatitis, lichen simplex chronicus, and extensive extra mammary Paget's disease [30]. Patch testing may be helpful in making the diagnosis of allergic contact dermatitis.

Successful treatment of contact dermatitis is dependent on the identification and removal of the causative irritant or allergen. Details of the patient's daily routine for hygiene (the use of soaps, detergents, douches, antifungal treatments, cleansing cloths, sprays, creams, and lotions) should be discussed, as well as their practices around the time of menses and intercourse. Proper vulvar care should be reviewed with these patients (and all patients with any vulvar disorder).

Topical steroids are used to decrease inflammation (triamcinolone 0.1% ointment twice daily for mild-to-moderate cases and clobetasol 0.05% ointment daily for severe cases). Ice packs (or bags of frozen peas) and antihistamines such as hydroxyzine can be used to help alleviate pruritus [27]. Amitriptyline 25 mg can be used to help prevent women from scratching in their sleep. An allergic response to a topical medication may be managed by a 2-week course of oral prednisone. Superimposed candidal infections should be treated with fluconazole, and bacterial infections should be treated with an oral antibiotic.

Lichen Simplex Chronicus

Lichen simplex chronicus (LSC) (Figure 9.5) of the vulva is an eczematous disorder characterized by pruritus and lichenification [23]. The condition is the end stage of an itch-scratch cycle and is also known as neurodermatitis, pruritus vulvae, squamous hyperplasia, and hyperplastic dystrophy. A variety of different inflammatory, irritant, and infectious insults can initiate pruritus, which starts the itch-scratch cycle. These include candidiasis, atopic dermatitis, and contact dermatitis [2]. The intense, chronic itching caused by these conditions leads the patient to repetitively rub and scratch the affected area. The skin responds by thickening and developing a coarse texture with increased skin markings. Vulvoscopic findings include lichenifcation, excoriations, pitting, and broken/absent pubic hair [33]. Histopathological examination shows hyperkeratosis, spongiosis, acanthosis, and a chronic dermal inflammatory infiltrate.

It is essential to break the itch-scratch cycle to effectively treat LSC. As in irritant and allergic contact dermatits, all irritant/allergen exposure must be eliminated. Secondly, it is necessary for women to stop scratching. This can be difficult as many women only scratch in their sleep. Oral amitriptyline (25 mg) at bedtime combined with application of ice very successfully relieves nighttime pruritus. Lastly, application of topical mid- or high-potency corticosteroids or topical calcineurin inhibitors are used to decrease the underlying inflammation [14, 33].

Additional Vulvar Dermatoses

The following diseases are much less common than the dermatoses discussed above. While a thorough discussion is beyond the scope of this chapter, we recommend that any sexual health practitioner should have a vulvar dermatology textbook in their reference library.

Aphthous Ulcers
Aphthous ulcers (AUs) are deep and painful vulvar ulcers (Figure 9.6). They are most commonly seen in adolescent Caucasian women. AU may be associated with Epstein–Barr virus or cytomegalovirus but are most commonly seen as a response to stress [34]. Vulvar AU can be associated with oral aphthae, which are commonly called canker sores. If a woman has recurrent oral and vulvar aphthae, the diagnosis is complex aphthosis. If a patient has a diagnosis of complex aphthosis, a practitioner must rule-out the diagnosis of Behcet's disease (see below).

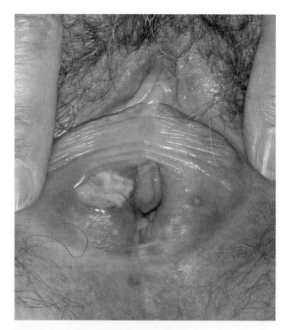

Figure 9.6 Aphthous ulcer in Behcet's disease.

Behcet's Disease
Behcet's disease (BD) (Figure 9.6) is a chronic, relapsing multisystem vasculitis with predominant involvement of the oral and vulvar mucosa. It has a worldwide distribution, but the prevalence is highest in Central Asia and the Far East (along the ancient Silk Route) [35]. Genetic, environmental, and immunological factors play a role in its pathogenesis. The International Study Group for Behcet's disease proposed the following criteria for its diagnosis: recurrent oral aphthae plus any two of recurrent vulvar aphthae, eye lesions (uveitis, iritis), skin lesions (erythema nodosum, acneiform nodules), and a positive pathergy test. Almost all organ systems can be affected, and vasculitis/thrombosis can result in blindness, arthritis, stroke, memory loss, and impaired speech [36].

Mucous Membrane Pemphigoid
Mucous membrane pemphigoid (MMP) is a rare autoimmune blistering disease primarily affecting mucosal surfaces. Blistering and scarring may occur in the eyes, mouth, esophagus, larynx, and on the vulva. Scarring can result in severe structural changes to the vulva that may mimic the findings of other inflammatory dermatologic disorders including LS and LP [26]. The diagnosis of MMP

is made by sending a biopsy for direct immunofluorescence studies to detect a deposition of C3 and IgG along the basement membrane.

Plasma Cell Vulvitis

Plasma cell vulvitis is a rare dermatologic condition of the vulva characterized by glistening, erythematous plaques [37]. Symptoms associated with plasma cell vulvitis include pruritis, dyspareunia, pain, and burning. Histologic examination reveals a lichenoid infiltrate that is composed of greater than 50% plasma cells.

Conclusion

The vulvar dermatoses discussed in this chapter may cause vulvar pruritis, pain, and scarring. They should be included in the differential diagnosis of any women with dyspareunia. It should be the goal of all practitioners who treat women with sexual pain to learn to recognize, diagnose, and manage these diseases.

References

1 Noller KL. (2004) Vulva: the forgotten pelvic organ. *Obstetrics and Gynecology* **104**, 913–14.

2 Foster DC. (2002) Vulvar disease. *Obstetrics and Gynecology* **100**, 145–63.

3 Goldstein AT, Marinoff SC, Christopher K, *et al.* (2005) Prevalence of vulvar lichen sclerosus in a general gynecology practice. *The Journal of Reproductive Medicine* **50**, 477–80.

4 Rouzier R, Haddad B, Deyrolle C, *et al.* (2002) Perineoplasty for the treatment of introital stenosis related to vulvar lichen sclerosus. *American Journal of Obstetrics and Gynecololgy* **186**, 49–52.

5 Smith YR, Haefner HK. (2004). Vulvar lichen sclerosus: pathophysiology and treatment. *American Journal of Clinical Dermatology* **5**, 105–25.

6 Goolamali SK, Barnes EW, Irvine WJ, *et al.* (1974) Organ-specific antibodies in patients with lichen sclerosus. *British Medical Journal* **4**, 78–79.

7 Harrington CI, Dunsmore IR. (1981) An investigation into the incidence of autoimmune disorders in patients with lichen sclerosus and atrophicus. *British Journal of Dermatology* **104**, 563–66.

8 Val I, Almeida G. (2005) An overview of lichen sclerosus. *Clinical Obstetrics and Gynecology* **48**, 808–17.

9 Leibowitch M, Neill S, Pelisse M, *et al.* (1990) The epithelial changes associated with squamous cell carcinoma of the vulva: a review of the clinical, histological, and viral findings in 78 women. *British Journal of Obstetrics and Gynaecology* **97**, 1135–39.

10 Gagne HM, Dalton VK, Haefner HK, *et al.* (2007) Vulvar pain and sexual function in patients with lichen sclerosus. *The Journal of Reproductive Medicine* **52**, 121.

11 Dalziel KL. (1995) Effect of lichen sclerosus on sexual function and parturition. *The Journal of Reproductive Medicine* **40**, 351–54.

12 Goldstein AT, Burrows LJ. (2007) Surgical treatment of clitoral phimosis caused by lichen sclerosus. *American Journal of Obstetrics and Gynecology* **196**, 126 e1-4.

13 Lorenz B, Kaufman RH, Kutzner SK. (1998) Lichen sclerosus: therapy with clobetasol propionate. *The Journal of Reproductive Medicine* **43**, 79–94.

14 Goldstein AT, Parneix-Spake A, McCormick CL, *et al.* (2007) Pimecrolimus cream 1% for treatment of vulvar lichen simplex chronicus: an open-label, preliminary trial. *Gynecologic and Obstetric Investigation* **64**, 180–86.

15 Virgili A, Lauriola MM, Mantovani L, *et al.* (2007) Vulvar lichen sclerosus: 11 women treated with tacrolimus 0.1% ointment. *Acta Dermato-Venereologica* **87**, 69–72.

16 Goldstein AT, Marinoff SC, Christopher K. (2004) Pimecrolimus for the treatment of vulvar lichen sclerosus: a report of 4 cases. *The Journal of Reproductive Medicine* **49**, 778–80.

17 Sideri M, Origoni M, Spinaci L, *et al.* (1994) Topical testosterone in the treatment of vulvar lichen sclerosus. *International Journal of Gynaecology and Obstetrics* **46**, 53–56.

18 Neill SM, Tatnall FM, Cox NH. (2002) Guidelines for the management of lichen sclerosus. *British Journal of Dermatology* **147**, 640–49.

19 Funaro, D. (2004) Lichen sclerosus: a review and practical approach. *Dermatologic Therapy* **17**, 28–37.

20 Moyal-Barracco M, Edwards L. (2004) Diagnosis and therapy of anogenital lichen planus. *Dermatologic Therapy* **17**, 38–46.

21 Cooper SM, Wojnarowska F. (2006) Influence of treatment of erosive lichen planus of the vulva on its prognosis. *Archives of Dermatology* **142**, 289–94.

22 Eisen D. (1999) The evaluation of cutaneous, genital, scalp, nail, esophageal, and ocular involvement in patients with oral lichen planus. *Oral Surgery, Oral Medicine, Oral Pathology, Oral Radiology and Endodontics* **88**, 431–36.

23 Ball SB, Wojnarowska F. (1998) Vulvar dermatoses: lichen sclerosus, lichen planus, and vulval dermatitis/lichen simplex chronicus. *Seminars in Cutaneous Medicine and Surgery* **17**, 182–88.

24 Lewis FM, Shah M, Harrington CI. (1996) Vulval involvement in lichen planus: a study of 37 women. *British Journal of Dermatology* **135**, 89–91.

25 Goldstein AT, Metz A. (2005) Vulvar lichen planus. *Clinical Obstetrics and Gynecology* **48**, 818–23.

26 Goldstein AT, Anhalt GJ, Klingman D, *et al.* (2005) Mucous membrane pemphigoid of the vulva. *Obstetrics and Gynecology* **105**, 1188–90.

27 Burrows, LJ, Shaw HA, Goldstein AT. (2008) The vulvar dermatoses. *The Journal of Sexual Medicine* **5**, 276–83.

28 Kirtschig G, Van Der Meulen AJ, Ion Lipan JW, *et al.* (2002) Successful treatment of erosive vulvovaginal lichen planus with topical tacrolimus. *British Journal of Dermatology* **147**, 625–26.

29 Byrd JA, Davis MD, Rogers RS, 3rd. (2004) Recalcitrant symptomatic vulvar lichen planus: response to topical tacrolimus. *Archives of Dermatology* **140**, 715–20.

30 Margesson LJ. (2004) Contact dermatitis of the vulva. *Dermatologic Therapy* **17**, 20–27.

31 Crone AM, Stewart EJ, Wojnarowska F, *et al.* (2000) Aetiological factors in vulvar dermatitis. *Journal of the European Academy of Dermatology and Venereology* **14**, 181–86.

32 Brenan JA, Dennerstein GJ, Sfameni SF, *et al.* (1996) Evaluation of patch testing in patients with chronic vulvar symptoms. *Australasian Journal of Dermatology* **37**, 40–43.

33 Lynch PJ. (2004) Lichen simplex chronicus (atopic/neurodermatitis) of the anogenital region. *Dermatologic Therapy* **17**, 8–19.

34 Huppert JS, Gerber MA, Deitch HR, *et al.* (2006) Vulvar ulcers in young females: a manifestation of aphthosis. *Journal of Pediatric and Adolescent Gynecology* **19**, 195–204.

35 Yesudian PD, Klafkowski J, Parslew R, *et al.* (2007) Tufted angioma-associated Kasabach–Merritt syndrome treated with embolization and vincristine. *Plastic and Reconstructive Surgery* **119**, 1392–93.

36 Reynolds, N. (2008) Vasculitis in Behcet's syndrome: evidence-based review. *Current Opinions in Rheumatology* **20**, 347–52.

37 Goldstein AT, Christopher K, Burrows LJ. (2005) Plasma cell vulvitis: a rare cause of intractable vulvar pruritis. *Archives of Dermatology* **141**, 789–90.

Hidradenitis Suppurativa

Jennifer M. Rhode,[1] *Angela S. Kueck,*[2] *Hope K. Haefner*[2]

[1] Wright-Patterson Medical Center, Dayton, OH, USA

[2] University of Michigan Medical Center, Ann Arbor, MI, USA

Introduction

Hidradenitis suppurativa (HS) is a chronic, relapsing inflammatory disease that involves the intertriginous regions such as the axillae, groin, inframammary, and anogenital regions [1]. HS is typified by chronicity, and patient and provider frustration. HS is believed to arise due to a defect in the terminal follicular epithelium. The initial process is abnormal cornification of the follicular infundibulum with follicular occlusion by keratin with subsequent active folliculitis. Secondary destruction of skin adnexae and the subcutis then develops. Abscesses form which may resolve spontaneously or progress into chronic cutaneous or subcutaneous tunneling (sinus tract formation) [2].

Historical Background

The French physician Alfred Velpeau first described HS in 1839 and reported it as an inflammatory process with superficial abscess formation affecting the axillary, mammary, and perianal regions [3]. The French surgeon Aristide Verneuil was the first to theorize a connection between HS and apocrine glands, naming the condition hidrosadenite phlegmoneuse [4, 5]. The term *hidradenitis suppurativa* is derived from "hidros" (sweat), "adeno" (gland), "itis" (inflammation), and "suppurativa" (pus forming).

Hidradenitis suppurativa has subsequently become classified as a member of the follicular occlusion tetrad,

Female Sexual Pain Disorders 1st edition. Edited by A. Goldstein, C. Pukall & I. Goldstein. © 2009 Blackwell Publishing, ISBN: 9781405183987.

along with acne conglobata and dissecting cellulitis of the scalp and pilonidal sinus [6, 7, 8]. In 1975, the follicular occlusion tetrad was formed by the addition of pilonidal sinus [8]. Plewig and Steger introduced the term acne inversa in 1989 based on overwhelming data supporting the follicular origin of the disorder [9].

Of historical note: Karl Marx was known to have suffered from an incapacitating skin disease. Recent review of his correspondence detailed lesions called "furuncles," "boils," and "carbuncles" that were persistent, recurrent, destructive, and site-specific consistent with HS [10]. It is hypothesized that the mental effects of this disabling disease may well have influenced Marx's work.

Epidemiology

Hidradenitis suppurativa is probably more common than is typically realized. The disease is frequently ignored or missed, leading to both patient's and health care provider's frustration [11]. The disease prevalence has been estimated at 1:100, 1:300, or 1:600, and as high as 4.1% based on objective findings in a young adult population [12–14].

There is no consensus regarding a relationship between HS and ethnicity. Some authors have suggested an increased frequency in African Americans [15–18], but others report no racial predilection [19]. The disorder is more common in women, with the female/male ratio ranging from 2:1 to 5:1 in most published series. The mean age of onset for men is 31.7 years and for women it is 26.4 years. Genitofemoral lesions are more commonly found in women, whereas the prevalence of axillary lesions does not differ significantly with gender [12].

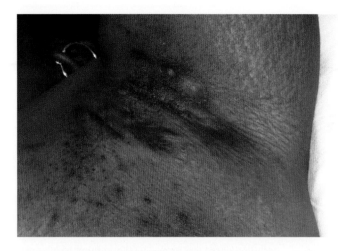

Figure 10.1 Hidradenitis suppurativa on the axilla.

Obesity tends to be more prevalent in patients with HS [20], although this has not been demonstrated in all studies [21]. It seems most likely that obesity is a secondary factor, aggravating the disease through mechanical trauma at skin folds rather than being a primary cause [22].

There is a high incidence of active smoking among HS patients compared with controls [23, 24]. No definitive causal mechanism has been determined; however, altered chemotaxis of polymorphic neutrophils might play a part [11].

Evidence from some families indicates transmission of HS occurs with single gene dominant inheritance [13, 25–27]. A recent genome-wide scan in a four-generation Chinese family mapped the chromosome location locus at chromosome 1p21.1–1q25.3 [28]. The female predominance found in most studies does argue against a purely

autosomal dominant inheritance, leading one to consider the possibility of hormonal influences on gene expression or the possibility of an X-linked chromosomal disease [11].

Hidradenitis suppurativa has been considered an androgen-dependent disorder [29]. Fifty percent of women report a flare-up before or during menses. Symptomatic improvement during pregnancy with postpartum flares is also often described. Numerous theories relating androgens to the pathogenesis of HS have been put forward, but none have achieved acceptance. Barth and Kealy studied apocrine glands, but they concluded that defects in these glands are not the primary cause of HS [30].

Diagnosis

The diagnosis of HS is primarily based on the clinical presentation. There are currently no recommended diagnostic tests. A biopsy is not required, unless used to exclude another diagnosis. A thorough history and physical exam is sufficient and should elicit the three main features of HS [31]:

1 Typical lesions (painful deep subcutaneous nodules, fibrotic sinus tracts).
2 Typical locations (axilla, perianal, and genital regions); Figures 10.1–10.3.
3 Relapses and chronicity.

Two methods (Hurley and Sartorius) currently exist to evaluate disease severity and guide treatment. Hurley

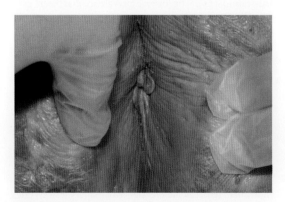

Figure 10.2 Hidradenitis suppurativa on the perianal tissue.

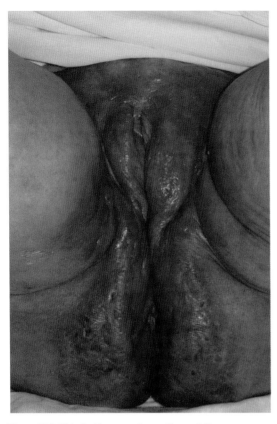

Figure 10.3 Hidradenitis suppurativa on the genitalia.

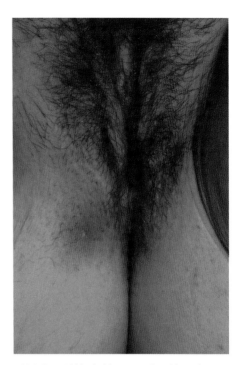

Figure 10.4 Stage I hidradenitis suppurativa with an abscess without sinus tract or cicatrization.

clinical staging [32] classifies patients in overall groups with early-stage disease benefiting from medical therapy and higher-stage disease requiring surgical intervention (Figures 10.4–10.6).

Stage I: One or more abscesses with no sinus tract or cicatrization.

Stage II: One or more wildly separated recurrent abscesses with a tract and scarring.

Stage III: Multiple interconnected tracts and abscesses throughout the entire affected area.

Sartorius [33] developed a scoring system for monitoring of disease severity in individual patients. A total score as well as scores of selected regions chosen for surgical or other intervention can be calculated and followed over time.

1 Anatomical region involved (three points per region involved).

2 Number and scores of lesions (points per lesion of all regions involved: nodules 2; fistulas 4; scars 1; others 1).

3 The longest distance between two relevant lesions (<5 cm, 2 points; <10 cm, 4 points; >10 cm, 8 points).

4 Are all lesions clearly separated by normal skin? (Yes, 0 points; No, 6 points).

The differential diagnosis includes other follicular infections such as carbuncles/furuncles or pilonidal cysts. Infected Bartholin's or epidermoid cysts and other chronic scarring conditions, such as tuberculosis and granuloma inguinale, may also be considered in HS. Crohn's disease may present with ulcerations, fistulae, and lesions in the perianal region, and must be excluded in patients with digestive symptoms. HS rarely involves the anal canal and does not track above the dentate line. An association between Crohn's disease and HS has been reported [34–37]. Squamous cell carcinomas may arise infrequently in HS, further emphasizing the need for close surveillance and biopsies of any suspicious lesions [38, 39]. Any excised tissue should be sent for pathology.

Unfortunately, HS is not a disease well known to health care providers, and patients may be referred to many specialists before a diagnosis is made and the proper treatment initiated. One series of 164 patients reported a mean delay

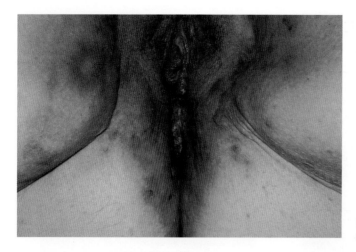

Figure 10.5 Stage II hidradenitis suppurativa with separated recurrent abscess with a tract and scarring.

in diagnosis of 7 years [40]. This can only compound the frustration and distress experienced by patients suffering from HS, and contributes to the negative impact on their quality of life.

Treatment

Treatment of HS involves a strategy of medical and surgical therapy to eliminate existing lesions and prevent the development of new lesions. Additionally, dealing with the patients' psychosocial issues is extremely important in this chronic, incurable condition. Initially, patients are instructed on reducing bacterial load by maintaining good hygiene, using warm baths, and wearing loose-fitting clothing [18]. Weight loss may be helpful if the patient is obese.

Medical Therapy

Early treatment consists of topical and systemic antibiotics used for their anti-inflammatory effects [31, 41]. Zinc has also been used in the treatment of HS [42]. Reducing androgen levels may reduce disease activity and the use of cyproterone acetate, finasteride, and spironolactone have been studied with some promise [43, 44]. Variable reports using isotretinoin, cyclosporine and steroids have shown only modest benefit in addition to their associated

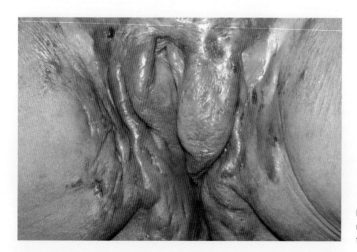

Figure 10.6 Stage III hidradenitis suppurativa with multiple interconnected tracts and abscesses throughout the entire affected area.

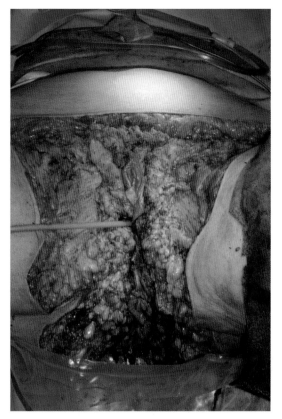

Figure 10.7 The appearance of the vulva immediately after a radical vulvectomy has been performed for stage III hidradenitis suppurativa.

that may significantly affect long-term sexual function and cosmesis if not addressed preoperatively. We recently reported our experience with five women with stage III vulvar HS who underwent radical excisions with skin grafting [50]. Our protocol involves a multidisciplinary approach using sexual counselors, nutritionists, and referrals to psychiatry if indicated.

Additionally, patients need to be prepared for a prolonged hospital stay, as well as given information on the use of wound VAC, hyperal, and a rectal tube to allow adequate healing. Overall, four out of our five patients were happy with the surgery, but all had depression. Hidradenitis suppurativa had a significant psychological impact on them. These issues must be addressed with all women prior to undertaking such a radical procedure.

A video demonstrating a radical procedure in one of our patients with stage III vulvar HS along with our protocol for pre- and postoperative management may be accessed at

http://www.med.umich.edu/obgyn/cvd/hidradenitis.asx

The surgery should be performed by an experienced surgeon with knowledge of skin grafting.

Figure 10.8 demonstrates the 1-year follow-up postoperative vulvar appearance of a patient who underwent radical vulvectomy with split thickness skin grafts. Figure 10.9 shows the healed thigh site from where the donor skin grafts were obtained.

side effects [45, 46]. Future prospects include anti-TNF agents that are being studied in Crohn's disease, rheumatoid arthritis, and other chronic inflammatory disorders [47]. Clearly, additional research is needed.

Surgical Management

For disease that is refractory to medical therapy and limited unroofing procedures, wide surgical excision may be required. Various surgical techniques have been described; however, the method utilized does not affect the local recurrence rate. Complete excision of the involved tissue is the most important factor in preventing recurrence [48, 49].

Figure 10.7 shows the appearance of the vulva immediately after a radical vulvectomy had been performed for stage III HS. Vulvar HS may require radical procedures

Psychosocial Issues

Hidradenitis suppurativa has been shown to cause particularly severe physical and psychosocial repercussions, especially with increasing duration and severity of disease [51]. It is imperative to keep in mind that an individual's morbidity is influenced by a myriad of confounding factors, including the symptoms caused by the condition, its visibility, and the person's coping ability [51]. Care must be taken to treat the whole person and not just the disease. Because HS preferentially affects intimate areas of the body, the disease has the connotation of socially unacceptable behavior or lack of hygiene. Its presence is often concealed, even from close relatives. Most of these patients seem to suffer in silence, as is poignantly reflected in the name chosen by the HS support group, "HIDE" [51].

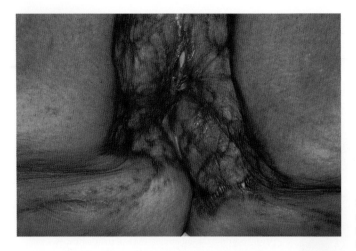

Figure 10.8 The postoperative vulvar appearance of a patient who underwent radical vulvectomy with split thickness skin grafts for stage III hidradenitis suppurativa, one year following her surgery.

There are a variety of assessment tools that can be utilized to gauge the extent of disease impact on an individual's well being. A subjective evaluation of pain from the worst lesion as chosen by the patient should be included with other routine vital signs. The Dermatology Life Quality Index [52] is a 10-question survey that provides a more in-depth assessment of disease impact. It also queries pain, but quantifies disease and treatment impact on activities and relationships as well. There is a maximum score of 30, with higher scores indicating a more significant adverse impact of the dermatologic condition. Other skin disease-specific quality of life measurement tools such as

Skindex and VQ-Dermato have also demonstrated that the impact of HS on quality of life is more significant than that found in other dermatologic conditions [53]. The Beck Depression Inventory [54] may provide valuable information on the impact of HS on the patient's mental health. Addressing and treating depression in addition to the physical manifestations of the disease process is integral to maximizing the individual's quality of life.

Assessing sexual function is likewise essential in understanding the complete extent of disease impact. The Female Sexual Distress Scale is a useful tool in identifying women who perceive they have a problem and in

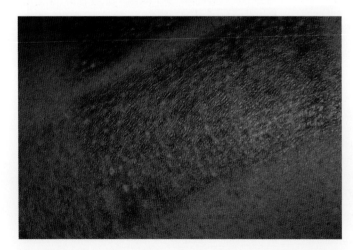

Figure 10.9 Healed area on thigh from which skin graft was obtained.

quantitatively measuring their sexually related personal distress [55]. The levels of sexual distress do not necessarily correlate with the level of depression as determined by the Beck Depression Inventory [50].

Utilizing a variety of these assessment tools will allow the provider to be cognizant of the full extent of disease impact and subsequently be able to intervene holistically and track the outcome of various interventions.

When extensive surgical intervention is required, thorough counseling regarding extent of surgery, healing time required, wound care requirements, postoperative appearance, as well as the likelihood of recurrence is needed. Psychological needs should be addressed prior to surgery. Discussion and counseling prior to surgery is also needed to encourage tobacco cessation.

Summary

Hidradenitis suppurativa is a debilitating disorder that may have severe physical and psychosocial repercussions. The disease is still poorly understood and delays in diagnosis are common. Medical treatments, while helpful, are not necessarily curative. In stage III disease, radical surgery may be successful; however, medical treatment should be considered following surgery to decrease recurrences. Chronic pain, depression, low sexual function, and poor quality of life are common occurrences in women with vulvar HS. The key to management is early diagnosis and control of the disease if possible. Early counseling for women may be beneficial, and careful surgical planning prior to radical excisions may provide women with some benefit and improvement in their quality of life.

References

1 Slade DE, Powell BW, Mortimer PS. (2003) Hidradenitis suppurativa: pathogenesis and management. *British Journal of Plastic Surgery* **56**, 451–61.

2 Parks RW, Parks TG. (1997) Pathogenesis, clinical features, and management of hidradenitis suppurativa. *Annals of the Royal College of Surgeons of England* **79**, 83–89.

3 Velpeau A. (1839) In: *Dictionnaire de medecine, un tepertoire general des sciences medicales sous la rapport theorique et practique*, 2nd ed. Vol. 2. Bechet Jeune, Paris, p. 91.

4 Verneuil A. (1854) Etudes sur les tumeurs de la peau et quelques maladies des glandes sudoripares. *Archives of General Medicine* **94**, 447–68, 693–705.

5 Verneuil A. (1864) De l'hidrosadenite phlegmoneuse et des abces sudoripares. *Archives of General Medicine* **114**, 537–57.

6 Brunsting HA. (1939) Hidradenitis suppurativa—abscess of apocrine sweat glands: a study of the clinical and pathologic features with a report of twenty-two cases and a review of the literature. *Archives of Dermatology and Syphilology* **39**, 108–120.

7 Pillsbury DM, Shelly WB, Kligman AM. (1956) Bacterial infections of the skin. In: *Dermatology*, 1st ed. Pillsbury DM (ed.) WB Saunders, Philadelphia, pp. 482–84, 489.

8 Plewig G, Kligman AM. (1975) *Acne: Morphogenesis and Treatment.* Springer-Verlag, Berlin, pp. 192–93.

9 Plewig G, Steger M. (1989) Acne inversa (alias acne triad, acne tetrad, or hidradenitis suppurativa). In: *Acne and Related Disorders*. Marks R, Plewig G (eds.) Martin Dunitz, London, pp. 345–57.

10 Shuster S. (2008) The nature and consequence of Karl Marx's skin disease. *British Journal of Dermatology* **158**, 1–3.

11 Jansen T, Altmeyer P, Plewig G. (2001) Acne inversa (alias hidradenitis suppurativa.) *Journal of the European Academy of Dermatology and Venereology* **15**, 532–40.

12 Jemec GBE, Heidenheim M, Nielsen NH. (1996) The prevalence of hidradenitis suppurativa and its potential precursor lesions. *Journal of the American Academy of Dermatology* **35**, 191–94.

13 Fitzsimmons JS, Guilbert PR, Fitzsimmons EM. (1985) Evidence of genetic factors in hidradenitis suppurativa. *British Journal of Dermatology* **113**, 1–8.

14 Harrison BJ, Mudge M, Hughes LE. (1989) The prevalence of hidradenitis suppurativa in South Wales. In: Marks R, Plewig G (eds.) *Acne and Related Disorders*. Martin Dunitz, London, pp. 365–66.

15 Homma H, Hans C. (1926) On apocrine sweat glands in white and Negro men and women. *Bulletin of the Johns Hopkins Hospital* **38**, 365.

16 Woolard HH. (1930) The cutaneous glands of man. *Journal of Anatomy* **64**, 415.

17 Bhatia NN, Berginan A, Broen EM. (1984) Advanced hidradenitis suppurativa of the vulva: a report of 3 cases. *The Journal of Reproductive Medicine* **29**, 436–40.

18 Paletta C, Jurkiewicz MJ. (1987) Hidradenitis suppurativa. *Clinics in Plastic Surgery* **14**, 383–90.

19 Banerjee AK. (1992) Surgical treatment of hidradenitis suppurativa. *British Journal of Surgery* **79**, 863–66.

20 Edlich RF, Silloway KA, Rodeheaver GT, *et al.* (1986) Epidemiology, pathology, and treatment of axillary hidradenitis suppurativa. *Journal of Emergency Medicine* **4**, 369–78.

21 Jemec GB, Heidenheim M, Nielsen NH. (1996) Hidradenitis suppurativa: characteristics and consequences. *Clinics in Experimental Dermatology* **21**, 419–23.

22 Lee RA, Yoon A, Kist J. (2007) Hidradenitis suppurativa: an update. *Advances in Dermatology* **23**, 289–306.

23 Konig A, Lehmann C, Rompel R, *et al.* (1999) Cigarette smoking as a triggering factor of hidradenitis suppurativa. *Dermatology* **198**, 261–64.

24 Freiman A, Bird G, Metelitsa AI, *et al.* (2004) Cutaneous effects of smoking. *Journal of Cutaneous Medicine and Surgery* **8**, 415–23.

25 Fitzsimmons JS, Fitzsimmons EM, Gilbert G. (1984) Familial hidradenitis suppurativa: evidence in favour of single gene transmission. *Journal of Medical Genetics* **21**, 281–85.

26 Fitzsimmons JS, Guilbert PR. (1985) A family study of hidradenitis suppurativa. *Journal of Medical Genetics* **22**, 367–73.

27 Von der Werth JM, Williams HC, Raeburn JA. (2000) The clinical genetics of hidradenitis suppurativa revisited. *British Journal of Dermatology* **142**, 947–53.

28 Gao M, Wang P, Cui Y, *et al.* (2006) Inversa acne (hidradenitis suppurativa): a case report and identification of the locus at chromosome 1p 21.1–1q25.3. *Journal of Investigative Dermatology* **126**, 1302–6.

29 Ebling FJG. (1986) Hidradenitis suppurativa: an androgen-dependent disorder. *British Journal of Dermatology* **115**, 259–62.

30 Barth JH, Kealey T. (1991) Androgen metabolism by isolated human axillary apocrine glands in hidradenitis suppurativa. *British Journal of Dermatology* **125**, 304–8.

31 Jemec GBE. (1988) The symptomatology of hidradenitis suppurativa in women. *British Journal of Dermatology* **119**, 345–50.

32 Hurley HJ. (1989) Axillary hyperhidrosis, apocrine bromhidrosis, hidradenitis suppurativa, and familial benign pemphigus: surgical approach. In: Roenigk RK, Roenigk HH (eds.) *Dermatologic Surgery*. Marcel Dekker, New York, pp. 729–39.

33 Sartorius K, Lapins J, Emtestam L, *et al.* (2003) Suggestions for uniform outcome variables when reporting treatment effects in hidradenitis suppurativa. *British Journal of Dermatology* **149**, 211–13.

34 Burrows NP, Jones RR. (1992) Crohn's disease in association with hidradenitis suppurativa. *British Journal of Dermatology* **126**, 523.

35 Ostlere LS, Langtr JA, Mortimer PS, *et al.* (1991) Hidradenitis suppurativa in Crohn's disease. *British Journal of Dermatology* **125**, 384–86.

36 Roy MK, Apleton MA, Delicata RJ, *et al.* (1997) Probable association between hidradenitis suppurativa and Crohn's disease: significance of epithelioid granuloma. *British Journal of Surgery* **84**, 375–76.

37 Church JM, Fazio VW, Lavery IC, *et al.* (1993) The differential diagnosis and co-morbidity of hidradenitis suppurativa and perianal Crohn's disease. *International Journal of Colorectal Disease* **8**, 117–19.

38 Short KA, Kalu G, Mortimer PS, *et al.* (2005) Vulval squamous cell carcinoma arising in chronic hidradenitis suppurativa. *Clinics in Experimental Dermatology* **30**, 481–83.

39 Manolitsas T, Biankin S, Jaworski R, *et al.* (1999) Vulval squamous cell carcinoma arising in chronic hidradenitis supurativa. *Gynecologic Oncology* **75**, 285–88.

40 Faye O, Bastuji-Garin S, Poli F, *et al.* (2006) Hidradenitis suppurativa: a clinical study of 164 patients. In: *Hidradenitis Suppurativa*. Jemec GBE, Revuz J, Leyden JJ (eds.) Springer-Verlag, Berlin, pp. 22–23.

41 Harrison BJ, Kumar S, Read GF, *et al.* (1985) Hidradenitis suppurativa: evidence for an endocrine abnormality. *British Journal of Surgery* **72**, 1002–4.

42 Brocard A, Knol AC, Khammari A, *et al.* (2007) Hidradenitis suppurativa and zinc: a new therapeutic approach. A pilot study. *Dermatology* **214**, 325–27.

43 Mortimer PS, Dawber RPR, Gales MA, *et al.* (1986) A double-blind cross-over trial of cyproterone acetate in females with hidradenitis suppurativa. *British Journal of Dermatology* **115**, 263–68.

44 Farrell AM, Randall VA, Vafee T, *et al.* (1999) Finasteride as a therapy for hidradenitis suppurativa [letter]. *British Journal of Dermatology* **141**, 1138–39.

45 Layton AM, Knaggs H, Taylor J, *et al.* (1993) Isotretinoin for acne vulgaris 10 years later: a safe and effective treatment. *British Journal of Dermatology* **129**, 292–96.

46 Buckley DA, Rogers S. (1995) Cyclosporin-responsive hidradenitis suppurativa. *Journal of the Royal Society of Medicine* **88**, 289–90.

47 Hanauer SB. (2004) Efficacy and safety of tumor necrosis factor antagonists in Crohn's disease: overiew of randomized clinical studies. *Reviews of Gastroenterologic Disorders* **4**, S18–S24.

48 Tanaka A, Hatoko M, Tada H, *et al.* (2001) Experience with surgical treatment of hidradenitis suppurativa. *Annals of Plastic Surgery* **47**, 636–42.

49 Rompel R, Petres J. (2000) Long-term results of wide surgical excision in 106 patients with hidradenitis suppurativa. *Dermatologic Surgery* **26**, 638–43.

50 Rhode JM, Burke WM, Cederna PS, *et al.* (2008) Outcomes of surgical management of stage III vulvar hidradenitis suppurativa. *The Journal of Reproductive Medicine* **53**, 420–28.

51 Von der Werth JM, Jemec GBE. (2001) Morbidity in patients with hidradenitis suppurativa. *British Journal of Dermatology* **144**, 809–13.

52 Finlay AY. (1997) Quality of life measurement in dermatology: a practical guide. *British Journal of Dermatology* **136**, 305–14.

53 Wolkenstein P, Loundou A, Barrau K, Auquier P, Revuz J, Quality of Life Group of the French Society of Dermatology. (2007) Quality of life impairment in hidradenitis suppurativa: a study of 61 cases. *Journal of the American Academy of Dermatologists* **56**, 621–23.

54 Beck AT, Ward CH, Mendelsohn M, *et al.* (1961) An inventory for measuring depression. *Archives of General Psychiatry* **4**, 561–71.

55 Derogatis LR, Rosen R, Leiblum S, *et al.* (2002) The Female Sexual Distress Scale (FSDS): initial validation of a standardized scale for assessment of sexually related personal distress in women. *Journal of Sexual and Marital Therapy* **28**, 317–30.

CHAPTER 11
Sexually Transmitted Infections (STIs)

Alison Mears, David Goldmeier

St Mary's Hospital, Imperial College Healthcare NHS Trust, London, UK

Introduction

A number of sexually transmitted infections (STIs) are associated with sexual pain in women, and we will discuss these under the headings of superficial and deep dyspareunia. In particular, ulcerative disease, vaginal discharges and vulvovaginitis, (see Chapter 15), and pelvic pain will be reviewed. In addition to dyspareunia, patient concerns about STIs include health anxieties about HIV, stigma, shame, and fertility issues [1]. Women with STIs are at significantly increased risk of transmitting and acquiring HIV and, surprisingly, may continue to have unprotected sex in spite of any symptoms including pain [2]. Treatment of the STIs, whether in syndromic fashion [3] or based on laboratory diagnosis, not only resolves pain but also decreases HIV transmission [4, 5].

Superficial Dyspareunia

Ulcerative Disease

Genital Herpes

Genital herpes (GH) is usually caused by herpes simplex type 2 (HSV-2), but herpes simplex type 1 (HSV-1) is an increasingly common isolate in the United States, probably as a result of lower rates of nonsexual acquisition of oral HSV in childhood and adolescence [6]. HSV-1 and HSV-2 are genotypically and phenotypically very similar, but

Female Sexual Pain Disorders 1st edition. Edited by A. Goldstein, C. Pukall & I. Goldstein. © 2009 Blackwell Publishing, ISBN: 9781405183987.

can be distinguished serologically [7]. In a recent survey, 17% of the United States population ages 14–49 showed positive-type specific antibody to type-2 herpes simplex [6]. Apart from causing local pain and dyspareunia, GH may cause marked psychological distress [8].

Viropathology

The virus gains entry into the genital mucosa by binding to the host cell surface. Molecular motor proteins then transport HSV up the sensory nerve fibers to the dorsal root ganglion [9] where latency is established. Reactivation results in transportation of virus back down the peripheral nerves to the skin and mucosa where typical lesions develop (not necessarily ending up in the site of initial entry). In many cases, the precipitating factors for reactivation cannot be identified, but local trauma (including sexual activity), dermatoses, fevers, and immunosuppression may initiate this event.

Clinical Presentations

Epidemiological studies suggest that as many as 90% of those who have type-specific antibodies to HSV-2 have never knowingly suffered a clinical outbreak [10]. However, in those individuals who are symptomatic, pain is an important symptom. Symptoms are more severe in a primary HSV-2 or HSV-1 infected woman who has not had HSV-1 in the past [11]. Clinically, primary HSV-1 and HSV-2 are indistinguishable. Fever, headache, malaise, and myalgia are reported in up to 70% of women with primary HSV-2 and appear in the first few days of the illness [12].

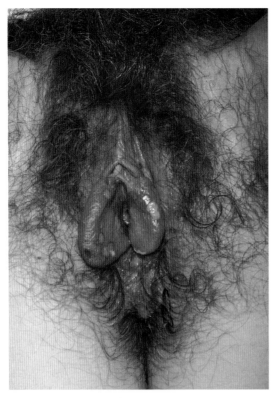

Figure 11.1 Primary genital herpes.

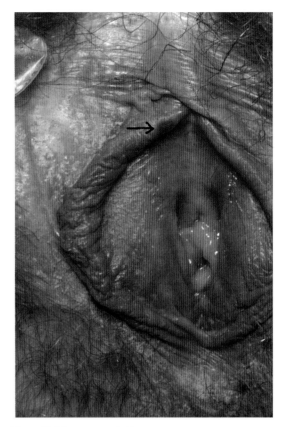

Figure 11.2 Recurrent genital herpes.

Classically, the lesions progress from erythematous papules, to vesicles, pustules, and then painful ulcers, which can coalesce (Figure 11.1). On moist mucosal surfaces they appear as ulcers without forming crusts as they would in the outer skin of the labia majora. Symptomatic lesions can appear anywhere on the genitalia from the introitus out to the upper thighs, perianal area, and buttocks [11]. Pain from these lesions may be severe and constant, with exacerbation at micturition and defecation if lesions are in the periurethral or perianal area, respectively. Untreated patients can develop new crops of lesions with pain persisting for up to 3–4 weeks [11]. Other complications of primary GH are acute urinary retention, sacral neuropathy, and meningitis.

About 25% of patients with a first clinical episode of HSV-2 have a mild clinical picture rather like that of a recurrence. These patients have preexisting HSV-2 antibodies, implying that they may not have acquired the infection from a recent partner [13].

Recurrences of GH are less common when the primary outbreak was with HSV-1 [14]. HSV-2 tends to recur sooner if the primary episode was prolonged, and 86% of women will have at least one recurrence after a year [15]. Recent data suggests that in the ensuing years, recurrence rates gradually decrease in most patients [16]. The lesions in recurrent GH tend to be fewer in number and less painful than first episodes with an average healing time of 5–10 days (Figure 11.2).

A proportion of patients exhibit a prodrome that usually manifests as itching, tingling, or pain in the sacral dermatomes or more specifically, in the area where the outbreak is about to appear. Some patients complain of a low mood at this time, which may be related to systemic cytokine release affecting their psychological state [8].

Atypical presentations include fissuring in genital dermatoses and postmenopausal atrophic genital mucosa.

Similar lesions may occur in healthy mucosa where the woman has genital arousal problems and is thus poorly lubricated. Some patients are quite severely psychologically disabled by recurrences of GH, often because of issues of poor self-esteem, reactive depression, and disclosure issues [17].

Diagnostic Testing

The clinical features of GH should strongly suggest the diagnosis. However, the diagnosis should be confirmed by testing the lesional material by viral tissue culture. This is about 80% sensitive in primary outbreaks and 50% in recurrent lesions [14]. Antibody staining will determine if the isolate is HSV-1 or HSV-2. The newer the lesional material (e.g., vesicles or pustules), the less likely there will be a false negative result.

Polymerase chain reaction (PCR) is up to four times more sensitive than culture and is being increasingly used by local hospital laboratories [18]. When local tests are negative, type-specific immunoglobulin G (IgG) testing of serum directed against glycoprotein G can be undertaken. The U.S. Food and Drug Administration (FDA) has licensed four such kits [19]. Clinical judgment is needed to ensure that a positive result relates to any clinical pathology.

Treatment

Antiviral agents underpin the treatment of GH. In primary and recurrent GH, the aims are to reduce viral reproduction, shorten time to healing, and decrease pain. The specific antivirals (aciclovir, valaciclovir, and famciclovir) and their dosing schedules are well presented in a recent paper [20]. Traditionally, suppressive therapy is given to women who have frequent recurrences. Their use has been shown to decrease rates of transmission of GH to partners [21]. Apart from antivirals, women should be counseled about the advantages of barrier contraception and the need to abstain from sex at the time of clinical outbreaks. Pain is best managed in the acute phase by the use of nonopiate analgesia and local anesthetic agents.

Other Less Common Ulcerative Disease

Ulcers may be caused by syphilis, chancroid, donovanosis, or lymphogranuloma venereum. An ulcer may contain more than one pathogen, and all of these conditions may enhance HIV transmission.

Syphilis

Syphilis is caused by *Treponema pallidum*. In the adult with ulcerative disease in North America, it is always acquired sexually. The average time to the appearance of a primary syphilitic ulcer or chancre is 3 weeks (9–90 days). The chancre is characteristically painless and indurated, but it can be painful and tender and may appear anywhere on the genital area. There is usually nontender local lymphadenopathy. Secondary syphilis usually commences 4–10 weeks after the appearance of the chancre and may cause, amongst its many other features, condylomata lata, which may be tender and appear as de-epithelialized genital warts [22]. Diagnosis by the nonspecialist is made by serology.

Chancroid

This condition is not common in North America. The combination of a painful genital ulcer and tender suppurative local lymphadenopathy should suggest chancroid, particularly if tests for syphilis and GH are negative. Laboratory diagnosis relies on special culture medium. No FDA-approved PCR tests are currently available.

Lymphogranuloma Venereum (LGV)

This is caused by *Chlamydia trachomatis* serovars L1-3. The most common clinical manifestation is tender inguinal and/or femoral lymphadenopathy (rarely with a "groove" between them). However, a tender genital ulcer at the site of inoculation may be present transiently. Nucleic acid amplification tests (NAAT) of ulcer or lymph node material are usually diagnostic. Very rarely, LGV causes vulvar elephantiasis [23].

Vaginal Discharge and Vulvovaginitis

Trichomoniasis

Trichomoniasis (TV) is the most common sexually transmitted infection worldwide. It is caused by a flagellated protozoan called *Trichomoniasis vaginalis*, which can infect the vagina, urethra, Skene's glands, and Bartholins glands [24–31]. Women with TV usually complain of a vaginal discharge (>50%) [32], vulvar itching, or dysuria [33], but some may be asymptomatic [34]. The vaginal discharge is classically frothy yellow-greenish (10–30%) but can vary in color and consistency and may indeed look normal [34]. Evidence of vulvitis or vaginitis is also common.

Diagnosis is usually made on microscopy of a sample from the posterior fornix; however, the sensitivity of this test is only 60–70% [5]. The gold standard test is still culture [35], although polymerase chain reaction (PCR) tests are being developed that are thought to be highly reliable (none approved by the FDA to date) [5, 36]. In-office rapid immunochromatographic assays for TV have recently become available.

Because TV commonly infects the uterine cavity, urethra, and paravaginal glands, it is imperative to give systemic medication. Cure rates with oral metronidazole are in the order of 90–95% [5]. True treatment failure is rare; however poor compliance with medication or re-infection is more common. Expert guidance should be sought in true treatment failure [5].

TV in pregnancy is associated with preterm labor and low birth weight. TV in a woman with HIV may increase her risk of transmitting HIV to a sexual partner or contracting HIV if exposed [37].

Partners should be screened and treated for TV. Follow-up is only necessary for women who remain symptomatic despite treatment [5].

Sexually Transmitted Causes of Pelvic Pain and Deep Dyspareunia

Acute Pelvic Inflammatory Disease (PID) and Its Complications

Introduction

PID is a condition characterized by endometriosis, parametritis, salpingitis, tuboovarian abscess, and pelvic peritonitis. *Chlamydia trachomatis* (CT) and *Neisseria gonorrhea* (NG) ascend from the vagina and cervix to the upper genital tract [38]. PID can vary greatly in severity from asymptomatic to generalised peritonitis and death (very rare). Indeed, many episodes are likely to go unnoticed, undiagnosed, or misdiagnosed due to the mild or nonspecific nature of the woman's symptoms. However, PID is a significant burden both to women's heath and

the economy. In the United States alone, it is estimated that every year over 1 million women have an episode of acute PID with more than 100,000 cases of subfertility occurring annually due to this condition. The average per person-lifetime cost of PID may be as high as $318,000 [39]. PID is an extremely important cause of preventable morbidity, particularly, reproductive ill health [40].

Both *Chlamydia trachomatis* and *Neisseria gonorrhea* have been proven as causal agents in PID [41]. The rates of both these infections continue to rise, particularly in the young, with the highest rates in the 15–19 age group. CT infections are more common than NG infections, and are the most common cause of PID in the United States, accounting for nearly 40% of all cases. The incidence of PID in women with untreated or inadequately treated CT can vary from 10% to 80% [42], but others feel the true rate is uncertain [43].

Not all women with an STI in the lower genital tract develop PID; host susceptibility may be genetically determined [44]. PID caused by NG is often more acute and severe in its presentation, but it is less likely to cause long-term sequelae when compared with chlamydial PID.

The role of other organisms such as *Mycoplasma genitalium*, anaerobes, *E. coli*, staphylococci, streptococci, and *H. influenzae* may also be important [45, 46]. The rates of bacterial vaginosis (BV) have been found to be higher in women with PID [47], and as many as one in seven women with BV have been shown to have subclinical PID on endometrial biopsy [48].

It was first thought that the oral contraceptive pill (OCP) might reduce the risk of PID by progesterone effects on the cervical mucus barrier, blocking the ascension of infection or by endometrial suppression. However, the recent PID Evaluation and Clinical Health (PEACH) study has concluded that the OCP does not reduce the risk of PID but simply lessens the clinical severity. So the OCP may have no effect on the true prevalence of PID and instead may simply reduce the prevalence and severity of symptomatic infection [49].

There have been many reports that vaginal douching may double the risk of PID [50], although a recent prospective observational study has found no such association [51].

Any breach of the cervical barrier can increase the risk of PID such as termination of pregnancy, recent intrauterine device insertion (less than 6 weeks), embryo transfer, or hysterosalpingography.

Other risk factors may be cigarette smoking [52] and sexual intercourse during menstruation. In the PEACH study, women carrying the HLA class II DQA*301 allele were found to have higher rates of gonococcal and chlamydial cervicitis, endometritis, and infertility [53].

Diagnosis and Investigation

Diagnosing PID can be difficult and imprecise [5] because the clinical picture can range from symptomatic to severely symptomatic and because the diagnostic tools lack sensitivity and specificity [54]. In view of its potentially serious complications if left untreated (see below), it is important to have a low threshold for diagnosing PID.

Symptoms suggestive of PID:

1 Lower abdominal pain.
2 Abnormal vaginal bleeding including postcoital bleeding, intermenstrual bleeding, and menorrhagia.
3 Deep dyspareunia.
4 Abnormal (cervical or vaginal) discharge.
5 Fever.
6 Dysuria.

Clinical signs suggestive of PID

1 Lower abdominal tenderness.
2 Adenexal tenderness and/or swelling.
3 Cervical motion pain.
4 Mucopurulent cervical discharge seen on speculum examination and/or contact bleeding on examination.
5 Fever (>38°C), although thought to be present in less than 40% of women.

The positive predictive value of a diagnosis based on these signs and symptoms varies depending on a number of factors, including the epidemiological characteristics of the group studied. There have been many attempts to define and standardize the clinical criteria used to diagnose PID. Jacobsen and Westrom's criteria in the 1960s had a 65% concordance with laparoscopy [55], and more recent attempts have not achieved a better sensitivity [56]. Diagnosing PID is certainly not an exact science, and too low a threshold for instigating treatment will inevitably result in an overdiagnosis of PID. However, the potential risks of treatment are far outweighed by the risks of a missed diagnosis.

Differential Diagnosis

It is imperative that pregnancy-related diagnoses are considered first in any sexually active woman and ruled out before any other diagnosis is made. The differential diagnoses below are by no means definitive.

Ectopic pregnancy
Ovarian cyst "event," e.g., torsion or rupture
Appendicitis
Irritable bowel syndrome
Endometriosis
Pelvic adhesions
Functional pain (i.e., no known physical cause)
Urinary tract infection
Inflammatory bowel disease
Mittelschmertz pain

Tests

Endocervical swabs for *Chlamydia trachomatis* and (NAAT test) and *Neisseria gonorrhea* (NAAT) and/or culture and antibiotic sensitivity (because NG is becoming increasingly resistant to a number of antibiotics) [57] should be taken, although the absence of infection does not exclude PID [5]. The absence of neutrophils (pus cells) in the vagina, as demonstrated on microscopy, has been shown by Yudin [58] to have a negative predictive value of 95% but a low positive predictive value.

An erythrocyte sedimentation rate or C-reactive protein, if raised, may assist in making the diagnosis of PID. If, however, the levels are normal, the patient can still have a mild to moderate case of PID [59].

Laparoscopy

Laparoscopy has long been thought of as the gold standard for diagnosing PID. However, this statement is not without contention [60, 61]. Practically, laparoscopy is not an option in the routine diagnosis of PID, but it does have an important role in selected cases (e.g., for women who have not responded to PID treatment, where a complication is suspected, or where the diagnosis is in doubt).

Other Investigations

Other tests include ultrasound scanning, transvaginal power Doppler sonography, and magnetic resonance imaging can all be used to diagnose PID in this setting. These modalities can be particularly helpful in monitoring

Table 11.1 Recommended antibiotic regimens for the treatment of PID [5].

Parenteral Regimen1	Parenteral Regimen 2
Cefotetan 2 g IV bid **OR** Cefoxitin 2 g IV qds **PLUS** Doxycycline 100 mg IV or PO bid	Clindamycin 900 mg IV tds **PLUS** Gentamicin loading dose IV/IM followed by maintenance dose tds

Oral Regimen 1	Oral Regimen 2	Oral Regimen 3
Ceftiraxone 250 mg IM stat **PLUS** Doxycycline 100 mg PO bid for 14 days **WITH OR WITHOUT** Metronidazole 500 mg bid for 14 days	Cefoxitin 2 mg IM stat with Probenecid 1 g stat **PLUS** Doxycycline 100 mg PO bid for 14 days **WITH OR WITHOUT** Metronidazole 500 mg bid for 14 days	Other parenteral third- generation cephalosporin (e.g., Cefotaxime) **PLUS** Doxycycline 100mg PO bid for 14 days **WITH OR WITHOUT** Metronidazole 500 mg bid for 14 days

severe cases and in looking for complications; also, in selected cases, they may negate the need for laparoscopy.

Management

Antibiotics

The principle of treatment is to cover for *Chlamydia trachomatis* and *Neisseria gonorrhea* and anaerobes. The Centers for Disease Control (CDC) recently changed their PID treatment recommendations based on data from the Gonococcal Isolate Surveillance Project (GISP), which is showing an increase in fluoroquinolone-resistant gonorrhea spreading across the United States [57].

Table 11.1 outlines the different recommended treatment regimens depending on severity. If PID is severe (or if oral treatment is not tolerated), parenteral antibiotics should be given and subsequently switched to oral treatment based on clinical findings.

Removal of *In Situ* Intrauterine Devices (IUDs)?

A European study has reported better short-term outcomes associated with removal of IUDs. However, the CDC guidelines do not recommend removal but do advocate close follow-up. If removal is to be contemplated, the pros and cons (i.e., risk of pregnancy) of doing so needs to be discussed with the patient. Removal may need to be accompanied by the provision of emergency contraception.

PID and Pregnancy

Although PID is uncommon in pregnancy (and should therefore prompt thorough investigation for other diagnoses), it is associated with poorer outcomes both for the mother and fetus. Therefore, hospital admission and parenteral antibiotics are advised, despite a paucity of evidence available regarding which antibiotics are most efficacious or safe [62].

PID in HIV Positive Patients

A number of studies have reported more severe symptoms and increased rates of complications in HIV-positive women [63]. However, more recent studies have found no such differences [5]. It is recommended that HIV positive patients be treated according to the protocol for HIV negative individuals until evidence dictates otherwise.

Partner Notification

Recent sexual partners should be offered tests for sexually transmitted infections. CDC guidelines recommend a look-back period of 60 days [5], whereas UK [64] and European guidelines [62] advise 6 months (this may differ depending on sexual history). Empirical treatment for NG and CT is also recommended regardless of symptoms, as contacts are often asymptomatic [5].

Outcomes/Complications

In the majority of patients, recovery is uneventful, and their fertility is usually well preserved [62]. However, severe disease can increase the risk of sub-fertility as can any delay in treatment [65]. A number of other sequelae may occur. In the short term, these consequences include tubo-ovarian abscess and perihepatitis (Fitz-Hugh-Curtis syndrome). This syndrome is characterized by the development of adhesions between the liver and the peritoneum, causing right upper quadrant pain. It is thought to occur in up to 10–20% of women with PID [66]. There is no evidence to support any specific treatment beyond that for PID [66].

Long-Term Complications

Tubal Infertility

This is usually the most feared complication by patients [67]. With each episode of PID, it is thought that the risk of subfertility doubles. Indeed, Westrom et al. found that after one episode, the rate was 8%, after two episodes the rate was 19.5%, and after three or more episodes the rate was 40% [68]. Of those who do conceive, studies have shown that previous PID is a risk factor for ectopic pregnancy [67], but absolute risk of ectopic pregnancy is still low (1%) [62].

Chronic Pelvic Pain (CPP) and Deep Dyspareunia

CPP can develop in up to 30% of women after an episode of PID [62]. Deep dyspareunia is also a common sequelae of PID. It should not be forgotten that the psychological effects of PID can be significant in some women.

Follow-up

All patients should be reviewed after 72 hr, and those in whom no clinical improvement has been made should be examined and hospitalised to undergo further investigation [5]. A further review is also recommended at 2–4 weeks.

Prevention

In light of the well-documented health burdens caused by *Chlamydia trachomatis* and the high rate of asymptomatic infection, many countries including the United States have introduced CT screening programs in men and women. The CDC recommends screening all sexually active women below the age of 26 for CT. Although the uptake is suboptimal at the present time, it is hoped that by reducing the undiagnosed pool of *Chlamydia*, this will significantly reduce the incidence of PID and subsequently its sequelae.

References

1 Arkell J, Osborn DP, Ivens D, *et al.* (2006) Factors associated with anxiety in patients attending a sexually transmitted infection clinic: qualitative survey. *International Journal of STD and AIDS* **17**, 299–303.
2 Nuwaha F, Kambugu F. (2000) Determinants for having sex while symptomatic among patients with sexually transmitted infections in Uganda. *African Journal of Health Sciences* **7**, 91–97.
3 Ballard RC. (1998) Syndromic case management of STDs in Africa. *African Health* **20**, 13–15.
4 Bell C, Richardson D, Wall M, *et al.* (2006) HIV-associated female sexual dysfunction: clinical experience and literature review. *International Journal of STD and AIDS* **17**, 706–9.
5 CDC Guidelines for Treating STIs. (2006) www.cdc.gov/std/treatment/.
6 Xu F, Sternberg MR, Kottir BJ, *et al.* (2006) Trends in herpes simplex virus type 1 and 2 seroprevalence in the United States. *Journal of the American Medical Association* **296**, 964–73.
7 Dolan A, Jamieson FE, Cunningham C, *et al.* (1998) The genome sequence of herpes simplex virus type 2. *Journal of Virology* **72**, 2010–21.
8 Goldmeier D, Garvey L, Barton S. (2008) Does chronic stress lead to increased rates of recurrences of genital herpes: a review of the psychoneuroimmunological evidence. *International Journal of STD and AIDS* **19**, 359–62.

9 Sodeik B, Ebersold MW, Helenius A. (1997) Microtubule–mediated transport of incoming herpes simplex virus 1 capsids to the nucleus. *Journal of Cell Biology* **136**, 1007–21.

10 Fleming DT, McQuillan GM, Johnson RE, *et al.* (1997) Herpes simplex virus type 2 in the United States, 1976–1994. *New England Journal of Medicine* **337**, 1105–11.

11 Corey L, Adams HG, Brown ZA, *et al.* (1983) Genital herpes simplex infections: clinical manifestations, course, and complications. *Annals of Internal Medicine* **98**, 958–72.

12 Corey L, Wald A. (1999) Genital herpes. In: Holmes KK, Sparling PF, Mardh P *et al.* (eds.) *Sexually Transmitted Diseases*, 3rd ed. McGraw-Hill, New York, pp. 285–312.

13 Bernstein D, Lovett M, Bryson Y. (1984) Serologic analysis of first episode nonprimary genital herpes simplex virus infection. *American Journal of Medicine* **77**, 1055–60.

14 Lafferty WE, Krofft S, Remington M, *et al.* (1987) Diagnosis of herpes simplex virus by direct immunofluorescence and viral isolation from samples of external genital lesions in a high prevalence population. *Journal of Clinical Microbiology* **25**, 323–26.

15 Benedetti JK, Corey L, Ashley R. (1994) Recurrence rates in genital herpes after symptomatic first–episode infection. *Annals of Internal Medicine* **131**, 14–20.

16 Crespi CM, Cumberland W, Wald A, *et al.* (2007) Longitudinal study of herpes simplex virus type 2 infection using viral dynamic modelling. *Sexually Transmitted Infections* **83**, 359–64.

17 Green J, Koscis A. (1997) Psychological factors in recurrent genital herpes. *Genitourinary Medicine* **73**, 253–58.

18 Strick LB, Wald A. (2006) Diagnostics for herpes simplex virus: is PCR the new gold standard? *Molecular Diagnosis and Therapy* **10**, 17–28.

19 Ashley RL. (2002) Performance and use of HSV type-specific serology test kits. *Herpes* **9**, 38–45.

20 Gupta R, Warren T, Wald A. (2007) Genital herpes. *Lancet* **370**, 2127–37.

21 Corey L, Wald A, Patel R, *et al.* (2004) Valacyclovir HSV Transmission Study Group. Once-daily valacyclovir to reduce the risk of transmission of genital herpes. *New England Journal of Medicine* **350**, 11–20.

22 Goldmeier D, Guallar C. (2003) Syphilis: an update. *Clinical Medicine* **3**, 209–11.

23 Gupta S, Ajith C, Kanwar AJ, *et al.* (2006) Genital elephantitis and sexually transmitted infections: revisited. *International Journal of STD and AIDS* **17**, 157–65.

24 Sosnik H, Sosnik K, Halon A. (2007) The pathomorphology of Bartholin's gland. Analysis of surgical data. *Polish Journal of Pathology* **58**, 99–103.

25 Tanaka K, Mikamo H, Ninomiya M, *et al.* (2005) Microbiology of Bartholin's gland abscess in Japan. *Journal of Clinical Microbiology* **43**, 4258–61.

26 Saul HM, Grossman MB. (1988) The role of *Chlamydia trachomatis* in Bartholin's gland abscess. *American Journal of Obstetrics and Gynecology* **158**, 76–77.

27 Davies JA, Rees E, Hobson D, *et al.* (1978) Isolation of *Chlamydia trachomatis* from Bartholin's ducts. *British Journal of Venereal Disease* **54**, 409–13.

28 Bleker OP, Smalbraak DJ, Schutte MF. (1990) Bartholin's abscess: the role of *Chlamydia trachomatis*. *Genitourinary Medicine* **66**, 24–25.

29 Hoosen AA, Nteta C, Moodley J, *et al.* (1995) Sexually transmitted diseases including HIV infection in women with Bartholin's gland abscesses. *Genitourinary Medicine* **71**, 155–57.

30 Haider Z, Condous G, Kirk E, *et al.* (2007) The simple outpatient management of Bartholin's abscess using the Word catheter: a preliminary study. *Australian and New Zealand Journal of Obstetric Gynecology* **47**, 137–40.

31 World Health Organization. Global Prevalence and incidence of selected curable sexually transmitted infections. WHO/HIV_AIDS/2001.02WHO/CDS/CSR/EDC2001.10, 2001

32 Hobbs MM, Sena AC, Swygard H, *et al.* (2008) *Trichomonas vaginalis* and trichomoniasis. In: Holmes KK, Sparling FP, Stamm WE *et al.* (eds.) *Sexually Transmitted Diseases*, 4th ed. McGraw-Hill, New York, pp. 771–93.

33 Fouts AC, Kraus SJ. (1980) *Trichomonas vaginalis*: re-evaluation of its clinical presentation and laboratory diagnosis. *Journal of Infectious Diseases* **141**, 137–43.

34 Wolner-Hanssen P, Kreiger JN, Stevens CE, *et al.* (1989) Clinical manifestations of vaginal trichomoniasis. *Journal of the American Medical Association* **264**, 571–76.

35 Schmid GP, Matheny LC, Zaidi AA, *et al.* Evaluation of six media for the growth of *Trichomonas vaginalis* from vaginal secretions. *Journal of Clinical Microbiology* **27**, 1230–33.

36 Mayta H, Gilman RH, Calderon MM, *et al.* (2000) 18S ribosomal DNA-based PCR for the diagnosis of *Trichomonas vaginalis*. *Journal of Clinical Microbiology* **38**, 2683–87.

37 Sorvillo F, Kernott P. (1998) *Trichomonas vaginalis* and amplification of HIV-1 transmission. *Lancet* **351**, 213–14.

38 Weström L, Eschenbach D. (2008) Pelvic inflammatory disease. In: Holmes KK, Sparling FP, Stamm WE, *et al.* (eds.) *Sexually Transmitted Diseases*. 4th ed. McGraw-Hill, New York, pp. 1017–50.

39 Yeh JM, Hook EW, Goldie SJ. (2003) A refined estimate of the average lifetime cost of pelvic inflammatory disease. *Sexually Transmitted Diseases* **30**, 369–78.

40 Department of Health. Summary and Conclusions of CMO's Expert Advisory Group on *Chlamydia trachomatis*. London: Department of Health; 2001.

41 Bevan CD, Johal BJ, Mumtaz G, *et al.* (1995) Clinical, laparoscopic, and microbiological findings in acute salpingitis: report on a United Kingdom cohort. *British Journal of Obstetrics and Gynaecology* **102**, 407–14.

42 Paavonen J, Puolakkainen M, Maukku M, *et al.* (1998) Cost–benefit analysis of first void urine *Chlamydia trachomatis* screening program. *Obstetrics and Gynecology* **92**, 292–98.

43 Risser WL, Risser JMH. (2007) The Incidence of pelvic inflammatory disease in untreated women infected with *Chlamydia trachomatis*: a structured review. *International Journal of STD and AIDS* **18**, 727–31.

44 Kimani J, Maclean IW, Bwayo JJ, *et al.* (1996) Risk factors for *Chlamydia trachomatis* pelvic inflammatory disease among sex workers in Nairobi, Kenya. *Journal of Infectious Diseases* **173**, 1437–44.

45 Simms I, Eastick K, Mallinson H, *et al.* (2003) Association between *Mycoplasma genitalium*, *Chlamydia trachomatis*, and pelvic inflammatory disease. *Sexually Transmitted Infections* **79**, 154–56.

46 Haggerty CL. (2008) Evidence for a role of *Mycoplasma genitalium* in pelvic inflammatory disease. *Current Opinion in Infectious Disease* **21**, 65–69.

47 Wiesenfeld HC, Hillier SL, Krohn MA, *et al.* (2003) Bacterial vaginosis is a strong predictor of *Neisseria gonorrhoea* and *Chlamydia trachomatis* infection. *Clinical Infectious Diseases* **36**, 663–68.

48 Wiesenfeld HC, Hillier SL, Krohn MA, *et al.* (2002) Lower genital tract infection and endometritis: insight on sub clinical pelvic inflammatory disease. *Obstetrics and Gynecology* **100**, 456–63.

49 Ness RB, Soper DE, Holley RL, *et al.* (2001) Hormonal and barrier contraception and the risk of upper genital tract disease in the PID Evaluation and Clinical Health (PEACH) study. *American Journal of Obstetrics and Gynecology* **185**, 121–27.

50 Scholes D, Daling JR, Stergachis A, *et al.* (1993) Vaginal douching as a risk factor for pelvic inflammatory disease. *Obstetrics and Gynecology* **81**, 601–05.

51 Ness RB, Hillier SH, Kip KE, *et al.* (2005) Douching, pelvic inflammatory disease, and incident gonococcal and chlamydial genital infection in a cohort of high-risk women. *American Journal of Epidemiology* **161**, 186–95.

52 Simms I, Stephenson JM. (2000) Pelvic inflammatory disease epidemiology: what do we know and what do we need to know. *Sexually Transmitted Infections* **76**, 80–87.

53 Ness RB, Brunham RC, Shen C, *et al.* (2004) Associations among human leukocyte antigen (HLA) class II DQ vari-

ants, bacterial STIs, endometritis and fertility among women with clinical pelvic inflammatory disease. *Sexually Transmitted Diseases* **31**, 301–04.

54 Morcos R, Frost N, Hnat M, *et al.* (1993) Laproscopic versus clinical diagnosis of acute pelvic inflammatory disease. *The Journal of Reproductive Medicine* **38**, 53–56.

55 Westrom L, Mardh PA. (1990) Acute pelvic inflammatory disease. In: Holmes KK, Mardh PA, *et al.* (eds.) *Sexually transmitted Diseases*. 2nd ed. McGraw-Hill, New York, pp. 593–543.

56 Pieper JF, Ness RB, Blume J, *et al.* (2001) Clinical predictors of endometritis in women with symptoms and signs of pelvic inflammatory disease. *American Journal of Obstetrics and Gynecology* **184**, 856–63.

57 MMWR, April 13, 2007, CDC. Updated recommended treatment regimens for gonococcal infections and associated conditions. http://www.cdc.gov/STD/treatment/2006/GonUpdateApril2007.pdf

58 Yudin MH, Hillier SL, Wiesenfeld HC. (2003) Vaginal polymorphonuclear leukocytes and bacterial vaginosis as markers for histological endometritis among women without symptoms of pelvic inflammatory disease. *American Journal of Obstetrics and Gynecology* **188**, 318–23.

59 Miettinen AK, Heinonen PK, Laippala P, *et al.* (1993) Test performance of erythrocyte sedimentation rate and C-reactive protein in assessing the severity of acute pelvic inflammatory disease. *American Journal of Obstetrics and Gynecology* **169**, 1143–49.

60 Molander P, Finne P, Sjoberg J, *et al.* (2003) Observer agreement with laparoscopic diagnosis of pelvic inflammatory disease using photographs. *Obstetrics and Gynecology* **101**, 875–80.

61 Sellors J, Mahony J, Goldsmith C, *et al.* (1991) The accuracy of clinical findings and laparoscopy in pelvic inflammatory disease. *American Journal of Obstetrics and Gynecology* **164**, 113.

62 Ross J, Judlin P, Nilas L. (2007) European guidelines for the management of pelvic inflammatory disease. *International Journal of STD and AIDS* **18**, 662–66.

63 Irwin KL, Moorman AC, O'Sullivan MJ, *et al.* (2000) Influence of human immunodeficiency virus on pelvic inflammatory disease. *Obstetrics and Gynecology* **95**, 525–34.

64 United Kingdom national guidelines for the management of pelvic inflammatory disease. Revised 2005 http://www.bashh.org/guidelines.asp.

65 Hillis SD, Joesoef R, Marchbanks PA, *et al.* (1993) Delayed care of pelvic inflammatory disease as a risk factor for impaired fertility. *American Journal of Obstetrics and Gynecology* **163**, 1503.

66 CEG (2005) *UK National Guideline on the Management of Pelvic Inflammatory Disease*. Clinical Effectiveness

Group (British Association for Sexual Health and HIV), http://www.bashh.org/guidelines.asp.

67 Paavonen J, Westrom, L. Eschenbach D. (2008) Pelvic inflammatory disease. In: Holmes KK, Sparling FP, Stamm WE, *et al.* (eds.) *Sexually Transmitted Diseases*, 4th ed. McGraw-Hill, New York, pp. 1017–50.

68 Westrom LV, Joesoef R, Reynolds G, *et al.* (1992) Pelvic inflammatory disease and fertility: a cohort study of 1844 women with laparoscopically verified disease and 657 control women with normal laparoscopic results. *Sexually Transmitted Diseases* **19**, 185–92.

CHAPTER 12
Generalized Vulvodynia

Andrew T. Goldstein,[1] *Caroline F. Pukall*[2]

[1] George Washington University School of Medicine and Health Sciences, Washington, DC, USA
[2] Queen's University, Kingston, Ontario, Canada

Introduction

In 2003, the International Society for the Study of Vulvovaginal Disease (ISSVD) issued new terminology for vulvar pain. It recognizes that vulvar pain can be attributed to definable conditions (e.g., those of infectious, dermatologic, neoplastic, or neurologic origin) and that it can also occur in the absence of physical findings (i.e., vulvodynia). Vulvodynia is "vulvar discomfort, most often described as burning pain, occurring in the absence of relevant visible findings or a specific, clinically identifiable, neurologic disorder" [1]. The pain of vulvodynia can be generalized or localized, and each pain presentation is further subdivided into provoked, unprovoked, or mixed temporal pain patterns [2]. Some authors believe that these distinctions are artificial, stating that many women have both localized and generalized pain [3]. This chapter will focus on the common subtype of generalized nonprovoked vulvodynia, termed *generalized vulvodynia* (GVD).

Epidemiology

In 1880, T.G. Thomas was the first to describe vulvar pain in the medical literature, characterizing it as "an abnormal sensitiveness; 'a plus state of excitability' in the diseased nerve" [4]. Until recently, however, little was known about the prevalence of chronic vulvar pain. In 2003, the authors of a landmark population-based study estimated the

Female Sexual Pain Disorders 1st edition. Edited by A. Goldstein, C. Pukall & I. Goldstein. © 2009 Blackwell Publishing, ISBN: 9781405183987.

prevalence of vulvodynia in an ethnically diverse sample of 4915 women and concluded that as many as 14 million women in the United States will experience chronic vulvar pain during their lifetime [5]. Contrary to earlier assessments, Caucasian and African-American women reported a similar lifetime prevalence; however, Hispanic women were 80% more likely to experience chronic vulvar pain than their Caucasian and African-American counterparts. Even if only a small percentage of these women have true vulvodynia, the number of women suffering from this pain is staggering. Unfortunately, at least 30% will suffer without seeking medical care [5].

Etiology

The etiology of GVD remains elusive, but it most likely occurs from a variety of sources and represents many different disease processes. In 2003, leaders at a National Institute of Health sponsored conference on vulvodynia concluded that GVD is described most accurately when conceptualized as a combined neuropathic pain process (e.g., pudendal neuralgia) and complex regional pain syndrome (CRPS), similar to other CRPSs (e.g., fibromyalgia, interstitial cystitis) [6]. As with patients with neuropathic pain, women with GVD exhibit dysesthesia (an abnormal, unpleasant pain sensation) characterized by allodynia (pain in response to a normally nonpainful stimulus), hyperpathia (pain in response to light touch), and hyperalgesia (increased response to a painful stimulus) [7].

In addition, like patients with CRPS, women with GVD exhibit enhanced systemic pain perception, a process likely due to central nervous system (CNS) sensitization [8], which develops when neuronal synapses within the CNS change in response to a persistent barrage of nociceptive impulses, thereby prolonging and amplifying pain perception [9]. In addition, women with GVD are more likely to have other CRPSs (e.g., interstitial cystitis) [10]; this co-occurrence may be due to "wind-up," in which there is progressively increasing activity in the dorsal horn cells of the spinal cord following repetitive activation of primary afferent C-fibers [11].

It has also been suggested that the nerves innervating the pelvis and vulva are especially prone to injury due to the complex anatomical structure of the pelvis and lower spine [12]. The vulva is innervated by the pudendal nerve originating from S2 to S4 and from the genitofemoral nerve arising from L1 to L2. The location and winding course of the pudendal nerve subjects it to potential injury through entrapment (in Alcock's canal), crush (e.g., falls on the buttocks, pressure from bicycle seats, hypertonus of the levator ani muscles), scarring (e.g., endometriosis), stretching (e.g., during childbirth), and infection (e.g., herpes) [12].

Perhaps consistent with pudendal nerve injury is the suggestion that women with GVD have pelvic floor muscle dysfunction. Although few studies have systematically investigated this issue, evidence indicates that affected women display abnormalities in resting amplitude; contractile amplitudes during tonic, phasic, and endurance contractions; and postcontractile pelvic floor muscle stability as compared with control women [13]. Supporting the involvement of the pelvic floor musculature is the improvement in pain and sexual function measures after electromyography-assisted pelvic floor muscle rehabilitation [14].

Although researchers have failed to find a consistent association between childhood victimization and GVD, one study demonstrated that women with chronic vulvar pain (including GVD and provoked vestibulodynia, or PVD) were more likely to have reported poor family social support and child physical abuse [15]. Theoretically, a stressor such as sexual abuse can lead to alternations in the pain pathways of the CNS [16]; however, this finding is in need of replication as several other controlled studies have failed to show this association [17].

Also, despite hints in the earlier literature of associations between psychosocial function and GVD such that psychological distress preceded the development of the pain, it is currently acknowledged that the presence of the pain of GVD and its associated disability leads to profound psychosocial ramifications including anxiety, depression, and disruption of interpersonal relationships [18–20].

Physical Examination

All women with vulvar pain should have a thorough physical examination with the goal of finding evidence of an identifiable disease that can cause vulvovaginal pain but would not be classified as vulvodynia (i.e. infections, trauma, dermatitis, interstitial cystitis, etc.). A thorough description of this exam can be found in Chapter 4.

Treatment

Unfortunately, most treatment recommendations for vulvodynia are not based on controlled trials. In addition, many studies do not distinguish between PVD and GVD. As such, this chapter will focus on treatments that are more applicable to GVD (PVD treatment is discussed in Chapter 8). For certain women displaying both types of symptoms, the treatments discussed in both chapters may be applicable.

Strategies to Minimize Vulvar Irritation

Most practitioners recommend numerous strategies to minimize vulvar irritation [21]. A common recommendation is to use 100% cotton underwear washed only in hot water to avoid irritation that may be caused by residual fabric detergents or softeners. Also, patients should be counseled to use mild soap for bathing without applying soap directly to the vulva because the interlabial sulci and vestibule can be easily cleaned with water and a gentle touch. Daily use of panty-liners can be irritating; unscented and dye-free cotton menstrual pads during menstruation are good alternatives. Adequate lubrication during intercourse is also suggested; for example, Slippery Stuff™ does not contain propylene glycol which can act as an allergen or irritant [22]. Rinsing the vulva after urination and gently patting the area dry after urination and bathing may also be helpful in some cases.

Topical Treatments

While topical treatments are more applicable to PVD, some women with GVD may benefit from them. Topical anesthetics may cause initial burning and stinging upon application; the discomfort lasts for a few minutes until the area is numb. The longer the ointment is on the area, the deeper the anesthesia. The most commonly prescribed anesthetic is lidocaine (Xylocaine™ jelly 2% or ointment 5%) [23]. The long-term use of overnight topical lidocaine has been proposed as a specific therapy for PVD, but may be useful for women with GVD, as it is theorized that the regular application of lidocaine interrupts repetitive activation of peripheral C-afferent nociceptors, thereby inhibiting the process of "wind-up" at the dorsal horn of the spinal cord [24]. However, several topical anesthetics may in fact sensitize the tissue and lead to unwanted outcomes (e.g., Benzocaine™); these should be avoided.

Topical therapies that patients describe as *not* having significant benefit for GVD are important to note in order to avoid side effects and symptom exacerbation. Theoretically, topical corticosteroids should improve the pain of GVD but they generally do not. In addition, their chronic use on the vulva may produce dermal atrophy or a steroid dermatitis, characterized by erythema and burning [22]. Topical antifungals are also often used, because early theories about the cause of vulvodynia included hypersensitivity to *Candida* species. However, such therapy generally does not improve vulvodynia. To the extent that these preparations provide some relief, it is most likely due to the soothing properties in the vehicle itself. Furthermore, these topical preparations may cause a superimposed irritant or allergic vulvovaginitis.

Oral Treatments

The CNS contains three primary areas associated with the processing of sensory input leading to the perception of pain [25]: (1) the ascending tracts starting at the dorsal horn neurons of the spinal cord; (2) cortical and subcortical pathways in the brain that translate nociceptive input into the conscious experience of pain; and (3) the descending pain system originating in the midbrain and terminating in the dorsal horn neurons of the spinal cord which modulate spinal sensitization. All three pathways can be potential targets in the treatment of GVD.

Tricyclic antidepressants (TCAs) are commonly used in the treatment of neuropathic pain conditions; as such, they have been used to treat vulvodynia [26]. TCAs inhibit the re-uptake of serotonin and norepinephrine in the descending pain system, which modulates the dorsal horn neurons, thereby limiting wind-up. TCAs frequently

used for the treatment of vulvodynia include amitriptyline (Elavil™), nortriptyline (Pamelor™), and desipramine (Norpramin™) [26]. The dosages of TCAs used for neuropathic pain and GVD are significantly less than those used for depression. When discussing TCAs with a patient, it is important for the clinician to emphasize that the TCAs are for the treatment of the pain rather than for depression. Facilitating the patient's understanding of her treatment avenue will ideally enhance compliance.

Amitriptyline is often used as a first-line agent, although many healthcare providers prefer nortriptyline and desipramine, as they tend to have fewer side effects than amitriptyline, although they are comparably dosed. All TCAs can cause dry mouth, somnolence, constipation, weight gain, and palpitation, and they are to be taken 2 hr before bedtime. Typically, TCAs are started at a low dose (5–25 mg in general, but use 5–10 mg for elderly patients) which is progressively increased (by 10–25 mg weekly, not to exceed 150 mg nightly) until symptomatic relief is obtained.

Other antidepressants have the potential to be used for pain control in GVD, although no studies have yet been published on their efficacy. Many providers have prescribed selective serotonin re-uptake inhibitors (SSRIs), but in general, they have not been shown to be effective for chronic pain syndromes [27]. A newer class of medications, the selective norepinephrine re-uptake inhibitors (SNRIs), may be more effective in treating GVD. Like TCAs, the SNRIs block the re-uptake of both serotonin and norepinephrine.

This combination down-regulates nociceptive impulses at the dorsal root ganglia, inhibiting wind-up and central sensitization. Currently, there are two SNRIs approved by the U.S. Food and Drug Adminstration (FDA): venlafaxine (Effexor XR™) and duloxetine (Cymbalta™). Duloxetine is approved for use in diabetic peripheral neuropathic pain and major depression; it may have an advantage over venlafaxine as it causes both serotonin and norepinephrine re-uptake inhibition at its lowest starting dose, whereas venlafaxine exhibits significant norepinephrine re-uptake inhibition only after higher doses have been achieved. Duloxetine is typically started at 30 mg daily and increased to 60 mg per day after one week. Venlafaxine is started at 37.5 mg daily and can be increased up to 300 mg daily over time. Side effects of both SNRIs include nausea, dizziness, somnolence, and fatigue. When discontinuing SNRIs, tapering is recommended [28].

With all of the antidepressants discussed, adequate time for a treatment trial must be given prior to abandoning them, as long as the side effects are tolerable. Often, significant pain relief is not seen until 4 or more weeks of use.

Gabapentin (Neurontin™) and pregabalin (Lyrica™) are anticonvulsants with unique effects on voltage-dependent Ca2+ channel currents at postsynaptic dorsal horn neurons. It is likely that both gabapentin and pregabalin interrupt an entire series of events that, if left unaltered, would lead to the development or maintenance of neuropathic pain. A large retrospective chart review of 152 women with GVD who used gabapentin showed that 64% had a least an 80% resolution of their pain [29]. However, in a study of 28 patients using pregabalin for GVD, only 12 patients (43%) reported at least a 25% improvement of their pain, and 10 patients (36%) discontinued the medication because of side effects [30].

Gabapentin is generally started at 300 mg daily and is increased by 300 mg every 3–7 days up to 3600 mg total daily dose. It is typically given in a three times a day dosing. Pregabalin is typically started at 75 mg twice daily and increased to 150 mg twice daily after one week. Patients can take up to 300 mg twice daily if they can tolerate the side effects and if pain control is not achieved at a lower dose. Both gabapentin and pregabalin tend to result in fewer side effects than the TCAs. Side effects include somnolence, dizziness, and, less commonly, gastrointestinal symptoms and mild peripheral edema. As with TCAs, it may take time to achieve adequate pain control; 3–8 weeks may be needed for titration to allow for tolerance to adverse effects. After the maximum tolerated dosage has been reached, 1–2 weeks of consistent medication usage should be allowed prior to giving a final assessment of pain improvement.

Injectable Therapies

A novel approach to the treatment of vulvodynia was recently published. In this prospective study, 27 women with PVD received intravestibular injections of 0.25% bupivacaine, pudendal nerve blocks of 0.25% bupivicaine, and caudal epidural injections of 0.2% ropivacaine [31]. The theory behind this study was that downregulation of nociceptive impulses at three points in the peripheral and central nervous systems would inhibit wind-up and central sensitization. Fifty-seven percent of the women described at least a 50% improvement in their symptoms. While this

study excluded women with GVD, it is possible that this treatment strategy may be beneficial for them.

Recently, the use of botulinum toxin A (Botox™) has been successfully used for the treatment of vulvodynia [32, 33]. Small clinical trials have shown significant reduction in pain scores in women with vulvodynia after intralevator injections of botulinum toxin A. This substance may reduce pain via several different mechanisms: its anticholinergic effects at neuromuscular junctions which may decrease pelvic floor muscle tone, and/or autonomic denervation, and/or inhibition of substance P and vasoactive intestinal peptide which combine to lower nociception [34]. In the author's (AG) experience, due to the high cost of botulinum toxin A, it is best used to augment pelvic floor physical therapy in women with recalcitrant levator ani hypertonicity.

Physical Therapy and Biofeedback

Physical therapy and biofeedback are commonly employed in the treatment of vulvodynia (see Chapter 13). Physical therapy is effective in lowering levator ani hypertonus, in normalizing and facilitating normal muscle tone, increasing pelvic floor strength, desensitizing local tissues, and improving vulvovaginal elasticity [35]. Biofeedback aids in the development of self-regulation strategies for coping with and reducing pain and it facilitates normal muscle tone and promotes muscle stability. Patients with vulvodynia typically have increased resting tone and decreased contractility of the pelvic floor muscles. With the aid of biofeedback, an individual can view their muscle tension on a display which, over time, allows them to develop voluntary control over their muscles. The time required for biofeedback and the frequencies of visits will vary with each person. Success rates in the 60–80% have been reported [36]. Physical therapists with experience in vulvodynia can be helpful in the interdisciplinary treatment of vulvodynia. They frequently complete a thorough evaluation and assessment of pelvic muscle tone, posture, mobility, and muscle strength [35] (see Chapter 6).

Psychological Aspects of GVD

The psychological impact of chronic pain is well documented; feelings of hopelessness, depression, and anxiety are common [17, 37]. These feelings can be compounded in vulvodynia, especially because the pain affects an intimate body area. This point is illustrated by the results of a randomized treatment outcome study that demonstrated that pain reduction does not necessarily lead to an increase in sexual function [38]. Therefore, in addition to treating the sensory aspect of pain, it is imperative to address associated psychosexual and relationship dysfunction.

Summary

Generalized vulvodynia is best understood as a peripheral and central neuropathic process. A rational treatment approach combines the reduction of irritating stimuli, peripheral nociceptive blockade with anesthetic, and central inhibition of the dorsal horn with oral medications. It is also imperative to address the associated pelvic floor dysfunction and the psychosocial ramifications of this chronic sexual pain syndrome. Therefore, it is essential to have an interdisciplinary team involving physicians, physical therapists, sexual therapists, and psychologists to adequately treat all aspects of GVD.

References

1 Haefner HK. (2007) Report of the International Society for the Study of Vulvovaginal Disease: terminology and classification of vulvodynia. *Journal of Lower Genital Tract Diseases* 11, 48–49.

2 Moyal-Barracco M, Lynch PJ. (2004) 2003 ISSVD terminology and classification of vulvodynia: a historical perspective. *The Journal of Reproductive Medicine* 49, 772–77.

3 Reed BD, Gorenflo DW, Haefner HK. (2003) Generalized vulvar dysesthesia vs. vestibulodynia: are they distinct diagnoses? *The Journal of Reproductive Medicine* 48, 858–64.

4 Thomas TG. (1880) *Practical Treatise on the Diseases of Women.* Henry C. Leason: Philadelphia, p. 145.

5 Harlow BL, Stewart EG. (2003) A population-based assessment of chronic unexplained vulvar pain: have we underestimated the prevalence of vulvodynia? *Journal of the American Medical Women's Association* 58, 82–88.

6 Edwards L. (2003) New concepts in vulvodynia. *American Journal of Obstetrics and Gynecology* 189, S24–S30.

7 Turner ML, Marinoff SC (1991). Pudendal neuralgia. *American Journal of Obstetrics and Gynecology* 165, 1233–2336.

8 Pukall CF, Strigo IA, Binik YM, *et al.* (2005) Neural correlates of painful genital touch in women with vulvar vestibulitis syndrome. *Pain* 115, 118–27.

9 Lawson, K. (2006) Emerging pharmacological therapies for fibromyalgia. *Current Opinion in Investigational Drugs* 7, 631–36.

10 Gordon AS, Panahian-Jand M, Mccomb F, *et al.* (2003) Characteristics of women with vulvar pain disorders: responses to a Web-based survey. *Journal of Sex and Marital Therapy* 29, 45–58.

11 Butrick CW. (2003) Interstitial cystitis and chronic pelvic pain: new insights in neuropathology, diagnosis, and treatment. *Clinical Obstetrics and Gynecology* 46, 811–23.

12 Robert R, Prat-Pradal D, Labat JJ, *et al.* (1998) Anatomic basis of chronic perineal pain: role of the pudendal nerve. *Surgical and Radiologic Anatomy* 20, 93–98.

13 Glazer HI, Jantos M, Hartmann EH, *et al.* (1998) Electromyographic comparisons of the pelvic floor in women with dysesthetic vulvodynia and asymptomatic women. *The Journal of Reproductive Medicine* 43, 959–62.

14 Glazer HI. (2000) Dysesthetic vulvodynia: long-term follow-up after treatment with surface electromyography–assisted pelvic floor muscle rehabilitation. *The Journal of Reproductive Medicine* 45, 798–802.

15 Harlow BL, Stewart WG. (2005) Adult-onset vulvodynia in relation to childhood violence victimization. *American Journal of Epidemiology* 161, 871–80.

16 Fenton BW. (2007) Limbic associated pelvic pain: a hypothesis to explain the diagnostic relationships and features of patients with chronic pelvic pain. *Medical Hypotheses* 69, 282–86.

17 Dalton VK, Haefner HK, Reed BD, *et al.* (2002) Victimization in patients with vulvar dysesthesia/vestibulodynia: is there an increased prevalence? *The Journal of Reproductive Medicine* 47, 829–34.

18 Tribó MJ, Andión O, Ros S, *et al.* (2008) Clinical characteristics and psychopathological profile of patients with vulvodynia: an observational and descriptive study. *Dermatology* 216, 24–30.

19 Arnold LD, Bachmann GA, Rosen R, *et al.* (2007) Assessment of vulvodynia symptoms in a sample of U.S. women: a prevalence survey with a nested case control study. *American Journal of Obstetrics and Gynecology* 196, 128 e1–6.

20 Masheb RM, Wang E, Lozano C, *et al.* (2005) Prevalence and correlates of depression in treatment-seeking women with vulvodynia. *Journal of Obstetrics and Gynecology* 25, 786–91.

21 Goldstein AT, Marinoff SC, Haefner HK. (2004) Vulvodynia: strategies for treatment. *Clinical Obstetrics and Gynecology* 48, 769–85.

22 Goldstein AT, Burrows L. (2008) Vulvodynia (CME). *Journal of Sex and Medicine* 5, 5–15.

23 Masheb RM, Wang E, Lozano C, *et al.* (2005) The vulvodynia guideline. *Journal of Lower Genital Tract Diseases* 9, 40–51.

24 Zolnoun DA, Hartmann KE, Steege JF. (2003) Overnight 5% lidocaine ointment for treatment of vulvar vestibulitis. *Obstetrics and Gynecology* 102, 84–87.

25 Lawson K. (2002) Tricyclic antidepressants and fibromyalgia: what is the mechanism of action? *Expert Opinion on Investigative Drugs* **11**, 1437–45.

26 Reed BD, Caron AM, Gorenflo DW, *et al.* (2006) Treatment of vulvodynia with tricyclic antidepressants: efficacy and associated factors. *Journal of Lower Genital Tract Diseases* **10**, 245–51.

27 Sindrup SH, Otto M, Finnerup NB, *et al.* (2005) Antidepressants in the treatment of neuropathic pain. *Basic Clinical Pharmacology and Toxicology* **96**, 399–409.

28 Gutierrez MA, Stimmel GL, Aiso JY. (2003) Venlafaxine: a 2003 update. *Clinical Therapy* **25**, 2138–54.

29 Harris G, Horowitz B, Borgida A. (2007) Evaluation of gabapentin in the treatment of generalized vulvodynia, unprovoked. *Journal of Reproductive Medicine* **52**, 103–6.

30 Aranda J. (2008) Treatment of vulvodynia with pregabalin. Presented at the International Society for the Study of Vulvovaginal Disease XIX World Congress Meeting, Alaska.

31 Rapkin AJ, McDonald JS, Morgan M. (2008) Multilevel local anesthetic nerve blockade for the treatment of vulvar vestibulitis syndrome. *American Journal of Obstetrics and Gynecology* **198**, 41 e1–5.

32 Yoon H, Chung WS, Shim BS. (2007) Botulinum toxin A for the management of vulvodynia. *International Journal of Impotence Research* **19**, 84–87.

33 Abbott JA, Jarvis SK, Lyons SD, *et al.* (2006) Botulinum toxin type A for chronic pain and pelvic floor spasm in women: a randomized controlled trial. *Obstetrics and Gynecology* **108**, 915–23.

34 Mahajan ST, Brubaker L. (2007) Botulinum toxin: from life-threatening disease to novel medical therapy. *American Journal of Obstetrics and Gynecology* **196**, 7–15.

35 Rosenbaum TY. (2007) Pelvic floor involvement in male and female sexual dysfunction and the role of pelvic floor rehabilitation in treatment: a literature review. *Journal of Sex and Medicine* **4**, 4–13.

36 Glazer HI, Rodke G, Swencionis C, *et al.* (1995) Treatment of vulvar vestibulitis syndrome with electromyographic biofeedback of pelvic floor musculature. *Journal of Reproductive Medicine* **40**, 283–90.

37 Brotto LA., Basson R, Gehring D. (2003) Psychological profiles among women with vulvar vestibulitis syndrome: a chart review. *Journal of Psychosomatic Obstetrics and Gynaecology* **24**, 195–203.

38 Bergeron S, Binik YM, Khalifé S, *et al.* (2001) A randomized comparison of group cognitive–behavioral therapy, surface electromyographic biofeedback, and vestibulectomy in the treatment of dyspareunia resulting from vulvar vestibulitis. *Pain* **91**, 297–306.

CHAPTER 13

Physical Therapy Treatment of Pelvic Floor Dysfunction

Amy Stein,[1] *Dee Hartmann*[2]

[1] Beyond Basics Physical Therapy, New York, NY, USA
[2] Dee Hartmann Physical Therapy for Women, Chicago, IL, USA

Introduction

Physical therapy (PT) has become an integral part of a multidisciplinary team approach for the treatment of pelvic floor dysfunction (PFD) and in the treatment of dyspareunia [1–3]. As such, this chapter examines PT treatment for pelvic floor muscle hypertonicity, visceral abnormalities (disorders of the bowel, bladder, urethra, and uterus), and musculoskeletal dysfunction.

Manual Therapy Techniques

Overview

Physical therapists use their hands to localize and treat tissue restrictions. With advanced training, they apply these skills not only to external structures (i.e., hip and low back musculature) but also to structures within the pelvis. Though the pelvic floor muscles are an integral part of pelvic function, they are influenced by the structures within the pelvic bowl (the viscera: urethra, bladder, uterus, rectum, and anus), ligaments, and fascia. Appropriate treatment addresses abnormalities in all of these structures, which allows for rehabilitation of the pelvic floor muscles.

In addition, it is not uncommon to see an imbalance in the muscles and fascia of the pelvic floor of a woman

with chronic vulvar pain. For example, pelvic floor hypertonicity can be driven by chronic low back and hip pain created by an abnormal balance of strength and tension between the muscles of the pelvis, hip, and lower back. Therefore, increased hip pain may cause an exacerbation in symptoms related to pelvic floor muscle hypertonus, including vulvar burning and introital dyspareunia. A skilled physical therapist will use the techniques discussed in this chapter to evaluate and correct these imbalances.

Myofascial Release

The myofascial system is a slightly mobile, continuous, laminated sheath of connective tissue that envelops all the somatic and visceral structures of the body. In addition, it covers visceral organs, muscles, bones, and nerves. In the healthy state, strength and mobility are largely influenced by myofascial control. In the unhealthy state (which may follow trauma, or result from poor posture, scarring, or inflammation), the fascial system can become restricted and adherent, thereby reducing flexibility and stability and creating chronic pain [4].

Myofascial release is a manual therapy technique that uses light stretch to cause increased blood flow. This technique has been shown to restore myofascial mobility, tissue hydration, and muscle length [4]. Women's health physical therapists have successfully utilized myofacial release to treat vulvodynia [2, 5–7], interstitial cystitis [8, 9], and dyspareunia [10]. In a study surveying women's health physical therapists, 96% used soft tissue mobilization and myofascial release to treat women with provoked vestibulodynia (PVD) [11].

Female Sexual Pain Disorders 1st edition. Edited by A. Goldstein,
C. Pukall & I. Goldstein. © 2009 Blackwell Publishing,
ISBN: 9781405183987.

Myofascial Trigger Point Release

Travell and Simons define a trigger point as a nodule within a palpably tight band of the muscle or fascia, which is exquisitely tender upon compression. Pressure applied to a trigger point will cause referred pain and tenderness [12]. In addition, trigger points can also disturb the proprioceptive, nociceptive, and autonomic functions of the affected region. Muscles containing trigger points are shortened, have limited range of motion, are weak and hypertonic, and present with a loss of coordination [9, 13, 14]. Studies have shown that trigger points are the key components of pain in up to 93% of patients presenting to a pain clinic [15].

Dyspareunia, as well as bladder and bowel dysfunction, can be a result of pelvic floor trigger points. Unfortunately, symptoms are highly variable and may include pain characterized as sharp, dull, achy, superficial, or deep [13, 14, 16, 17]. Trigger points typically occur in muscle because of trauma, repetitive overuse, or inflammation [16]. Trigger points associated with pelvic pain have been well documented in the following muscles: levator ani, obturator internus, coccygeus, abdominals, gluteals, adductors, piriformis, quadratus lumborum, paraspinals, iliotibial band/tensor fascia lata, quadriceps, and hamstrings [18]. Trigger points in the posterior pelvis typically refer pain to the rectum, anus, coccyx, and sacrum, while trigger points in the anterior pelvis create genital pain.

Trigger points can go unrecognized until a skilled practitioner locates them and recreates the patient's symptoms. Manual therapies used to eliminate trigger points include skin rolling, strumming, and stripping of the affected muscle fibers. Physical therapists also use stretching, proprioceptive neuromuscular facilitation (i.e., contract/relax and reciprocal inhibition), active release techniques, and other muscle energy techniques to help facilitate muscle relaxation and lengthening. Trigger point injections and intramuscular injections of botulinum toxin type A can also be used to augment manual release techniques [19].

Weiss found an 83% reduction in symptoms, including a decrease in neurogenic bladder inflammation, central sensitization, and pelvic floor hypertonicity through manual release of myofascial trigger points [8]. In addition, Anderson et al. reported a 72% improvement in chronic pelvic pain and urinary symptoms using a combination of myofascial trigger point release of the pelvic floor muscles and paradoxical relaxation [20].

Visceral Manipulation

Visceral manipulation is a physical therapy technique used to improve tissue and organ mobility. The technique allows for the diagnosis and treatment of adhesions, fixations, and spasm in the viscera of the thorax, abdomen, and pelvis. The benefits of this technique are improved tissue metabolism, increased serotonin production, vasodilatation, and improved function of the respiratory and digestive systems [21]. For example, symptoms of an overactive bladder (urinary urgency/frequency, and pain) may be caused by excessive tone within the pelvic floor muscles, bladder, and urethra. If the bladder or urethra is in spasm, the surrounding muscles will respond with reflexive splinting. Manual release of the pelvic floor muscles will be beneficial but short-lived unless the abnormal tone in the viscera (bladder and urethra) is also treated. In the clinical experience of the authors, effective treatment includes releasing tension in both the musculoskeletal and the visceral systems simultaneously.

When visceral manipulation was used to treat women with generalized vulvodynia (GVD) or PVD, there was a 71% improvement in overall symptoms and a 62% improvement in sexual function (i.e., decreased dyspareunia, increased intercourse frequency, and increased desire) [11]. In addition, the American Society for Colposcopy and Cervical Pathology published Vulvodynia Guidelines that included visceral manipulation in its multidisciplinary approach to treating women with vulvar pain [3]. When women's health physical therapists were surveyed, 33% reported having utilized visceral manipulation for treatment of women with PVD [11].

Neural Mobilization

The nervous system, from its origin in the brain to its most distal nerve endings in the extremities, also requires mobility. When the cervical spine is flexed or extended, it causes increase neural tension throughout the entire nervous system. If there are restrictions (e.g., disc herniation, spinal stenosis, myofascial restrictions, and muscle spasm) and nerve mobility is impeded, there will be an adverse increase in neural tension which can lead to neuropathic pain.

Adverse neural tension due to physiological abnormalities can be a major factor in pelvic pain [22], resulting in nerve irritation and subsequently, nerve pain (neuralgia) in any or all areas supplied by the affected nerve. Neuralgia manifests as itching, burning, tingling, cold sensations, sharp and shooting pain, as well as spasms of the innervated muscles [23]. It can result from adhesions, hypertonic or shortened muscles, biomechanical abnormalities (e.g., narrowing of a foramen or canal where the nerve travels), myofascial trigger points, or connective tissue restrictions surrounding the nerve.

In reference to pelvic pain, these physiological or biomechanical changes could be the result of a traumatic fall or injury, abdominal, pelvic or thigh surgery, traumatic childbirth, emotional or physical abuse, hormonal imbalances, or skeletal malalignment [22]. The nerves that innervate the pelvic floor muscles can also refer pain to the somatic and visceral nervous systems. The afferents of these nerves converge at the dorsal horn of the spinal cord, thereby affecting the visceral organs as well as resulting in a neuropathic pain pattern. This convergence exists in the form of viscerosomatic reflexes, in which dysfunction in the viscera is expressed as somatic dysfunction, and somatovisceral reflexes, in which dysfunction at the surface of the body is reflexively conveyed to the viscera [24].

Joint Mobilization

Joint mobilization is a passive manual therapy technique applied to joints and their adjacent soft tissues that is used to normalize range of motion and decrease pain. Joint normalization can be a component of a treatment regimen for pelvic pain and dyspareunia. Pelvic floor dysfunction or vulvovaginal pain may arise from an anterior pelvic tilt, leg length/pelvic postural asymmetry, loss of hip range of motion, and lumbar joint dysfunction [25]. Because of common innervation, it is not unusual to find abnormalities in the lumbar vertebrae, joint capsules, discs, hip joints, and ligaments. In the women's health PT survey, joint mobilization was used by 78% of those responding in treating women with PVD [11].

Therapeutic Exercise

Spinal ("Core") Stabilization

In the last decade, physical therapists have focused on the neuromuscular mechanisms underlying lumbopelvic dysfunction and the concomitant incontinence, respiratory dysfunction, and low back and pelvic pain. Recent research suggests that lumbopelvic dysfunction is a result of altered motor control between the larger support musculature (e.g., erector spinae, latissumus dorsi, resctus abdominus, gluteals) and the weaker, smaller trunk stabilizers (also known as the core structures: transverses abdominis, pelvic floor, and multifidus muscle) and the respiratory diaphragm. The outgrowth of this work has led to the use of the term *core stabilization*. The goal of core stabilization is to renew the balance and strength at the body's pelvic base [26].

It is not uncommon for women with PFD to have weakness and imbalance throughout their core structures. Pelvic and abdominal dysfunction, including increased tone and/or weakness and/or a diastasis recti (a separation of the right and left rectus abdominus muscles), can cause core instability and dysfunctional postures. According to Howard, faulty postures are those positions that increase stress to joints and use excessive muscle activity [27]. A dysfunctional pelvic posture can result in the formation of trigger points, hypertonicity, and pelvic pain [25, 27]. When creating a treatment plan, therapeutic exercises should address these musculoskeletal abnormalities and should include strengthening and lengthening where indicated, postural corrections, diastasis recti correction, and pelvic floor retraining. Specific examples of core exercises include, but are not limited to, transverse abdominus isometric contractions, pelvic tilts, oblique crunches, bridging, quadruped with opposite arm and leg raise, hip external and internal rotation exercises, squats, pelvic floor exercises, and the plank.

Pelvic Floor Retraining

Pelvic floor retraining involves the active renewal of neuromuscular control over the pelvic floor muscles and may include strengthening of muscular weakness, down-training of muscular tension, and re-coordinating of overall muscular control. The majority of the research on pelvic floor retraining has been on urinary and fecal incontinence rather than vulvar pain or dyspareunia. Some studies have shown success with treating chronic pain and PFD without the use of biofeedback [2, 5, 6, 10, 28].

When reviewing the PT treatment approach of women with chronic pelvic tension, it is evident that manual techniques (contract/relax, reciprocal inhibition, proprioceptive neuromuscular facilitation) augment the process of pelvic floor retraining [9]. There are divergent thoughts on how to address pelvic floor hypertonicity from an exercise perspective. One philosophy is that overactivated muscles should not be further stressed by active exercise, and that down-training should be the focus until pain-free range of motion is achieved and contractile activity is normalized [29].

The other ideology is that the normalization of the strength and length of the pelvic floor muscles is necessary for full pelvic floor function (sphincteric control, visceral support, sexual function, etc.). Physiologically, a muscle that is in a weakened and shortened state needs increased blood flow, improved active range of motion, and normalization of strength to restore optimal function. Both approaches appear to be successful and no studies have proven one method as superior to the other.

Surface electromyography (biofeedback), when used on a daily basis, has been shown to be an effective treatment for pelvic floor hypertonicity [30]. However, this study only addressed the pelvic floor retraining aspect without adjunctive manual therapies. Some experts, however, believe that biofeedback should not be recommended as an independent modality [1]. As many as 66% of physical therapists use biofeedback for women with PVD [11].

Dilators and vibrators can also aid in pelvic floor retraining. A set of graduated vaginal dilators can help women begin to overcome both the physical and psychological stressors of introital penetration. By gradually increasing the diameter of the dilator, pelvic floor tension is relaxed as the introitus is stretched. Dilators can also be used to perform self-trigger point release therapy. The presence of the dilator provides proprioception to the musculature during exercise, augmenting improved pelvic floor contraction and relaxation.

Vaginal dilatation can also diminish the anxiety of penetration as the woman has complete control of vaginal entry [2, 6, 10, 31]. Vibrators can also be used on the perineum to facilitate tissue relaxation and desensitization, and for clitoral stimulation. These exercises should be given under the guidance of a skilled professional experienced in the treatment of sexual dysfunction such as a certified sex therapist, a women's health physical therapist, or a sexual medicine physician.

Behavioral Therapies

Behavioral therapy is a necessary adjunct to pelvic floor muscle rehabilitation, as it helps to break the cycle of dysfunction and pain. Education and training focus on proper motor control of the pelvic floor. An example of this would be training to actively relax the pelvic floor to initiate voiding (releases tension of the urinary sphincters) and with intercourse (helps to increase the diameter of the introitus) rather than allowing the reflexive splinting or "tensing" due to the fear of pain. Another example would be to utilize this same active relaxation throughout the day in order to terminate a chronic holding pattern. The learned response of elongating and relaxing the pelvic floor can occur during PT and include verbal cuing, manual therapy, and digital or mechanical biofeedback.

The operant learning model and cognitive behavioral therapy are also used for behavioral training [2, 5]. Other behavioral modifications include scheduled voiding, urge control, normalization of bowel function, pain charts, avoidance of triggers, and patient education.

Additional Modalities

Electrical stimulation applied in various wave forms can be used both externally and internally at the pelvis to improve proprioception and contractile function of the pelvic floor and to decrease sensitization to pain [6]. Fitzwater has reported success with pelvic floor electrical stimulation in reducing levator ani hypertonicity and pain [32]. Muscle strengthening and pain reduction also occurred with pelvic stimulation in women with PVD [6, 33]. It has been reported that 42% of physical therapist use electrical stimulation to treat PVD [11].

Therapeutic ultrasound provides deep heat via transmission of sound waves into tissue. It is often used to treat the localized pain of dyspareunia from episiotomy or perineal injury following vaginal birth [34]. Of practicing physical therapists, 37% use ultrasound to treat vulvar pain [11].

Conclusion

Physical therapy has become an essential part of the armamentarium in the clinical management of women with sexual health problems. By providing physical strategies to lessen pelvic floor hypertonicity or increase pelvic floor strength or correct imbalances in the strength and tension of non-pelvic floor muscle, women with sexual pain disorders will frequently benefit from physical therapy.

References

1 Bo K, Berghmans B, Morkved S, *et al.* (eds.) (2007) *Evidence-Based Physical Therapy for the Pelvic Floor.* Elsevier, Philadelphia.

2 Bergeron S, Lord MJ. (2003) The integration of pelvi-perineal reeducation and cognitive–behavioural therapy in the multidisciplinary treatment of the sexual pain disorders. *British Association for Sexual and Relationship Therapy* **18**, 135–41.

3 Haefner HK, Collins ME, Davis GD, *et al.* (2005) The vulvodynia guideline. *Journal of Lower Genital Tract Disease* **9**, 40–51.

4 Barnes JF. (2006) Myofascial release approach. *Massage.*

5 Pukall CF, Smith KB, Chamberlain SM. (2007) Provoked vestibulodynia. *Women's Health* **3**, 583–92.

6 Bergeron S, Brown C, Lord MJ. (2002) Physical therapy for vulvar vestibulitis syndrome: a retrospective study. *Journal of Sex and Marital Therapy* **28**, 183–92.

7 Hartmann EH, Nelson CA. (2001) The perceived effectiveness of physical therapy treatment on women complaining of chronic vulvar pain and diagnosed with either vulvar vestibulitis syndrome or dysesthetic vulvodynia. *Section on Women's Health, APTA* **25**, 13–18.

8 Weiss JM. (2001) Pelvic floor myofascial trigger points: manual therapy for interstitial cystitis and the urgency–frequency syndrome. *Journal of Urology* **166**, 2226–31.

9 FitzGerald MP, Kotarinos R. (2003) Rehabilitation of the short pelvic floor: treatment of the patient with the short pelvic floor. *International Urogynecology Journal* **14**, 269–75.

10 Rosenbaum TY. (2007) Pelvic floor involvement in male and female sexual dysfunction and the role of pelvic floor rehabilitation in treatment: a treatment review. *The Journal of Sexual Medicine* **4**, 4–13.

11 Hartmann D, Strauhal MJ, Nelson CA. (2007) Treatment of women in the United States with localized, provoked vulvodynia: practice survey of women's health physical therapists. *The Journal of Reproductive Medicine* **52**, 48–52.

12 Travell J, Simons D. (1983) *Myofascial Pain and Dysfunction: The Trigger Point Manual, Volume 1. The Upper Extremities.* Williams & Wilkins, Baltimore.

13 FitzGerald MP, Kotarinos R. (2003) Rehabilitation of the short pelvic floor: background and patient evaluation. *International Urogynecology Journal and Pelvic Floor Dysfunction* **14**, 261–68.

14 Bernstein AM, Philips HC, Linden W, *et al.* (1992) A psychophysiological evaluation of female urethral syndrome: evidence for a muscular abnormality. *Journal of Behavioural Medicine* **15**, 299–312.

15 Jantos M. (2007) Understanding chronic pelvic pain. *Pelviperineology*, **26**.

16 Weiss JM. (2000) Chronic pelvic pain and myofascial trigger points. *The Pain Clinic* **2**, 13–18.

17 Schmidt RA, Vapnek JM. (1991) Pelvic floor behaviour and interstitial cystitis. *Seminars in Urology* **9**, 154.

18 Travell JG, Simons DG. (1992) *Myofascial Pain and Dysfunction: The Trigger Point Manual, Volume 2. The Lower Extremities.* Williams & Wilkins, Baltimore, pp. 110–131.

19 Abbott JA, Jarvis SK, Lyons SD, *et al.* (2006) Botulinum toxin type A for chronic pain and pelvic floor spasm in women: a randomized controlled trial. *Obstetrics and Gynecology* **108**, 915–23.

20 Anderson R, Wise D, Sawyer T, *et al.* (2005) Integration of myofascial trigger point release and paradoxical relaxation training treatment of chronic pelvic pain in men. *Journal of Urology* **174**, 155–60.

21 Barral JP, Mercier P. (2005) *Visceral Manipulation.* Eastland Press, Seattle.

22 Weiss J, Prendergast S. (2003) Screening for musculoskeletal causes of pelvic pain. *Clinical Obstetrics and Gynecology* **46**, 773–82.

23 Butler D. (1991) *Mobilization of the Nervous System.* Churchill Livingston, Melbourne.

24 Mein EA, Richards DG, McMillin DL, *et al.* (2000) Physiological regulation through manual therapy. *Physical Medicine and Rehabilitation: State of the Art Reviews* **14**, 27–42.

25 King Baker PK. (1993) Musculoskeletal origins of chronic pelvic pain. *Obstetrics and Gynecology Clinics of North America* **20**, 719–43.

26 Whitaker J. (2006) Motor control of lumbopelvic region: implications for pelvic floor dysfunction. Lecture notes. International Pelvic Pain Society Meeting, Birmingham, AL.

27 Howard F, Perry P, Carter J, *et al.* (2000) *Pelvic Pain: Diagnosis and Management.* Lippincott Williams & Wilkins, Philadelphia.

28 Reissing ED, Brown C, Lord MJ, *et al.* (2005) Pelvic floor muscle function in women with vulvar vestibulitis syndrome. *Journal of Psychosomatic Obstetrics and Gynecology* **26**, 107–13.

29 Laycock J, Haslam J. (eds.) (2002) *Therapeutic Management of Incontinence and Pelvic Pain.* Springer-Verlag, London.

30 Glazer HI, Jantos M, Hartmann EH, *et al.* (1998) Electromyographic comparisons of the pelvic floor in women with dysesthetic vulvodynia and asymptomatic women. *The Journal of Reproductive Medicine* **43**, 959–62.

31 Fisher KA. (2007) Management of dyspareunia and associated levator ani muscle. *Physical Therapy* **87**, 935–41.

32 Fitzwater JB, Kuehl TJ, Schrier JJ. (2003) Electrical stimulation in the treatment of pelvic pain. *The Journal of Reproductive Medicine* **48**, 573–77.

33 Nappi RE, Ferdeghini F, Abbiati I, *et al.* (2003) Electrical stimulation (ES) in the management of sexual pain disorders. *Journal of Sex and Marital Therapy* **29**, 103–110.

34 Hay-Smith EJ. (2004) Therapeutic ultrasound for postpartum perineal pain and dyspareunia. *Cochrane Database System Review* **2**, CD000945.

CHAPTER 14
Interstitial Cystitis and Dyspareunia

Nadya M. Cinman, Chad Huckabay, Robert M. Moldwin

The Smith Institute for Urology, Long Island Jewish Medical Center, New York, NY, USA

Introduction

Interstitial cystitis/painful bladder syndrome (IC/PBS) is a condition characterized by pelvic pain, pressure, or discomfort related to the bladder filling, and is typically associated with a persistent urge to void, or urinary frequency, in the absence of infection or other pathology [1]. The prevalence is 30–300 per 100,000 population; however, this statistic may grossly underestimate the frequency of the disorder given the variability of how IC/PBS is characterized and identified [2].

Because the presenting symptoms of IC/PBS are variable, it is frequently confused with endometriosis (see Chapter 19), recurrent urinary tract infections, overactive bladder, irritable bowel syndrome (see Chapter 21), generalized vulvodynia (GVD) (see Chapter 12), and vestibulodynia (PVD) (see Chapter 8) [3-6]. The female-to-male ratio of people diagnosed with IC/PBS is approximately 10:1 [7].

Etiology

The etiology of IC/PBS remains incompletely understood, which has resulted in debate as to what characterizes the disorder. It has become clear that IC/PBS is heterogeneous condition with multiple etiologies, the components of which act in combination to cause the symptoms of IC/PBS [8]. It is likely that structural, neurologic, immunologic, genetic, infectious, environmental, dietary, and psychological factors all play a role in IC/PBS.

Female Sexual Pain Disorders 1st edition. Edited by A. Goldstein, C. Pukall & I. Goldstein. © 2009 Blackwell Publishing, ISBN: 9781405183987.

The most commonly accepted hypothesis of the pathogenesis of IC focuses on an abnormality of bladder mucosal integrity [9]. Normally, the epithelium of the bladder is protected by the glycosaminoglycan (GAG) layer which prevents penetration by ions and toxic substances. If the bladder is subject to repeated insult or injury, the GAG layer can become damaged and more permeable. This increased permeability permits potassium to leak through the bladder mucosa and causes irritation of the underlying nerves, resulting in neurogenic pain and inflammation. Mast cell activation (see Chapter 27) leads to the release of histamine and other inflammatory mediators, increasing pain and tissue damage [10]. There is further degradation of the GAG layer, leading to a vicious cycle of pain and inflammation [11].

It also appears that IC/PBS is similar to other chronic visceral pain syndromes, such as GVD [12]. Substance P, an inflammatory mediator, is found in high concentrations in the bladder mucosa and urine of women with IC/PBS. Substance P stimulates the unmyelinated C-afferent nerve fibers which, in turn, stimulates the dorsal horn of the spinal cord [8]. Persistent activation of the dorsal horn leads to activation of the N-methyl-D-aspartate (NMDA) receptors, resulting in a wind-up phenomenon in which the dorsal horn neurons are disinhibited. This disinhibition is the pathophysiology underlying allodynia and hyperpathia. Lastly, normally afferent nerves can become efferent, leading to a neurogenic inflammation in the bladder mucosa that perpetuates the pain cycle [8].

Diagnosis

The diagnosis of IC/PBS begins with thorough history outlined in Chapter 4. A urinalysis and culture are the

Table 14.1 PUF questionnaire.

The Pelvic Pain and Urinary/Frequency (PUF) Patient Symptom Scale

Please circle the answer that best describes how you feel for each question.

	0	1	2	3	4	Symptom Score	Bother Score
1. How many times do you go to the bathroom during the day?	3–6	7–10	11–14	15–19	20+		
2a. How many times do you go to the bathroom at night?	0	1	2	3	4+		
2b. If you get up at night to go to the bathroom, does it bother you?	Never	Mildly	Moderate	Severe			
3. Are you currently sexually active? Yes___ No___							
4a. If you are sexually active, do you now or have you ever had pain or symptoms during or after sexual intercourse?	Never	Occasionally	Usually	Always			
4b. If you have pain, does it make you avoid sexual intercourse?	Never	Occasionally	Usually	Always			
5. Do you have pain associated with your bladder or in your pelvis (vagina, lower abdomen, urethra, perineum, testes, or scrotum)?	Never	Occasionally	Usually	Always			
6. Do you have urgency after going to the bathroom?	Never	Occasionally	Usually	Always			
7a. If you have pain, is it usually...		Mild	Moderate	Severe			
7b. Does your pain bother you?	Never	Occasionally	Usually	Always			
8a. If you have urgency, is it usually...		Mild	Moderate	Severe			
8b. Does your urgency bother you?	Never	Occasionally	Usually	Always			

Symptom Score (1, 2a, 4a, 5, 6, 7a, 8a) =

Bother Score (2b, 4b, 7b, 8b) =

Total Score (Symptom Score + Bother Score) =

initial diagnostic tests in the work-up of IC/PBS. If hematuria is present, urine should be sent for cytology. The physical exam should focus on the abdomen and pelvis, with palpation of the anterior vaginal vault along the course of the urethra, bladder neck, and bladder fundus. The pelvic floor musculature should be examined as thoroughly outlined in Chapter 6.

There are several validated scales that can be useful in the diagnosis of IC/PBS. In addition, these scales can quantify the severity of IC/PBS and its impact on sexual function. The Pelvic Pain and Urgency/Frequency Scale (PUF) is a short, self-assessment questionnaire that combines symptom and bother scores [13] (Table 14.1). The symptom score includes the assessment of daytime and nighttime urinary frequency, urinary urgency, pain with sexual activity, and pain location. The bother score quantifies the degree of discomfort related to the variables comprising the symptom score.

The PUF scale has been validated in a large multicenter study, including both urologic and gynecologic patients with chronic pelvic pain (CPP) [13, 14]. Women without IC/PBS generally have PUF scores less than 4. A score of 12–15 is suggestive of IC/PBS, whereas a score greater than 15 is associated with a very strongly likelihood of having IC/PBS. In a study of 334 patients with IC/PBS and 48 controls, 84% of women with PUF scores greater than 15 had a positive potassium sensitivity test (PST; see below). While degree of discomfort is thoroughly assessed and quantified in the PUF questionnaire, bother related to sexual issues is limited to one question on dyspareunia [13].

The O'Leary–Sant Symptom and Problem Index (OSSOI) can differentiate IC/PBS from other urinary disorders. The OSSOI may be used as a screening tool for IC/PBS, but it appears to be most helpful in gauging changes in clinical state over time. The OSSOI does not independently have high enough sensitivity and specificity to warrant its use as the sole diagnostic tool of IC/PBS [15].

Another multidimensional self-report questionnaire that may be used to assess the impact of IC/PBS on sexual function is the Female Sexual Distress Scale (FSDS) [16]. The FSDS is a self-report screening tool shown to be a valid and reliable measure for assessing sexually related personal distress in women. The FSDS consist of 12 items that relate to feelings such as sexual distress, unhappiness, guilt, frustration, stress, inferiority, worry, inadequacy, regretful, embarrassment, dissatisfaction, and anger during the past 30 days. Each item is scored as never (0), rarely (1), occasionally (2), frequently (3), and always (4). Women with high distress associated with their sexual health problem, such as sexual pain, will score high on this measure. Longitudinal scores are useful to assess improvement or worsening of the distress over time [16].

A procedure called the PST is useful in the diagnosis of IC/PBS [17]. Initially, sterile saline is instilled through a catheter in an empty bladder. The patient then rates her sensations of urinary frequency and pain. The bladder is then emptied and a solution containing potassium is instilled [18]. Again, the patient rates her symptoms. If she experiences increased pain with the potassium solution, the test is positive, indicating that the diagnosis of IC/PBS is highly likely. A positive PST has been observed in 78% of women with symptoms of IC/PBS but is positive in only 4% of healthy controls [13].

Cystoscopy with hydrodistention is a useful diagnostic tool, but it is not required when making the diagnosis of IC/PBS [19]. Glomerulations (petechial hemorrhages) are found in 95% of women with IC/PBS. Ulcerations of the bladder mucosa (Hunner's ulcers) are found in only 5–10% of women with IC/PBS [20].

Treatment of IC/PBS

A range of therapeutic interventions, including pharmacologic modalities, are recommended for the management of IC/PBS. Initial treatment should include patient education and behavior modification. The practice of keeping voiding diaries detailing the frequency, volume of voided urine, time of urination, and associated symptoms should be encouraged. Recording such information may help to identify foods and behaviors that cause an exacerbation of symptoms.

Given the complexity of IC/PBS, a multifaceted medical treatment regimen is recommended in targeting the various pathophysiologic aspects of the disorder [9]. Current pharmacologic treatment recommendations include several concurrent treatments, each addressing different disease mechanisms. In addition, there is evidence that early recognition and treatment of IC/PBS leads to a more rapid relief of symptoms [21].

Medication to restore the protective barrier between the bladder and urine which counteract dysfunctional epithelium include pentosanpolysulfate sodium (PPS) (Elmiron®) or intravesical heparin (with or without lidocaine) [8]. To date, PPS is the only oral medication approved by U.S. Food and Drug Administration (FDA) for use in the treatment of patients with IC/PBS.

More recently, oral PPS has been used in combination with intravesical instillation of PPS and this combination was shown to be a safe and effective therapeutic option [22]. In addition, inhibition of mast cell activation is achieved by the use of hydroxyzine (Atarax®) [23]. In addition, the use of amitriptyline (Elavil®), nortriptyline (Pamelor®), or other tricyclic antidepressants is recommended to treat the neuropathic pain component of IC/PBS [23, 24] (see Chapter 26 on the role of neurologist). Likewise, gabapentin and pregabalin are anticonvulsants that may be used to decrease the neuropathic pain component of IC/PBS [9]. Several treatments used to reduce IC/PBS symptoms (e.g., antidepressants) may exacerbate female sexual dysfunction (Table 14.2).

A recently published study examined whether patients with IC/PBS treated with an intravesical therapeutic solution of lidocaine, heparin, and sodium bicarbonate experienced an alteration in the quality and frequency of dyspareunia [25]. Sexually active patients were treated with this solution three times a week for 3 weeks. Follow-up occurred 3 weeks later with the administration of the Objective Rating of Improvement of Symptom scale. Sixty-five percent of the patients reported improvement greater than 50%. There was significantly less nocturia, more voided volume of urine, and improvement in PUF scores. In addition, over half the patients reported resolution of dyspareunia [25].

As with other chronic regional pain syndromes, a multidisciplinary approach to the treatment of IC/PBS is necessary. Pelvic floor physical therapy or biofeedback (see Chapter 13) can be used to address the pelvic floor muscle dysfunction that frequently accompanies IC/PBS [26].

Table 14.2 Medications and female sexual dysfunction.

Medications that cause disorders of desire	Medications that cause disorders of arousal
Psychoactive medications	Anticholinergics
Antipsychotics	Antihistamines
Barbiturates	Antihypertensives
Benzodiazepines	Psychoactive medications
SSRIs	Benzodiazepines
Lithium	SSRIs
TCAs	Monoamine oxidase inhibitors
Antihypertensivesmedications	TCAs
Cholesterol-lowering agents	
Beta blockers	**Medications that cause**
Clonidine (Catapres)	**orgasmic dysfunction**
Digoxin	Methyldopa (Aldomet)
Spironolactone (Aldactone)	Amphetamines
Danazol (Danocrine)	Antipsychotics
GnRH agonists (e.g., Lupron,	Benzodiazepines
Synarel)	SSRIs
Oral contraceptives	Narcotics
Histamine H_2-receptor blockers	Trazadone (Desyrel)
Promotility agents	TCAs
Indomethacin (Indocin)	
Ketoconazole (Nizoral)	
Phenytoin sodium (Dilantin)	

Adapted from Ref. 41.

Key: SSRIs = selective serotonin reuptake inhibitors; TCAs = tricyclic antidepressants.

Some patients may benefit from cognitive behavior therapy and sex therapy (see Chapter 23) to treat concurrent anxiety, depression, and sexual dysfunction [27]. Additional therapies include sacral neuromodulation [28] and botulinum toxin type A injections [29]; hydrodistention may be useful in some patients [30].

IC/PBS and Sexual Dysfunction

Recent reports of IC/PBS have included dyspareunia as one possible presenting symptom [31]. The inclusion of dyspareunia secondary to underlying bladder pathology has not traditionally been recognized, and to date, it has not been widely addressed in the peer-reviewed literature. In fact, pelvic pain of bladder origin continues to be widely diagnosed as a gynecologic entity, often as endometriosis, GVD, or PVD. While these entities individually may be a source of dyspareunia, they may coexist with IC/PBS

[32]. Pelvic floor dysfunction, a condition of hypertonicity and spasm of the pelvic floor muscles (see Chapters 6, 13, and 35), is a common source of sexual pain during or after sexual relations. Pelvic floor dysfunction accompanies IC/PBS in 75% of patients [33].

In one study of women with IC/PBS, 94% reported varying degrees of lower abdominal, urethral, lower back, and vestibular or vaginal pain [8]. Seventy-five percent of women with IC/PBS state that sex exacerbates their urinary and pain symptoms [33]. Over time, the dyspareunia associated with IC/PBS becomes chronic, and threatens libido, arousal, and orgasm.

Salonia et al. [34] compared women with urinary incontinence and/or lower urinary tract symptoms and matched controls without urinary symptoms to determine the prevalence of female sexual dysfunction. Findings demonstrated that women with urinary incontinence/lower urinary tract symptoms demonstrated greater levels of sexual dysfunction. In a British study, 30% of members of an IC/PBS support group indicated that IC/PBS made a considerable impact on their sexual relationships. Sexual dysfunction was identified as one of the strongest predictors of poorer quality of life in women with refractory IC/PBS [35].

Peters et al. [36] used self-assessment questionnaires in women with IC/PBS and control women to identify predisposing factors and comorbidities. On all domains, women with IC/PBS scored worse than controls. Women with IC/PBS reported significantly greater pelvic pain, more fear of pain, and more pain with intercourse during adolescence and adulthood as compared with control women. Before the diagnosis, 86% of the women with IC/PBS recalled having moderate to high sexual desire versus 78% of the controls. After the diagnosis, however, only 40% reported sexual desire in the moderate to high range. Before the diagnosis of IC/PBS, the rate of frequent or very frequent orgasm was similar between both groups, but this percentage was significantly lower postdiagnosis. In terms of the FSDS, women with IC/PBS scored in the sexually distressed range. Interestingly, in both groups, as age increased FSDS score decreased, indicating that less distress was associated with increasing age.

It is possible that recurrent episodes of dyspareunia initiate fear of pain that may lead to a reflex hypertonicity of pelvic floor musculature (i.e., vaginismus) (see Chapter 35). This reaction may cause increased dyspareunia and mechanical trauma to the vestibular mucosa or

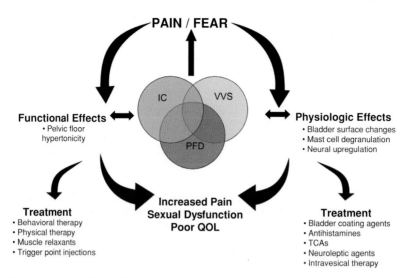

Figure 14.1 The vicious cycle between dyspareunia and sexual dysfunction. The symptomatic overlap between IC/PBS, VVS, and PFD, with pain and fear potentiating the worsening of symptoms as well as the physiologic and functional response to pain.

KEY: TCAs = tricyclic antidepressants; IC/PBS = interstitial cystitis/painful bladder syndrome; VVS = vulvar vestibulitis syndrome, currently termed *provoked vestibulodynia*; PFD = pelvic floor dysfunction.

urethra [37]. Noxious stimuli activate the pain system, and repeated episodes of noxious stimuli may transform nociceptive pain to neuropathic pain. The repeated instances of pain result in a chronic pain condition, with an associated alteration in sexual function (Figure 14.1).

In patients with IC/PBS, depression, use of poor coping strategies, impaired social relationships, and genitourinary/pelvic pain are associated with poor quality of life [38, 39]. Michael et al. [40] collected multidimensional measures of quality of life in a cohort of women with and without IC/PBS. After adjusting for age, women with IC/PBS had significantly lower quality of life scores in four of seven domains (i.e., self-image, bodily pain, vitality, and self-esteem). Relative to a group of women with rheumatoid arthritis, women with IC/PBS did not report restrictions of physical function, but demonstrated impaired vitality and mental health.

Conclusion

IC/PBS and sexual dysfunction are often comorbid. As with other chronic regional pain syndrome, IC/PBS should be treated within a biopsychosocial model. Medical treatments should focus on the multiple components

of this pain syndrome, including reducing local inflammation and decreasing neuropathic pain. Physical therapy should be used to address concurrent pelvic floor dysfunction. Cognitive-behavior therapy and sex therapy should address the psychosexual distress that often accompanies IC/PBS.

References

1 Chancellor MB. (2007) A Multidisciplinary Consensus Meeting on IC/PBS: Outcome of the Consensus Meeting on Interstitial Cystitis/Painful Bladder Syndrome, February 10, 2007, Washington, DC. *Reviews in Urology* **9**, 81–83.

2 Jones CA, Nyberg L. (1997) Epidemiology of interstitial cystitis. *Urology* **49**, 2–9.

3 Porru D, Politano R, Gerardini M, *et al.* (2004) Different clinical presentation of interstitial cystitis syndrome. *International Urogynecology Journal of Pelvic Floor Dysfunction* **15**, 198–202.

4 McCormack WM. (1990) Two urogenital sinus syndromes: interstitial cystitis and focal vulvitis. *The Journal of Reproductive Medicine* **35**, 873–76.

5 Heitkemper M, Jarrett M. (2005) Overlapping conditions in women with irritable bowel syndrome. *Urologic Nursing* **25**, 25–30.

6 Bogart LM, Berry SH, Clemens JQ. (2007) Symptoms of interstitial cystitis, painful bladder syndrome, and similar diseases in women: a systematic review. *Journal of Urology* **177**, 450–56.

7 Curhan GC, Speizer FE, Hunter DJ, *et al.* (1999) Epidemiology of interstitial cystitis: a population-based study. *Journal of Urology* **161**, 549–52.

8 Butrick CW. (2003) Interstitial cystitis and chronic pelvic pain: new insights in neuropathology, diagnosis, and treatment. *Clinical Obstetrics and Gynecology* **46**, 811–23.

9 Evans RJ. (2002) Treatment approaches for interstitial cystitis: multimodality therapy. *Reviews in Urology* **4**, S16–S20.

10 Theoharides TC, Cochrane DE. (2004) Critical role of mast cells in inflammatory diseases and the effect of acute stress. *Journal of Neuroimmunology* **146**, 1–12.

11 Marshall K. (2003) Interstitial cystitis: understanding the syndrome. *Alternative Medicine Review* **8**, 426–37.

12 Moldwin RM, Sant GR. (2002) Interstitial cystitis: a pathophysiology and treatment update. *Clinical Obstetrics and Gynecology* **45**, 259–72.

13 Parsons CL, Dell J, Stanford EJ, *et al.* (2002) Increased prevalence of interstitial cystitis: previously unrecognized urologic and gynecologic cases identified using a new symptom questionnaire and intravesical potassium sensitivity. *Urology* **60**, 573–78.

14 Nickel JC. (2004) Interstitial cystitis: a chronic pelvic pain syndrome. *Medical Clinics of North America* **88**, 467–81.

15 O'Leary MP, Sant GR, Fowler FJ, Jr, *et al.* (1997) The interstitial cystitis symptom index and problem index. *Urology* **49**, 58–63.

16 Derogatis LR, Rosen R, Leiblum S, *et al.* (2002) The Female Sexual Distress Scale (FSDS): initial validation of a standardized scale for assessment of sexually related personal distress in women. *Journal of Sex and Marital Therapy* **28**, 317–30.

17 Parsons CL. (2004) Diagnosing chronic pelvic pain of bladder origin. *The Journal of Reproductive Medicine* **49**, 235–42.

18 Parsons CL, Greenberger M, Gabal L, *et al.* (1998) The role of urinary potassium in the pathogenesis and diagnosis of interstitial cystitis. *Journal of Urology* **159**, 1862–67.

19 Evans RJ, Sant GR. (2007) Current diagnosis of interstitial cystitis: an evolving paradigm. *Urology* **69**, 64–72.

20 Denson MA, Griebling TL, Cohen MB, *et al.* (2000) Comparison of cystoscopic and histological findings in patients with suspected interstitial cystitis. *Journal of Urology* **164**, 1908–11.

21 Forrest JB, Dell JR. (2007) Successful management of interstitial cystitis in clinical practice. *Urology* **69**, 82–86.

22 Davis EL, El Khoudary SR, Talbott EO, *et al.* (2008) Safety and efficacy of the use of intravesical and oral pentosan polysulfate sodium for interstitial cystitis: a randomized double-blind clinical trial. *Journal of Urology* **179**, 177–85.

23 Moldwin RM, Evans RJ, Stanford EJ, *et al.* (2007) Rational approaches to the treatment of patients with interstitial cystitis. *Urology* **69**, 73–81.

24 Dimitrakov J, Kroenke K, Steers WD, *et al.* (2007) Pharmacologic management of painful bladder syndrome/interstitial cystitis: a systematic review. *Archives of Internal Medicine* **167**, 1922–29.

25 Welk BK, Teichman JM. (2008) Dyspareunia response in patients with interstitial cystitis treated with intravesical lidocaine, bicarbonate, and heparin. *Urology* **71**, 67–70.

26 Peters KM, Carrico DJ. (2006) Frequency, urgency, and pelvic pain: treating the pelvic floor versus the epithelium. *Current Urology Reports* **7**, 450–55.

27 Jackson JL, O'Malley PG, Kroenke K. (2006) Antidepressants and cognitive-behavioral therapy for symptom syndromes. *CNS Spectrums* **11**, 212–22.

28 Peters KM, Feber KM, Bennett RC. (2007) A prospective, single-blind, randomized crossover trial of sacral vs. pudendal nerve stimulation for interstitial cystitis. *BJU International* **100**, 835–39.

29 Giannantoni A, Porena M, Costantini E, *et al.* (2008) Botulinum A toxin intravesical injection in patients with painful bladder syndrome: 1-year follow-up. *Journal of Urology* **179**, 1031–34.

30 Ottem DP, Teichman JM. (2005) What is the value of cystoscopy with hydrodistension for interstitial cystitis? *Urology* **66**, 494–99.

31 Whitmore K, Siegel JF, Kellogg-Spadt S. (2007) Interstitial cystitis/painful bladder syndrome as a cause of sexual pain in women: a diagnosis to consider. *The Journal of Sexual Medicine* **4**, 720–27.

32 Ottem DP, Carr LK, Perks AE, *et al.* (2007) Interstitial cystitis and female sexual dysfunction. *Urology* **69**, 608–10.

33 Weiss JM. (2001) Pelvic floor myofascial trigger points: manual therapy for interstitial cystitis and the urgency–frequency syndrome. *Journal of Urology* **166**, 2226–31.

34 Salonia A, Zanni G, Nappi RE, *et al.* (2004) Sexual dysfunction is common in women with lower urinary tract symptoms and urinary incontinence: results of a cross-sectional study. *European Urology* **45**, 642–48.

35 Nickel JC, Tripp D, Teal V, *et al.* (2007) Sexual function is a determinant of poor quality of life for women with treatment refractory interstitial cystitis. *Journal of Urology* **177**, 1832–36.

36 Peters KM, Killinger KA, Carrico DJ, *et al.* (2007) Sexual function and sexual distress in women with interstitial cystitis: a
case-control study. *Urology* **70**, 543–47.

37 Graziottin A. (2006) *Sexual Pain Disorders: Dyspareunia and
Vaginismus.* Blackwell, Oxford, UK.

38 Rothrock NE, Lutgendorf SK, Kreder KJ. (2003) Coping
strategies in patients with interstitial cystitis: relationships
with quality of life and depression. *Journal of Urology* **169**,
233–36.

39 Rothrock NE, Lutgendorf SK, Hoffman A, *et al.* (2002) Depressive symptoms and quality of life in patients with interstitial cystitis. *Journal of Urology* **167**, 1763–67.

40 Michael YL, Kawachi I, Stampfer MJ, *et al.* (2000) Quality of
life among women with interstitial cystitis. *Journal of Urology*
164, 423–27.

41 Abramowicz M. (1992) Drugs that cause sexual dysfunction:
an update. *The Medical Letter on Drugs and Therapeutics* **34**,
73–78.

CHAPTER 15
Vulvovaginitis

Jack D. Sobel
Wayne State University School of Medicine, Detroit, MI, USA

Introduction

Vulvovaginal inflammation is a common, frequently curable cause of dyspareunia (Table 15.1). The purpose of this chapter is to review infectious causes of vulvovaginitis while excluding cervicitis and upper genital tract inflammation, both of which can cause sexual pain, especially deep dyspareunia.

Vaginitis and Dyspareunia

Transient vaginal symptoms, which are temporary and mild, are extremely common. More severe and persistent symptoms usually prompt some action on the part of the woman; she may either visit a health care provider or self-treat with topical over-the-counter (OTC) symptom-relieving agents or a topical antimycotic without having received a medical evaluation or diagnosis. Vulvovaginal symptoms, including vaginal discharge, are among the 25 most common reasons for a physician in a private office to receive a consultation in the United States [1]. As indicated in Table 15.1, vulvovaginitis is only found in approximately 40% of women with vulvovaginal symptoms and in over 25% of women attending sexually transmitted infection (STI) clinics.

While the mechanism of dyspareunia encountered in the presence of vulvovaginal disease usually results from friction, pressure, and irritation of sensitized and inflamed nerve fibers, other mechanisms undoubtedly exist. In virtually all women with vulvovaginitis, symptoms of burning and irritation may either begin or continue after intercourse and may last for hours or days. Vulvovaginitis may also be associated with pelvic floor dysfunction (see Chapter 13), a factor frequently missed by practitioners.

It should be emphasized that "reasonable expectations" should be addressed with the patient at the initial visit. Given that many vulvovaginal disorders are long-standing and multifactorial in their etiology, they will most likely not be resolved immediately and in some cases may never be completely resolved. Symptoms of severe vulvovaginitis, especially due to *Candida* species, do not disappear in a matter of a day or two but may take up to 2 weeks to dissipate, especially with regards to intercourse.

Recurrent vaginitis (more than four episodes per year), especially candidiasis, can result in frequent, painful sexual relations with each "flare," followed by a progressive healing period until the patient's baseline subjective feelings and comfort are restored. Not surprisingly, frequent vaginitis results in frequent pain/discomfort which can stress an intimate relationship. Thus, for many reasons, breaking the vicious cycle of repeated recurrent infections is a major goal of treatment. Unfortunately, some women never return to their baseline function and represent a major challenge in pain management. Complete control of the underlying infection is often not achieved due to inadequate treatment measures.

Bacterial Vaginosis

Epidemiology

Bacterial vaginosis (BV) is the most common cause of vaginitis in women of childbearing age [2]. BV has been diagnosed in 17–19% of women who seek gynecologic care in family practice or student health care settings [2].

Female Sexual Pain Disorders 1st edition. Edited by A. Goldstein, C. Pukall & I. Goldstein. © 2009 Blackwell Publishing, ISBN: 9781405183987.

Table 15.1 Differential diagnosis of vulvovaginitis.*

Infectious Vulvovaginitis
Vulvovaginal candidiasis
Bacterial vaginosis
Trichomoniasis
Mixed infections
Genital herpes
Group A streptococcus
Desquamative inflammatory vaginitis (DIV) (??)
Vaginal fistula (rectovaginal, vesicovaginal)

Noninfectious
Estrogen deficiency
    atrophic vaginitis
    atrophic vestibulitis
Desquamative inflammatory vaginitis
Erosive lichen planus
Lichen simplex chronicus
Contact dermatitis /chemical irritant
Allergic vaginitis/vulvitis
Dermatosis
    eczema
    psoriasis
Pemphigus/pemphigoid syndromes
Idiopathic vestibulitis syndrome
Cytolytic vaginosis (??)

* Does not include causes of cervicitis.
(??) indicates that controversy exists for these conditions

It has also been observed in 16–29% of pregnant women, and its prevalence increases considerably among symptomatic women in STI clinics, ranging from 24% to 37% [2]. Although *Gardnerella vaginalis*, one of the predominant organisms found in BV, has been found in 10–31% of virgin adolescent girls, it is still found significantly more often among sexually active women, reaching a prevalence of 50–60% in some populations at risk for infection [3]. Epidemiologic study has revealed that intrauterine devices, intravaginal pessaries, smoking, and douches were found to be more common in women with BV. BV is significantly more common in blacks and lesbians, and in women with a multiple number of sexual partners in the prior 12 months [2].

Pathogenesis

BV is the result of massive overgrowth of mixed, predominantly anaerobic flora, including peptostreptococci, *Bacteroides*, *Gardnerella vaginalis*, *Mobiluncus*, and genital mycoplasmas [4]. With BV, there is little inflam-

mation; the disorder represents a disturbance of the vaginal microbial ecosystem rather than a true infection of the tissues. The overgrowth of mixed flora is associated with a loss of the normal *Lactobacillus*-dominated vaginal flora. No single bacterial species is responsible for BV.

Two factors support the role of sexual transmission of BV: (1) the higher prevalence of BV among sexually active young women than among sexually inexperienced women, and (2) the observation that BV-associated microorganisms are isolated more often from the urethras of male partners of women with BV [2]. On the other hand, treatment of male partners does not result in reduced recurrence of BV in females.

The cause of the anaerobic overgrowth—including *Gardnerella*, *Mycoplasma*, and *Mobiluncus* species—that results in BV is unknown. Theories include increased substrate availability, increased pH, and loss of the restraining effects of the predominant *Lactobacillus* flora in the vagina. Women without BV are colonized by hydrogen peroxide–producing strains of lactobacilli, whereas women with BV have reduced numbers of lactobacilli, and the lactobacillus species that are present lack the ability to produce hydrogen peroxide [4, 5]. The hydrogen peroxide produced by lactobacilli may inhibit the pathogens associated with BV.

Accompanying the bacterial overgrowth in BV is the increased production of amines by anaerobes. These amines produce the typical fishy odor of BV. It is likely that amines together with the organic acids found in the vagina are cytotoxic, resulting in exfoliation of vaginal epithelial cells, creating the vaginal discharge typical of BV. *Gardnerella vaginalis* attaches avidly to exfoliated epithelial cells, especially at an alkaline pH. The adherence of *Gardnerella* organisms results in formation of the pathognomonic clue cells seen on a wet mount.

Clinical Features

As many as 50% of women with BV are asymptomatic. An abnormal malodorous vaginal discharge (often described as "fishy") is usually detected, the odor often appearing after unprotected coitus. Examination reveals a nonviscous, grayish-white, adherent discharge. Pruritus, dysuria, and dyspareunia are rare.

Until recently, BV had largely been considered only a nuisance. However, there is substantial evidence that serious obstetric and gynecologic sequelae may occur (Table 15.2), even with asymptomatic disease. Untreated

Table 15.2 Complications of bacterial vaginosis.

Obstetric
Chorioamnionitis
Premature rupture of membranes
Preterm labor and delivery
Low birth weight
Amniotic fluid infections
Postpartum endometritis

Gynecologic
Tubal infertility
Pelvic inflammatory disease
Postabortal pelvic inflammatory disease
HIV transmission/acquisition/susceptibility
Postsurgical infection
Urinary tract infection
Cervical intraepithelial neoplasia
Mucopurulent endocervicitis
Strong association with STIs (trichomoniasis, gonorrhea, chlamydia, herpes simplex virus, human papillomavirus)

BV has been reported to be associated with increased clinical exacerbations of genital herpes and increased HIV transmission [6].

Diagnosis

Signs and symptoms cannot reliably diagnose BV. The diagnosis is made by the presence of at least three of the following Amsel criteria: (1) an adherent, white, nonfloccular, homogenous discharge; (2) a positive amine test, with release of fishy odor on addition of 10% KOH to vaginal secretions; (3) a vaginal pH > 4.5; and (4) the presence of clue cells on light microscopy (the most reliable predictor). These criteria are simple, reliable, and easy to test.

At least 20% of observed epithelial cells should be clue cells, the exfoliated vaginal squamous epithelial cells covered with *G. vaginalis*, for this finding to be of diagnostic significance. The fishy odor may be apparent during the physical examination or the "whiff" (i.e., amine) test. A Gram stain of vaginal secretions is valuable in making the diagnosis, with a sensitivity of 93% and specificity of 70% [7].

Although cultures for *G. vaginalis* are positive in almost all cases of BV, the organism also may be detected in 50–60% of women who do not meet the diagnostic criteria for the disease [7]. Vaginal cultures are not used to diagnose BV.

Management

Poor efficacy has been observed in the treatment of BV with triple sulfa creams, erythromycin, fluoroquinolone, ampicillin, tetracycline, acetic acid gel, and providone–iodine vaginal douches [8]. The most successful oral therapy is metronidazole. Multiple divided-dose regimens of metronidazole at 800–1200 mg/day for 1 week achieved clinical cure rates in excess of 90% immediately and of approximately 80% at 4 weeks [8]. Although single-dose therapy with 2 g of metronidazole achieved similar immediate clinical response rates, higher recurrence rates have been reported. The beneficial effect of metronidazole results primarily from its antianaerobic activity and its hydroxymetabolites.

Topical therapy with 2% clindamycin (once daily for 7 days) cream or suppositories, or metronidazole gel 0.75% (once daily for 5 days) has been shown to be as effective as oral metronidazole in eliminating BV without the side effects of the oral medication. Single-dose vaginal clindamycin in a bioadhesive preparation is also available.

In the past, asymptomatic BV was not treated because patients often improved spontaneously over several months. However, the growing evidence linking asymptomatic BV with numerous obstetric and gynecologic complications involving the upper reproductive tract has prompted a reassessment of this policy, especially with the availability of convenient topical therapies [6].

Asymptomatic BV should be treated before pregnancy, in women with cervical abnormalities, and before elective gynecologic surgery. Routine screening and treatment for asymptomatic BV in pregnancy is controversial. Some controlled studies have shown that treatment of BV with topical clindamycin and oral metronidazole may reduce preterm labor and prematurity, but only in women with a past history of preterm labor. At present, this category of women seems most suited for screening [9]. Despite indirect evidence of its sexual transmission, no study has documented reduced recurrence rates of BV in women whose partners have been treated with a variety of regimens, including metronidazole. Accordingly, most clinicians do not routinely treat the male partners of affected women.

After treatment with oral metronidazole, symptoms of BV recur within 3 months in approximately 30% of patients who initially respond [7]. The reasons for such recurrence are unclear; possibilities include reinfection or vaginal relapse due to failure to eradicate the offending organisms and concurrent failure of the *Lactobacillus*-dominant vaginal flora to reestablish itself. Management of symptoms of acute BV during relapse includes treatment with oral or vaginal metronidazole or topical clindamycin, usually prescribed for a longer (10–14 days) period than the initial treatment regimen.

A recent study found that long-term suppressive maintenance therapy with twice weekly metronidazole gel (0.75%) is an effective prophylaxis, but long-term cure occurred in < 50% [10]. Attempts to prevent relapse by use of exogenous *Lactobacillus* preparations have been reasonably successful but remain controversial [11].

Trichomoniasis

Epidemiology

Studies estimate that 3–5 million American women contract trichomoniasis annually, with a worldwide distribution of approximately 180 million cases each year [12]. The prevalence of trichomoniasis correlates with the overall level of sexual activity of the group of women studied, with the disease diagnosed in approximately 5% of women in family-planning clinics, 13–25% of women in gynecology clinics, 50–75% of sex workers, and 7–35% of women in STI clinics. Recent surveys indicate a decline in the incidence of trichomoniasis in many industrialized countries [12].

Pathophysiology

Sexual transmission is the dominant method of introduction of *Trichomonas vaginalis* into the vagina [7]. The organism was found in 70% of urethral cultures of men who had had sexual contact with infected women within the previous 48 hr. Women with trichomoniasis also show a high prevalence of gonorrhea, and both diseases are significantly associated with the use of nonbarrier contraceptive methods.

Recurrent trichomoniasis is common and indicative of a lack of significant protective immunity. Nevertheless, an immune response to *T. vaginalis* does develop, as indicated by low titers of serum antibody, but this information is not sufficient for diagnostic serology. Antitrichomonal immunoglobulin A has been detected in vaginal secretions, but a protective role for it has not been defined. The periurethral and Skene's glands are infected in most

patients, and *T. vaginalis* organisms can be seen in the urine.

Clinical Features

The severity of *Trichomonas* infection in women ranges from an asymptomatic carrier state to severe acute inflammatory disease [13]. Foul-smelling vaginal discharge is reported by 50–75% of women with trichomoniasis; however, the discharge is not always malodorous. Pruritus occurs in 25–50%. Other symptoms include dyspareunia, dysuria, and urinary frequency of micturition. Lower abdominal pain occurs in fewer than 10% of patients and should alert the physician to the possibility of concomitant pelvic inflammatory disease (see Chapter 20). Symptoms of acute trichomoniasis often appear during or immediately after menstruation. Although its duration is controversial, the incubation period has been estimated to range from 3 to 28 days [13].

Vulvar findings may be absent but are typically characterized in severe cases by diffuse vulvar erythema (10–33%), edema, and a profuse purulent vaginal discharge [11]. The discharge is often described as yellow–green and frothy, but can also be white. The vaginal walls are erythematous and, in severe cases, may have a granular appearance. Punctate hemorrhages (colpitis macularis) of the cervix may give it a "strawberry-like" appearance which is apparent to the naked eye in only 1–2% of patients, but seen in 45% patients upon colposcopy [13].

The clinical course of trichomoniasis in pregnancy is identical to that in the nonpregnant state; when untreated, the disease is associated with premature rupture of membranes and prematurity. Trichomoniasis facilitates transmission of HIV and metronidazole therapy dramatically reduces free HIV virus in vaginal secretions [14].

Diagnosis

None of the clinical features of *Trichomonas* vaginitis is sufficiently specific to allow a diagnosis of trichomonal infection based on signs and symptoms alone [7]. A definitive diagnosis requires demonstration of the organism. The vaginal pH is markedly increased (usually above 5.0). On saline microscopy, an increase in polymorphic nuclear leukocytes (PMNLs) is almost invariably present. The ovoid trichomonal parasites are slightly larger than PMNLs and are best recognized by their motility. A wet mount is positive in only 40–80% of cases. The Gram stain is of little value and although trichomonads are often seen on Pap smears, this method has a sensitivity of only 60–70% when compared with saline preparation microscopy, and false-positive results have been reported.

Several culture methods for *T. vaginalis* are available (Diamond's medium preferred), and growth is usually detected within 48 hr. Culture is now recognized as the most sensitive method for detecting the presence of trichomonads (95% sensitivity) and should be considered in patients with vaginitis in whom one finds an increased pH and PMNLs but the absence of motile trichomonads. A two-chambered plastic bag culture system (InPouch: Biomed Diagnostic, San Jose, CA) is equivalent to Diamond's medium for detection of *T. vaginalis*. Polymerase chain reaction (PCR) technology is extremely sensitive but not available commercially. OSOM Trichomonas Rapid Test, a new point-of-care antigen-based diagnostic test (Genzyme Diagnostics, Cambridge, MA) has high sensitivity and specificity, and is rapid and user-friendly [15].

Management

Treatment is based on the 5-nitroimidazole class of drugs (metronidazole, tinidazole, and ornidazole), all of which have similar efficacy [8]. Oral therapy is preferred to topical vaginal therapy because of the frequency of infection of the urethra and periurethral glands, which provide sources for reinfection. Treatment consists of oral metronidazole 500 mg twice daily for 7 days, which produces a cure rate of 95%. Similar results have been obtained with a single dose of oral metronidazole 2 g, which produced cure rates of 82–88% [8]. The latter cure rate increases to >90% when sexual partners are treated simultaneously [7]. The advantages of single-dose therapy include better patient compliance, a lower total dose, a shorter period of alcohol avoidance, and possibly, decreased subsequent *Candida* vaginitis infection.

Patients who do not respond to an initial course of treatment often respond to an additional standard 7-day course of therapy. Some patients are refractory to repeated courses of therapy even when compliance is assured and sexual partners are known to have been treated. If reinfection is excluded, these rare patients may have strains of *T. vaginalis* that are resistant to metronidazole. Increased doses of metronidazole and a longer duration of therapy are necessary to cure these refractory cases of the disease; patients should be given maximum tolerated doses of oral metronidazole of 2–4 g/day for 10–14 days. Considerable success has been observed in the treatment of resistant trichomonal infections with oral tinidazole [16]. Most investigators use high-dose tinidazole at 1–4 g/day for 14 days [17]. Rare patients who do not respond to nitroimidazoles can be treated with topical paromomycin.

Side effects of metronidazole include an unpleasant or metallic taste, nausea (10%), transient neutropenia (7.5%), and a disulfiram-like effect when alcohol is ingested [8]. Long-term and high-dose therapy increases the risk of neutropenia and peripheral neuropathy. Superinfection with *Candida* may occur.

Vulvovaginal Candidiasis

Epidemiology

In the United States, *Candida* is the second most common cause of vaginal infection [1, 18]. It is estimated that 75% of women experience at least one episode of vulvovaginal candidiasis (VVC) during their childbearing years, and approximately 40–50% experience a second attack. Five to eight percent of adult women suffer from recurrent, often intractable *Candida* vaginitis [18].

Candida is isolated from the genital tract of approximately 15–20% of asymptomatic, healthy women of childbearing age [18]. The natural history of asymptomatic colonization is unknown; however, studies suggest that vaginal carriage continues for several months and perhaps for years. Several factors are associated with increased rates of asymptomatic vaginal colonization with *Candida*, including pregnancy (30–40%), use of oral contraceptives, uncontrolled diabetes mellitus, and frequent visits to STI clinics. The rarity of isolating *Candida* from premenarchal girls, the lower prevalence of postmenopausal *Candida* vaginitis, and the possible association of VVC with hormone-replacement therapy emphasize the hormonal dependence of this condition [19].

Pathogenesis

Infecting Organisms

Between 85% and 90% of yeasts isolated from the vagina are strains of *Candida albicans*. The remainder belong to other species, the most common of which is *Candida glabrata*. Non-*albicans Candida* species are less virulent but still capable of inducing vaginitis, and they are often more resistant to conventional therapy than is *C. albicans* [18]. VVC caused by non-*albicans Candida* species, particularly *C. glabrata*, is increasing [20]. *Candida* organisms gain access to the vaginal lumen and secretions predominantly from the adjacent perianal area. This finding is borne out by epidemiologic typing studies.

Host Factors

Candida vaginitis is seen predominantly in women of childbearing age, and only in the minority of cases can a precipitating factor be identified to explain the transformation from asymptomatic carriage of *Candida* organisms to symptomatic vaginitis in individual patients [19]. High levels of reproductive hormones during pregnancy result in higher glycogen content in the vaginal environment and provide an excellent carbon source for the growth and germination of *Candida*. Estrogens enhance vaginal epithelial cell avidity for the adherence of *Candida*. Several studies have shown increased VVC associated with oral contraceptive use [21] and uncontrolled diabetes mellitus. Glucose tolerance tests have been recommended for women with recurrent VVC, but their yield is low and such testing is not justified in otherwise healthy premenopausal women.

Symptomatic VVC is often observed during or after courses of systemic or vaginal antibiotic therapy. Antibiotics are responsible for approximately 20% of sporadic *Candida* vaginitis episodes [22]. All antimicrobial agents can cause this complication, likely by eliminating the normally protective vaginal bacterial flora. The natural flora of the vagina provides a colonization-resistant mechanism to prevent *Candida* from germinating, primarily by *Lactobacillus* species [23].

Other factors that contribute to an increased incidence of *Candida* vaginitis include the use of tight, poorly ventilated clothing which increases perineal moisture and temperature. Chemical contact, local allergy, and hypersensitivity reactions also may predispose to symptomatic *Candida* vaginitis.

Candida may cause cell damage and resulting inflammation by direct hyphal invasion of epithelial tissue. It is possible that proteases and other hydrolytic enzymes of the organism facilitate its cell penetration with resultant inflammation, mucosal swelling, erythema, and exfoliation of vaginal epithelial cells. The characteristic nonhomogenous vaginal discharge of VVC consists of a conglomerate of hyphal elements and exfoliated nonviable epithelial

cells, with few PMNLs. *Candida* also may induce symptoms by hypersensitivity or allergic reaction, particularly in women with idiopathic recurrent VVC.

Pathogenesis of Recurrent and Chronic *Candida* Vaginitis

Careful evaluation of women with recurrent vaginitis usually fails to reveal any precipitating or causal mechanism for such disease [19]. Although sexual transmission of *Candida* organisms occurs via vaginal intercourse and orogenital contact, the role of sexual reintroduction of yeast as a cause for recurrent vulvovaginal candidiasis is doubtful. Recurrent VVC frequently occurs in celibate women, whereas only the minority of male partners of affected women has been colonized with *Candida*. Although most studies aimed at treating male partners of infected women have not reduced the frequency of recurrent episodes of vaginitis, others have achieved reduction in recurrent VVC by treating the colonized male partners of such patients [24].

Vaginal relapse implies incomplete eradication or clearance of *Candida* from the vagina with antimycotic therapy. According to this concept, *Candida* organisms persist in small numbers in the vagina, causing their continued carriage. Whether recurrence is caused by vaginal reinfection or relapse, women with recurrent VVC differ from those with infrequent episodes of such infection in their inability to tolerate small numbers of *Candida* reintroduced into or persisting in the vagina. Host factors responsible for frequent episodes of VVC are not clearly delineated and more than one mechanism may be at work. Recurrent VVC is rarely caused by antimicrobial drug resistance [19, 25].

Women who are seropositive for HIV have higher vaginal colonization rates with *Candida* than do seronegative women, but reports of severe recurrent VVC are largely unsubstantiated. Recurrent VVC in the absence of other risk factors for HIV infection does not indicate HIV testing [25].

Clinical Features

The most frequent symptom of VVC is vulvar pruritus, because vaginal discharge is inconsistently present and often minimal [18]. Although typically described as having a cottage cheese–like character, the discharge may vary from watery to homogenously thick. Vaginal soreness, irritation, vulvar burning, dyspareunia, and external dysuria are commonly present. Odor, if present, is minimal and nonoffensive. Examination frequently reveals erythema and swelling of the labia and vulva, often with discrete pustulopapular peripheral lesions. The cervix appears normal, and vaginal mucosal erythema with an adherent whitish discharge is present. Characteristically, symptoms are worst during the week before the onset of menses and are somewhat relieved with the onset of menstrual flow.

Diagnosis

The relative lack of specificity of symptoms and signs of VVC precludes a diagnosis that is based only on history and physical examination. Most patients with symptomatic VVC may be diagnosed readily on the basis of a simple microscopic examination of vaginal secretions. A wet mount or saline preparation has a sensitivity of 40–60%. The 10% KOH preparation is more sensitive in diagnosing the presence of germinated yeast. A normal vaginal pH (4.0–4.5) is found in *Candida* vaginitis; a pH finding higher than 4.5 suggests the possibility of BV, trichomoniasis, or a mixed infection [18].

Although routine fungal cultures are usually unnecessary, in patients who test negative for *Candida* by microscopy, cultures should be obtained in symptomatic patients to confirm the diagnosis and avoid empirical therapy. There is no reliable serologic technique for the diagnosis of symptomatic *Candida* vaginitis and no reliable rapid antigen detecting tests are available commercially.

Management

Topical Agents for Acute *Candida* Vaginitis

Antimycotic creams, vaginal tablets, suppositories, and coated tampons (Table 15.3) are widely available. There is little evidence to suggest that the formulation of a topical antimycotic influences its clinical efficacy in vulvovaginal candidiasis [26]. In the presence of extensive vulvar inflammation, a topical cream preparation together with a topical steroid for severe inflammation is useful.

Azoles achieve clinical mycologic cure rates (~85–90%). Although many studies have compared the clinical efficacy of the various azoles, there is little evidence that any one azole agent is superior to the others [26, 27]. Topical azoles are free of local and systemic side effects; nevertheless, the initial application of topical agents is not infrequently accompanied by local burning and discomfort.

There has been a major trend toward shorter courses of treatment of VVC with progressively higher doses of antifungal agents, culminating in highly effective single-dose topical regimens. Although short-course regimens are effective for mild and moderate vaginitis, cure rates for severe and complicated vaginitis are lower.

Oral systemic azoles available for the treatment of VVC include ketoconazole (400 mg bid for 5 days), itraconazole (200 mg/day for 3 days or bid for 1 day), and fluconazole (150-mg single dose) [27–29]. All of these oral regimens achieve clinical cure rates in excess of 80%. Women generally prefer oral treatment regimens because of their convenience and lack of local side effects. Hepatotoxicity with ketoconazole precludes its widespread use in VVC [26].

VVC is classified as either uncomplicated or complicated based on its likelihood of being cured clinically and mycologically with short-course therapy. Uncomplicated VVC, which represents the most common form of vaginitis, is caused by highly sensitive strains of *C. albicans*. When of mild to moderate severity, it responds well to all topical or oral antimycotic therapy (including single-dose therapy), with cure rates exceeding 90% [27]. In contrast, patients with complicated VVC have either an organism, host factor, or severity of infection that dictates more intensive and prolonged treatment that lasts 7–14 days [28]. Most infections with non-*albicans* species of *Candida* respond to conventional topical or oral antifungal agents provided they are administered for a sufficient period. Vaginitis caused by *C. glabrata* often fails to respond to azoles and may require treatment with vaginal capsules of boric acid at 600 mg/day or flucytosine cream for 14 days [30].

Treatment of Recurrent VVC

The management of recurrent VVC is directed at its control rather than its cure, and requires long-term maintenance therapy with a suppressive prophylactic regimen. The clinician should first confirm the diagnosis of recurrent VVC before initiating treatment. Uncontrolled diabetes must be managed, and the use of corticosteroids and other immunosuppressive agents should be discontinued when possible. Unfortunately, no underlying or predisposing factor can be identified in most women with recurrent VVC. Because of the chronicity of therapy for recurrent VVC, oral treatments are most useful; the best suppressive prophylaxis has been achieved with weekly

Table 15.3 Therapy for vaginal candidiasis.

Drug	Formulation	Dosage Regimen
Topical Agents		
Butoconazole*	2% cream	5 g/day for 3 days
Clotrimazole*	1% cream	5 g/day for 7–14 days
		100 mg vaginal tablets, 1 tablet/day for 7 days
		100 mg vaginal tablets, 2 tablet/day for 3 days
		500 mg vaginal tablet, 1 tablet, single dose
Miconazole*	2% cream	5g/day for 7 days
		100 mg vaginal suppository, 1 suppository/day for 7 days
		200 mg vaginal suppository, 1 suppository/day for 3 days
		1200 mg vaginal suppository, 1 suppository, single dose
Econazole	—	150 mg vaginal tablet, 1 tablet/day for 3 days
Fenticonazole	2% cream	5 g/day for 7 days
Tioconazole*	2% cream	5 g/day for 3 days
	6.5% cream	5 g, single dose
Terconazole	0.4% cream	5 g/day for 7 days
	0.8% cream	5 g/day for 3 days
		80 mg vaginal suppository, 80 mg/day for 3 days
Nystatin	—	100,000 U vaginal tablets, 1 tablet/day for 14 days
Oral Agents		
Ketoconazole	—	200 mg bid for 5 days
Itraconazole	—	200 mg daily for 3 days
Fluconazole	—	150 mg single dose
		150 mg × 2 days for seven days

* Drugs available over the counter, without prescription.

fluconazole orally at a dose of 150 mg [31]. An effective topical prophylactic regimen consists of weekly vaginal suppositories of clotrimazole in a dose of 500 mg [18, 28].

Noninfectious Vaginitis and Vulvitis

Women often present with acute or chronic vulvovaginal symptoms of noninfectious etiology. These symptoms are indistinguishable from those of infectious syndromes but are most commonly confused with those of acute *Candida* vaginitis. Noninfectious causes of vaginitis and vulvitis include physical and chemical irritants, and allergens responsible for immunologic acute and chronic hypersensitivity reactions, including contact dermatitis.

There is a long list of topical agents that are responsible for local inflammatory reactions and symptoms, and many more have yet to be defined. Depending on the site of contact, symptoms may be vaginal or vulvar. A noninfectious mechanism may coexist with or follow an infectious process and should be considered when (1) the three common infectious causes of vulvovaginal symptoms, as well as hormone deficiency, are excluded, (2) the vaginal pH and saline content are normal, and (3) KOH microscopy and a yeast culture are negative.

Unfortunately, given the anticipated 20% colonization rates in normal asymptomatic women, a positive yeast culture sometimes reflects the presence of an "innocent bystander" organism rather than the cause of a patient's vulvovaginal symptoms. The only logical way of establishing the role of *Candida* in this context is to treat the patient with an oral antifungal agent and assess the clinical response.

When a local chemical, irritant, or allergic reaction is suspected as the cause of vaginitis and/or vulvitis, a detailed inquiry into possible causal factors is essential.

Offending agents or behaviors should be eliminated whenever possible, including the avoidance of chemical irritants and allergens (e.g., soaps, detergents). The immediate management of severe vulvovaginal symptoms of noninfectious etiology should not rely on topical corticosteroids, which are rarely the solution to such symptoms; moreover, high-potency steroid creams often cause intense burning. Local relief measures include sodium bicarbonate sitz baths and oral antihistamines.

References

1 Kent HL. (1991) Epidemiology of vaginitis. *American Journal of Obstetrics and Gynecology* **165**, 1168–76.

2 Morris M, Nicoll A, Simms I, *et al.* (2001) Bacterial vaginosis: a public health review. *British Journal of Obstetrics and Gynecology* **108**, 439–50.

3 Joesoef MR, Schmid G. (2005) Bacterial vaginosis. *Clinical Evidence* **13**, 1968–78.

4 Hill GB. (1969) Microbiology of bacterial vaginosis. *American Journal of Obstetrics and Gynecology* **169**, 450–54.

5 Eschenbach DA, Davick PR, Williams BL, *et al.* (1989) Prevalence of hydrogen peroxide producing *Lactobacillus* species in normal women and women with bacterial vaginosis. *Journal of Clinical Microbiology* **27**, 251–56.

6 Myer L, Denny L, Telerant R, *et al.* (2005) Bacterial vaginosis and susceptibility to HIV infection in South African women: a nested case-control study. *Journal of Infectious Diseases* **192**, 1372–80.

7 Holmes KK. (1990) Lower genital tract infections in women: cystitis, urethritis, vulvovaginitis, and cervicitis. In: Holmes KK, Mardh P-A, Sparling PF, *et al.* (eds.) *Sexually Transmitted Diseases*, 2nd ed. McGraw-Hill, New York.

8 Centers for Disease Control and Prevention. (2002) 2002 Sexually transmitted diseases treatment guidelines. *MMWR Morbid Mortal Weekly Rep*ort **51**, 22.

9 Hauth JC, Goldenberg RL, Andrews WW, *et al.* (1995) Reduced incidence of preterm delivery with metronidazole and erythromycin in women with bacterial vaginosis. *New England Journal of Medicine* **333**, 1732–36.

10 Sobel JD, Ferris D, Schwebke J, *et al.* (2006) Suppressive antibacterial therapy with 0.75% metronidazole vaginal gel to prevent recurrent bacterial vaginosis. *American Journal of Obstetrics and Gynecology* **194**, 1283–89.

11 Larsson PG, Stray-Pedersen B, Ryttig KR, *et al.* (2008) Human lactobacilli as supplementation of clindamycin to patients with bacterial vaginosis reduce the recurrence rate; a 6-month, double-blind, randomized, placebo-controlled study. *BMC Womens Health* **15**, 8.

12 Sutton M, Sternberg M, Koumans EH, *et al.* (2007) The prevalence of *Trichomonas vaginalis* infection among reproductive-age women in the United States, 2001–2004. *Clinical Infectious Diseases* **45**, 1319–26.

13 Wolner-Hanssen P, Krieger JN, Stevens CE, *et al.* (1989) Clinical manifestations of vaginal trichomoniasis. *Journal of the American Medical Association* **261**, 571–76.

14 Wang CC, McClelland RS, Reilly M, *et al.* (2002) The effect of treatment of vaginal infections on shedding of human immunodeficiency virus type 1. *Journal of Infectious Diseases* **183**, 1017–22.

15 Sobel JD. (2005) What's new in bacterial vaginosis and trichomoniasis? *Infectious Disease Clinics of North America* **19**, 387–406.

16 Sobel JD, Nyirjesy P, Brown W. (2001) Tinidazole therapy for metronidazole-resistant vaginal trichomoniasis. *Clinical Infectious Diseases* **33**, 1341–46.

17 Hager WD. (2004) Treatment of metronidazole-resistant *Trichomonas vaginalis* with tinidazole: case reports of three patients. *Sexually Transmitted Diseases* **31**, 343–45.

18 Sobel JD. (1993) Candidal vulvovaginitis. *Clinical Obstetrics and Gynecology* **36**, 153–65.

19 Sobel JD. (2007) Vulvovaginal candidosis. *Lancet* **369**, 1961–71.

20 Spinillo A, Capuzzo E, Egbe TO, *et al.* (1995) Torulopsis glabrata vaginitis. *Obstetrics and Gynecology* **85**, 993–98.

21 Foxman B. (1996) Epidemiology of vulvovaginal candidiasis: risk factors. *American Journal of Public Health* **80**, 329–31.

22 Spinillo A, Capuzzo E, Acciano S, *et al.* (1999) Effect of antibiotic use on the prevalence of symptomatic vulvovaginal candidiasis. *American Journal of Obstetrics and Gynecology* **180**, 14–17.

23 Hooton TM, Roberts PL, Stamm WF. (1994) Effects of recent sexual activity and use of a diaphragm on the vaginal microflora. *Clinical Infectious Diseases* **19**, 274–78.

24 Spinillo A, Carrato L, Pizzoli G. (1992) Recurrent vulvovaginal candidiasis: results of a cohort study of sexual transmission and intestinal reservoir. *The Journal of Reproductive Medicine* **37**, 353–57.

25 Lynch ME, Sobel JD. (1994) Comparative in vitro activity of antimycotic agents against pathogenic yeast isolates. *Journal of Medical and Veterinary Mycology* **32**, 267–74.

26 Reef S, Levine WC, McNeil MM, *et al.* (1995) Treatment options for vulvovaginal candidiasis, background paper for development of 1993 STD treatment recommendations. *Clinical Infectious Diseases* **20**, 580–90.

27 Watson MC, Grimshaw JM, Bond CM, *et al.* (2002) Oral versus intravaginal imidazole and triazole antifungal agents for the treatment of uncomplicated vulvovaginal candidiasis (thrush): a systematic review. *British Journal of Obstetrics and Gynaecology* **109**, 85–95.

28 Sobel JD, Faro S, Force R, *et al.* (1998) Vulvovaginal candidiasis: epidemiologic, diagnostic, and therapeutic considerations. *American Journal of Obstetrics and Gynecology* **178**, 203–11.

29 Sobel JD, Brooker D, Stein GE, *et al.* (1995) Single oral dose fluconazole compared with clotrimazole in topical therapy of *Candida* vaginitis: Fluconazole Vaginitis Study Group. *American Journal of Obstetrics and Gynecology* **172**, 1263–68.

30 Sobel JD, Chaim W, Nagappan V, *et al.* (2003) Treatment of vaginitis caused by *Candida glabrata*: use of topical boric acid and flucytosine. *American Journal of Obstetrics and Gynecology* **189**, 1297–1300.

31 Sobel JD, Wiesenfeld HC, Martens M, *et al.* (2004) Maintenance fluconazole therapy for recurrent vulvovaginal candidiasis. *New England Journal of Medicine* **351**, 876–83.

CHAPTER 16
Noninfectious Vaginitis

Ahinoam Lev-Sagie,[1] Paul Nyirjesy[2]

[1] Weill Medical College of Cornell University, New York, NY, USA
[2] Drexel University College of Medicine, Philadelphia, PA, USA

Introduction

A variety of vaginal disorders, some infectious, others noninfectious, cause dyspareunia. This chapter reviews the two most common causes of noninfectious vaginitis—atrophic vaginitis and desquamative inflammatory vaginitis (DIV.)

Vaginal Atrophy and Atrophic Vaginitis

While dyspareunia affects 10–15% of premenopausal women, it is a presenting complaint in up to 39% of postmenopausal women [1]. In postmenopausal women, dyspareunia is attributed mainly to dryness resulting from vaginal atrophy. Atrophic vaginitis, defined here as symptomatic vaginal atrophy, is believed to be the most common cause of vulvovaginal symptoms in menopausal women and affects 10–40% [2]. However, only about 25% of symptomatic patients seek medical help.

Etiology of Vaginal Atrophy

Vaginal atrophy results from inadequate estrogen levels in the vagina. This occurs most commonly with menopause and aging, but can result in younger women due to hypothalamic amenorrhea, hyperprolactinemia, lactation, and usage of antiestrogenic medications [2]. Occasionally, usage of extra-low dose contraceptive pills [1] and cancer therapy [2] may cause similar symptoms.

Female Sexual Pain Disorders 1st edition. Edited by A. Goldstein, C. Pukall & I. Goldstein. © 2009 Blackwell Publishing, ISBN: 9781405183987.

During the reproductive years, estrogen plays a major role in maintaining the normal vaginal environment. This includes a thickened, rugated vaginal surface, increased blood flow and lubrication, lactobacillus-dominant flora, and a low (< 4.5) pH [2, 3]. With estrogen withdrawal during menopause, significant changes occur in the vagina, resulting in the tissue becoming pale, thin, and less flexible. Blood flow diminishes, secretions decrease, and pH increases [2, 3]. Vaginal flora changes from a lactobacillus-dominant flora to one with primarily anaerobic gram-negative rods and gram-positive cocci [4]. These changes may affect a woman's well-being, particularly when it comes to sexual activity.

Although all menopausal women undergo the same hormonal changes, only 10–40% of them will become symptomatic. There is limited ability to predict which women will develop symptoms [2]. The effect of estradiol on the vagina at the molecular level was recently studied [5]: differentially expressed mRNA transcripts in vaginal biopsies were determined by microarray analysis in women with vaginal atrophy before and after estradiol treatment. This study found evidence for estrogen-mediated regulation of over 3,000 genes involved in vaginal-tissue remodeling. It is possible that the variation in vaginal symptoms between menopausal women may result from genetic polymorphisms that mediate processes such as estrogen metabolism and expression of estrogen receptors in this tissue.

Sexual Dysfunction in Vaginal Atrophy

Data from the Yale Midlife Study indicated that 77% of menopausal women reported loss of sex drive, 58% had vaginal dryness, and 39% suffered from dyspareunia [6]. The physiological changes occurring in vaginal atrophy expose menopausal women to potential dyspareunia in several ways. Vaginal dryness causes increased friction during intercourse. The thin vaginal walls are friable and become prone to mechanical damage and formation of petechiae, ulcerations, and tears with sexual activity. With long-standing estrogen deficiency, the vagina may become shorter, narrower, and less elastic. All of these changes increase the likelihood of trauma, infection, and pain. Furthermore, changes occurring with aging, such as subcutaneous fat loss and decreased skin lipid production, can result in slower healing after injury. Lastly, age-dependent hypotonia or hypertonia of the pelvic floor muscles can also contribute to dyspareunia [7].

In addition to the physical changes occurring with estrogen depletion, sexual dysfunction in this population is influenced by the coexistence of decreased libido, decreased sexual arousal, and psychosocial factors. In general, premenopausal women have enough lubrication- and, even in the absence of arousal, can accommodate vaginal penetration without pain [1]. In contrast, vaginal engorgement and lubrication that accompanies sexual arousal may be decreased in patients with vaginal atrophy [8].

In postmenopausal women, dyspareunia may result from a pre existing arousal disorder that was unidentified until "unmasked" by estrogen depletion [8]. Psychosocial factors in this age group, including depression, anxiety, partner disability, poor overall health, and changes in so-cial status, can contribute to dyspareunia [7]. Avoidance of intercourse by symptomatic women may further contribute to vaginal shrinkage and loss of elasticity, which in turn can lead to additional barriers to future acts of sexual intimacy. Thus, it is essential that health care providers address both physiologic and psychological factors when treating patients with vaginal atrophy and sexual dysfunction.

Diagnosis of Atrophic Vaginitis

Patients with atrophic vaginitis may complain of vaginal dryness, dyspareunia, itching, discharge, pain [2], and irritative urinary symptoms. Symptoms are usually progressive and do not resolve spontaneously [2]. Although secretions are typically decreased, patients may note an abnormal yellow or watery discharge [3]. Vaginal bleeding may occur with severe atrophy [2].

Signs vary with the degree of atrophy. Loss of connective tissue substance results in shrinkage of the labia majora. The labia minora may disappear completely, and the introital opening is often diminished. The vagina has a pale, dry, nonrugated appearance, and submucosal petechial hemorrhages may be visualized [9]. The vaginal dimensions decrease, and the fornices may become obliterated, making the cervix flush with the vault [2, 9].

In general, the diagnosis is made by identifying characteristics changes on physical examination, noting an elevated vaginal pH, and finding parabasal cells on saline microscopy (Figure 16.1 and Table 16.1). Interestingly, the degree of atrophic changes as measured by microscopy

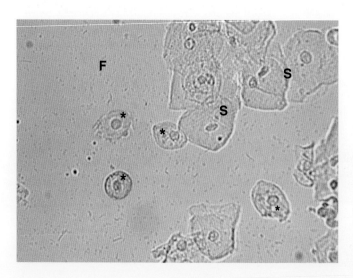

Figure 16.1 Microscopic findings in atrophic vaginitis. Normal superficial cells (S) are replaced by parabasal cells (*), which are smaller, rounder, and have a large nucleus. Vaginal flora (F) is scant, with a relative absence of lactobacilli. A maturation index, where a cytopathologist quantifies the percentage of immature vaginal epithelial cells, can aid in the diagnosis if a provider is unable to recognize intermediate and parabasal cells.

Table 16.1 Comparison between atrophic vaginitis, DIV and ELP.

	Atrophic vaginitis	Desquamative inflammatory vaginitis	Erosive vaginal lichen planus
Symptoms			
Discharge	−\+ (watery /yellow)	+ + ++ (purulent)	+ + ++ (purulent)
Dryness	+ + +	−	−
Irritation/burning	++	+ + +	+ + +
Dyspareunia	++	+ + +	+ + +
Other	Itching, irritative urinary symptoms	Pruritus, malodor	Itching
Signs	Labial atrophy; epithelial thinning; loss of rugae; pale, dry appearance; submucosal petechial hemorrhages; fornices obliteration	Purulent discharge; erythema; ecchymotic spots; colpitis macularis.	White, lacy, reticulated margins; erosions; purulent discharge; intravaginal synechiae; vaginal narrowing, stenosis, or obliteration.
Laboratory findings			
pH	>4.5	>4.5	>4.5
Whiff test	Negative	Negative	Negative
Microscopy	Predominantly parabasal/intermediate EC*; scant flora, ↓ lactobacilli.	Multiple PMNs; ↓ squamous EC*; ↑ parabasal EC*; lactobacilli absent; ↑ cocci.	Multiple PMNs, multiple mononuclear cells, parabasal cells, variable flora.
Extra-vaginal manifestations	No	No	Yes

*EC-epithelial cells; PMNs-polymorphonuclear leukocytes.

does not correlate with symptoms [10]. Unfortunately, measuring serum estrogen levels does not aid in the diagnosis of atrophic vaginitis. Although the findings above establish an accurate diagnosis, symptoms alone dictate the need for treatment.

Treatment

Expert consensus opinion [2] recommends nonhormonal vaginal lubricants and moisturizers, as well as ongoing sexual activity, as first-line therapy for symptomatic vaginal atrophy. Regular coitus provides protection from atrophy, presumably by increasing the blood flow to the pelvic organs. However, from a practical point of view, painful intercourse is difficult to sustain. Lubricants are useful for relieving dryness during intercourse and are preferred by women who do not want to or cannot use hormones. Few controlled studies have assessed their effect and their long-term therapeutic effect is undocumented. One moisturizer, Replens, was shown to be as effective as local estrogen treatment in improving cytopathologic characteristics and vaginal moisture [11], and it achieved equivalent improvement of vaginal symptoms [12].

Despite these data, consensus opinion is that estrogen therapy, both systemic and topical, gives a more complete response than lubricants and moisturizers [2, 11]. Because the overall dose of estrogen is lower and is associated with less systemic absorption than oral or transdermal preparations, topical estrogen is generally considered safer and can be less concerning to patients. The most common side effects include vaginal bleeding, breast pain, nausea, and perineal pain. With topical estrogen therapies (Table 16.2), atrophic changes, including those observed with microscopy, rapidly and markedly reverse themselves. When it comes to choosing between various topical therapies, in the absence of adequate studies comparing commercially available and compounded options, individualized therapy is suggested [3].

Desquamative Inflammatory Vaginitis (DIV)

DIV is an uncommon clinical syndrome characterized by diffuse exudative inflammation of the vagina, profuse purulent discharge, and dyspareunia. Although the first description of DIV was published more than 50 years ago,

Table 16.2 Choices for vaginal therapy in AV.

	Product	Brand name	Dosing
Non-estrogen	Vaginal moisturisers	Replens	Every 2–3 days
Estrogen	Estradiol 0.01% vaginal cream	Estrace vaginal cream	2–4 g/day for 1–2 weeks, then 1 g/day
	Conjugated estrogen (0.625 mg/g) cream	Premarin vaginal cream	0.5–2 g/day
	Estradiol (0.025 mg) tablet	Vagifem	1/day for 2 weeks, then twice a week
	Estradiol (2 mg) vaginal ring	Estring	One ring every 3 months
	Estradiol (0.05 mg/day or 0.1 mg/day) vaginal ring	Femring[1]	One ring every 3 months

Adapted from North American Menopause Society [2].
[1]The Femring should be viewed as systemic therapy.

only a few small studies have been published since, and much about this condition remains poorly understood.

DIV was first described by Scheffey et al. in 1956, in a single patient [13]. Subsequently Gardner [14] described a series of eight patients with classic complaints and physical findings, defined the clinical and cytological characteristics of this type of vaginitis, and named the condition DIV. In his primary description, Gardner stated that "in many respects, this vaginitis resembles atrophic vaginitis, although it appears in women with normal estrogen levels."

Although this statement reflects some of the overlap that may exist between DIV and atrophic vaginitis, it is unclear how estrogen levels were measured in Gardner's study. In 1994, Sobel [15] described a group of 51 patients with DIV, both pre- and postmenopausal, identified epidemiologic characteristics, and suggested intravaginal clindamycin as a treatment. As Sobel found DIV in patients with a hypo-estrogenic state as well as in those with preserved ovarian function [15], it is clear that DIV is a separate entity from AV.

Epidemiology

Although DIV is considered rare, its occurrence in the general population is unknown. Its prevalence among patients presenting to referral practices for chronic vulvovaginal problems varies between 0.7% [15] and 8% [16]. DIV tends to be chronic, with the mean duration of symptoms >31 months and it affects mostly Caucasian women (94%) [15]. Although DIV is found over a broad age range, it is encountered primarily in older women. In Sobel's series [15], the mean age was 41.8 years old, and 37% of the patients were menopausal. Although most of these

menopausal patients were receiving hormonal therapy at presentation, many of them were not on hormonal therapy when the symptoms began. Low estrogen was also described as a precipitating factor in an additional 35% of the patients as they were either perimenopausal, lactating, or on anti-estrogenic treatment.

Etiology

The etiology of DIV is poorly understood. Factors such as vaginal flora alteration, changes in hormonal status, and association with other dermatoses occur in women with DIV, but their causal relationship is unclear. The microscopic findings in vaginal secretions indicate an inflammatory state with alteration of vaginal flora (Figure 16.2). Vaginal biopsies, when taken, reveal nonspecific features of an inflammatory reaction [15]. In general, Gram stain of vaginal secretions shows an absence of lactobacilli and an increase in Gram-positive cocci [14, 15]. Group B streptococci were found in 44% of the cases studied but is not considered the cause of DIV [15]. Cultures for traditional pathogenic organisms are generally negative [17].

Because the majority of patients are hypo-estrogenic, estrogen deficiency seems to play a role in the pathogenesis of DIV, by means of a mechanism that has yet to be defined. However, a lack of estrogen alone does not seem to be the true cause of DIV because affected women do not improve with estrogen alone.

DIV may, at times, accompany various dermatoses, including erosive lichen planus (ELP), pemphigus vulgaris, and mucous membrane pemphigoid. In the absence of extravaginal manifestations or a clear-cut biopsy result, ELP is often indistinguishable from DIV. Whether DIV is a

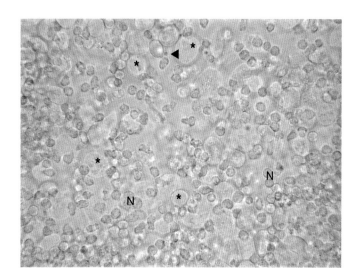

Figure 16.2 Microscopic findings in DIV. This wet mount shows a high number of PMNs (N), an under-representation of mature squamous cells, an increase in the number of immature, parabasal cells (*), an absence in lactobacilli, and a coccoid flora (arrow). (Courtesy of Jack Sobel, MD, Wayne State University School of Medicine, Detroit, MI.)

separate entity or is in reality undiagnosed vaginal ELP is a source of active debate among specialists [17–19]. Murphy and Edwards [20] suggest that some inflammations may be caused by ELP, whereas others may indeed be an idiopathic subset of DIV. Sobel [15] defined his patients as having isolated DIV, without any characteristics typical to ELP. Table 16.1 highlights the similarities and differences between atrophic vaginitis, DIV, and ELP.

Diagnosis

The most common manifestation of DIV is a copious, purulent vaginal discharge. Among women suffering from DIV, 90% of sexually active patients complain of dyspareunia. As DIV is primarily a vaginal condition, the pain occurs mainly with thrusting. However, when DIV causes vestibular inflammation or erosions, patients may have introital dyspareunia as well. Some patients may not complain of dyspareunia because they have ceased having intercourse due to the abnormal discharge. Other symptoms include vulvovaginal burning and irritation [15].

Patients may exhibit findings of vulvar erythema and introital ecchymotic spots. Vaginal examination reveals diffuse erythema and a purulent yellow or green vaginal discharge in all patients. Some patients may have ecchymotic spots on the upper third of the vagina or on the cervix. Similar to atrophic vaginitis, the pH is elevated and microscopy shows parabasal cells, but the presence of many polymorphonuclear leukocytes (PMNs) and

a heavy coccoid flora establishes the diagnosis of DIV (Figure 16.2) [3].

The differential diagnosis for DIV includes other disorders causing purulent vaginitis. These include infectious vaginitis such as trichomoniasis and Group A streptococcal vaginitis, dermatologic disorders such as ELP, mucosal blistering disorders, mucous membrane pemphigoid, and vulvo-gingival syndrome. It is therefore essential to examine the mouth and eyes as part of the evaluation [17], and to perform bacterial cultures specifically for Group A streptococci and cultures or polymerase chain reaction (PCR) for trichomonas prior to initiating therapy. Purulent vaginitis can also result from usage of chemical irritants, such as fluorouracil for genital warts [21]. Because of the similarities between atrophic vaginitis and DIV, the two entities may be difficult to distinguish from each other. With atrophic vaginitis the epithelial surface remains intact, and response to local estrogen therapy is usually rapid. Thus, failure to reverse the abnormal appearance of the vulvar vestibule or vagina and consequent symptoms with topical estrogen therapy constitutes a diagnostic test [22].

Treatment

There are no controlled studies of therapies for DIV. Treatment consists of either antibiotic or corticosteroid therapy. In 1994, Sobel [15] described the use of intravaginal clindamycin to treat DIV. In this retrospective study, which occurred prior to the approval of 2% vaginal clindamycin cream, Sobel evaluated 51 patients who had received 14 days of 200 mg clindamycin suppositories. Overall, there was an improvement in > 95% of cases, with a relapse rate of 30%. In the authors' clinical experience, a two-week course of 2% clindamycin cream, 5 g administered nightly, works similarly to the clindamycin suppositories described by Sobel. It is thought that the effect of clindamycin on DIV may be due to its potent anti-inflammatory properties [22].

Some practitioners consider corticosteroids to be the drug of choice for DIV. The use of intravaginal hydrocortisone, alone or in combination with clindamycin, has been suggested [22]. The suggested protocol is daily use of 4–5 g of 10% hydrocortisone cream inserted intravaginally. The regimen is well-tolerated and highly effective; a dramatic clinical response can be expected within 2 weeks in patients with mild to moderate vaginitis [22]. The duration of therapy remains undetermined, and there are no additional published studies analyzing the response rates to various therapies in DIV patients. With both topical clindamycin and hydrocortisone, most experts will retreat patients who relapse, generally with a longer course of therapy.

Finally, postmenopausal patients with DIV may show a suboptimal response because of associated AV. This can happen even in women receiving systemic hormone therapy. The addition of once- or twice-weekly intravaginal estrogen preparations is often helpful and may be required to maintain remission [15].

Summary

Atrophic vaginitis and DIV are the most common noninfectious causes of vaginitis. Some similarities exist between these two separate entities, potentially complicating or delaying appropriate diagnosis and intervention. Left untreated, both types of vaginitis can result in years of vulvovaginal discomfort and dyspareunia, resulting in a negative impact on quality of life. As the number of menopausal women is expected to rise, practitioners can expect to see an increase in the number of women with symptomatic vaginal atrophy. Because many affected women may not volunteer their symptoms, a thorough history, addressing both physiologic and psychological factors, is critical to the successful treatment of these patients. It is therefore essential for health care providers who treat this population to be familiar with these entities and their treatment modalities.

References

1 Graziottin A. (2003) Etiology and diagnosis of coital pain. *Journal of Endocrinological Investigation* **26**, 115–21.
2 NAMS: North American Menopause Society. (2007) The role of local vaginal estrogen for treatment of vaginal atrophy in postmenopausal women: 2007 position statement of the North American Menopause Society. *Menopause* **14**, 357–69.
3 Nyirjesy P. (2007) Postmenopausal vaginitis. *Current Infectious Disease Reports* **9**, 480–84.
4 Hillier SL, Lau RJ. (1997) Vaginal microflora in postmenopausal women who have not received estrogen replacement therapy. *Clinical Infectious Diseases* **25**, S123–26.
5 Cotreau MM, Chennathukuzhi VM, Harris HA, *et al.* (2007) A study of 17β-estradiol-regulated genes in the vagina of postmenopausal women with vaginal atrophy, *Maturitas* **58**, 366–76.
6 Sarrel PM. (1990) Sexuality and menopause. *Obstetrics and Gynecology* **75**, 26S–30S.
7 Graziottin A, Leiblum SR. (2005) Biological and psychosocial pathophysiology of female sexual dysfunction during the menopausal transition. *The Journal of Sexual Medicne* **2**, 133–45.
8 Kovalevsky G. (2005) Female sexual dysfunction and use of hormone therapy in postmenopausal women. *Seminars in Reproductive Medicine* **23**,180–87.
9 Johnston SL, Farrell SA, Bouchard C, *et al.* (2004) The detection and management of vaginal atrophy. *Journal of Obstetetrics and Gynaecology Canada* **26**, 503–15.
10 Davila GW, Singh A, Karapanagiotou I, *et al.* (2003) Are women with urogenital atrophy symptomatic? *American Journal of Obstetrics and Gynecology* **188**, 382–88.
11 Bygdeman M, Swahn ML. (1996) Replens versus dienestrol cream in the symptomatic treatment of vaginal atrophy in postmenopausal women. *Maturitas* **23**, 259–63.
12 Nachtigall LE. (1994) Comparative study: Replens versus local estrogen in menopausal women. *Fertility and Sterility* **61**, 178–80.
13 Scheffey LC, Rakoff AE, Lang WR. (1956) An unusual case of exudative vaginitis (hydrorrhea vaginalis) treated with local hydrocortisone. *American Journal of Obstetrics and Gynecology* **72**, 208–11.
14 Gardner HL. (1968) Desquamative inflammatory vaginitis: a newly defined entity. *American Journal of Obstetrics and Gynecology* **102**, 1102–05.
15 Sobel JD. (1994) Desquamative inflammatory vaginitis: a new subgroup of purulent vaginitis responsive to topical 2%

clindamycin therapy. *American Journal of Obstetrics and Gynecology* **171**, 1215–20.

16 Nyirjesy P, Peyton C, Weitz MV, *et al.* (2006) Causes of chronic vaginitis: analysis of a prospective database of affected women. *Obstetrics and Gynecology* **108**, 1185–91.

17 Murphy R. (2004) Desquamative inflammatory vaginitis. *Dermatologic Therapy* **17**, 47–49.

18 Edwards L. (1992) Desquamative vulvitis. *Dermatologic Clinics* **10**, 325–37.

19 Pelisse M. (1989) The vulvo-vaginal-gingival syndrome. A new form of erosive lichen planus. *International Journal of Dermatology* **28**, 381–84.

20 Murphy R, Edwards L. (2004) Sterile inflammatory vaginitis: what is it? *The Journal of Reproductive Medicine* **11**, 933.

21 Sobel JD. (2000) Nontrichomonal purulent vaginitis: clinical approach. *Current Infectious Diseases Report* **2**, 501–5.

22 Sobel JD. (2003) Erosive vulvovaginitis. *Current Infectious Diseases Report* **5**, 494–98.

CHAPTER 17
Pudendal Neuralgia

Philip W.H. Peng,[1,3] *Stanley J. Antolak, Jr.,*[2] *Allan S. Gordon*[3]

[1] Toronto Western Hospital, University of Toronto, Toronto, Ontario, Canada

[2] Center for Urologic and Pelvic Pain, Lake Elmo, MN, USA

[3] Wasser Pain Management Center, University of Toronto, Toronto, Ontario, Canada

Definition

Chronic pelvic pain involving the sensory distribution of the pudendal nerve is termed *pudendal neuralgia*. Perineologists (perineology is a neologism which means the study of the perineum) [1] use the term *pudendal neuropathy*, which encompasses a spectrum of clinical presentations suggestive of pudendal nerve dysfunction including hyperesthesia, hypoesthesia, and urinary and fecal incontinence. The confirmatory test for pudendal neuropathy is an increase in pudendal nerve terminal motor latencies [2]. In contrast, pudendal *neuralgia* represents another aspect of pudendal nerve dysfunction, which is characterized by *pain* in the territory innervated by the pudendal nerve (Figure 17.1) [3]. In patients with neuropathic pain, electrophysiological testing will exclude some patients who can potentially benefit from pain management [4–6].

Clinical Presentation

There are no published data on the prevalence of pudendal neuralgia. It is more common in females, with a female/male ratio of 2.5:1 [3, 7, 8]. The mean age of presentation is in the sixth decade of life but ranges from 25 to 80 years old.

The pertinent clinical feature is pain in the territory innervated by the pudendal nerve. This includes the anterior and posterior urogenital areas (vulva, clitoris, and perianal

Female Sexual Pain Disorders 1st edition. Edited by A. Goldstein, C. Pukall & I. Goldstein. © 2009 Blackwell Publishing, ISBN: 9781405183987.

area) [3, 4, 7]. The pain may be unilateral or bilateral. The classic presentation includes pain that is exacerbated with sitting. Pain may be alleviated (or diminished) by standing, lying on the nonpainful side, or sitting on a toilet seat. However, this relationship with posture may not be readily apparent, probably due to the process of central sensitization. The onset is typically gradual and the pain is usually described as severe burning and aching, and may be associated with a foreign body sensation in the rectum or vagina. Bowel and bladder disturbances are not common.

In those patients presenting with perineal pain, the most common finding is pain when the examiner applies pressure against the ischial spine during a rectal or vaginal examination. Sensory testing of the perineum may reveal hypoesthesia, hyperalgesia, or allodynia.

Anatomy

The pudendal nerve is formed from the anterior rami of the second, third, and fourth sacral nerves (S2, S3, and S4). Exiting the pelvis through the greater sciatic foramen, the pudendal nerve is accompanied by the internal pudendal artery on its medial side and travels dorsal to the sacrospinous ligament abutting the attachment of the latter to the ischial spine (Figure 17.2a). At this level, the nerve is situated between the sacrospinous and sacrotuberous ligament (interligamentous plane) [3, 9, 10–12]. The nerve then swings ventrally to enter the pelvis through the lesser sciatic foramen and enters Alcock's canal [12]. Alcock's canal is the fascial tunnel formed by the duplication of the obturator internus muscle under the plane of the

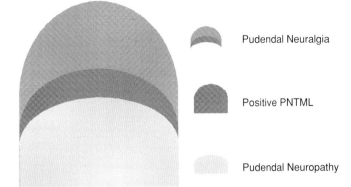

Figure 17.1 Different ways of looking at pudendal nerve syndrome. A subset of patients with pudendal neuralgia may have abnormalities in PNTML. PNTML–pudendal nerve terminal motor latency.

levator ani muscle on the lateral wall of ischiorectal fossa (Figure 17.2b).

The pudendal nerve subsequently gives off three terminal branches: the dorsal nerve of the clitoris, the inferior rectal nerve, and the perineal nerve, providing the sensory branches to the skin of the perianal area, labia majora, and clitoris. It also innervates the external anal sphincter (inferior rectal nerve) and deep muscles of the urogenital triangle (perineal nerve) [12, 13]. The path of the pudendal nerve between the sacrotuberous and the sacrospinous

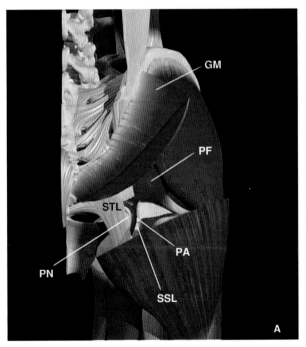

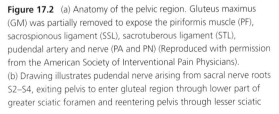

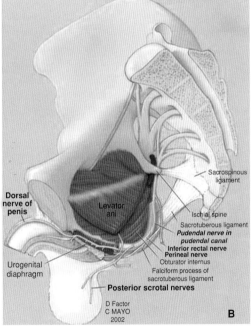

Figure 17.2 (a) Anatomy of the pelvic region. Gluteus maximus (GM) was partially removed to expose the piriformis muscle (PF), sacrospionous ligament (SSL), sacrotuberous ligament (STL), pudendal artery and nerve (PA and PN) (Reproduced with permission from the American Society of Interventional Pain Physicians). (b) Drawing illustrates pudendal nerve arising from sacral nerve roots S2–S4, exiting pelvis to enter gluteal region through lower part of greater sciatic foramen and reentering pelvis through lesser sciatic foramen. Pudendal nerve gives rise to inferior rectal nerve, perineal nerve, and dorsal nerve of penis or clitoris. Inferior rectal nerve arises from pudendal nerve before entering Alcock's canal. Note the location of falciform process of sacrotuberous ligament, which is possible site for pudendal nerve entrapment. (Reprinted from Ref. 10 with permission of the Mayo Foundation for Medical Education and Research.)

ligaments, or through Alcock's canal, makes it susceptible to entrapment as it is fixed in these locations [3, 8]. The course of the dorsal nerve of the penis under the subpubic arch or sulcus nervi dorsalis penis exposes the nerve to compression by the nose of the saddle of the bicycle [14]. The configuration of the nerve across the pelvis simulates a hammock hanging in the pelvis, resulting in susceptibility of the nerve to stretch during vaginal delivery [15].

Etiology

In most patients, the onset of symptoms is gradual and no causative factors can be identified. However, a few conditions are known to be associated with pudendal neuralgia.

Bicycle riding is well known to be associated with genital numbness and perineal pain secondary to pudendal nerve compression and/or stretch injury [16]. The pressures that are applied on the perineum of the cyclists by the saddle nose have been shown to be above the threshold pressure known to cause ischemic injury [16, 17]. The severity of the neuronal damage is dictated mainly by the duration of the pressure, rather than the amount of pressure.

Vaginal childbirth may significantly alter pudendal nerve conduction patterns [18]. The dorso-ventral course of the pudendal nerve crossing the base of the pelvis makes it susceptible to stretch injury during fetal descent. A 3D computer-simulated vaginal delivery study demonstrated that the strain on the inferior rectal nerve and the perineal branch to the anal sphincter reaches 35% and 33%, respectively, far exceeding the 15% strain threshold known to cause permanent damage in peripheral nerves [19–20].

Orthopedic procedures requiring the use of the traction table can result in pudendal nerve injury secondary to direct pressure of the countertraction device on the pudendal nerve [20, 21]. Other conditions that may be associated with pudendal neuralgia are pelvic fracture, colpopexy (vaginal vault suspension procedures) [22], pelvic radiation [23], and intense athletic activities [24].

Diagnosis of Pudendal Neuralgia

The diagnosis of pudendal neuralgia is based on clinical symptoms: chronic debilitating perineal pain that is usually exacerbated in the seated position and relieved by standing [3]. Other tests are helpful in formulating the diagnosis and include pudendal nerve terminal motor latency testing (PNTMLT), quantitative sensory testing,

and pudendal nerve block. Because nerve blocks are both diagnostic and therapeutic, they will be described in both the diagnosis and management sections. Magnetic resonance imaging (MRI) is generally not very useful except to exclude some rare structural abnormalities around the course of the pudendal nerve.

Neurophysiologic Testing

Several neurophysiologic tests can confirm the presence of pudendal "neuropathy." These include sensory-evoked potentials, motor-evoked potentials, and bulbocavernosus latency testing [25, 26]. Electromyography of the external urethral and anal sphincters as well as the bulbocavernosus and ischiocavernosus muscles may show denervation and reinnervation [27]. The quantitative sensory test (QST) called the warm detection threshold (WDT) is a sensitive test for pudendal neuropathy [28]. It uses the NTE-2A Thermosensory Tester (Physitemp, Inc., Clifton, NJ) and follows a stepping algorithm [29].

The three branches of the pudendal nerve are measured bilaterally. Failure to detect warm temperature properly is indicative of neuropathy. The PNTMLT uses a St. Mark's surface electrode (Alpine Biomed, Fountain Valley, CA) [30]. A prolonged PNTMLT (>2.2 msec) is specific for motor neuropathy; however, the sensitivity of this test is limited because it measures only one branch of the pudendal nerve. Dysesthesias may be reproduced by both temperature and electronic test stimuli and indicate neuropathy. Findings may include evocation of subjective pain, bladder pressure or urgency, and rectal pain. The QST and PNTMLT are both practical for use in the clinician's office.

Pudendal Nerve Block

As with other neuralgias arising from a peripheral nerve, nerve blockade is crucial in both diagnosis and treatment [31]. Various pudendal nerve injection techniques have been described via different routes: transvaginal (TV) [32], transperineal [33, 34] and transgluteal (TG). The TG approach is the most popular approach and permits blockade at the ischial spine and in Alcock's canal. In addition, the TG approach can be guided by different imaging techniques: fluoroscopy [3], computed tomography (CT) [35, 36], or ultrasonography [37, 38].

Typically, after performing a diagnostic block at the ischial level, a second block at Alcock's canal is performed. At this level, a CT-guided block is the only technique that can reliably guide the needle into the canal. In clinical practice, the injection of both local anesthetic and steroid allows the pudendal nerve block to serve as both a diagnostic and therapeutic intervention.

In every patient, a baseline sensory test must be established before the nerve block. A diary for the pain score both at rest and sitting down is important for the patient to document the pain relief. A second and even third block is advisable to confirm the consistency of response because of the possibility of placebo effect. Patients who do not develop temporary pain relief despite exhibiting a sensory block in the perineum following a series of pudendal nerve blocks should be re-evaluated for another diagnosis.

Management of Pudendal Neuralgia

Patients with pudendal neuralgia can be managed with a stepwise approach: modification of activities, pharmacological measures, physical therapy, pudendal nerve block, and surgical management.

Modification of Activities

In patients with pudendal neuralgia, perineal pain is aggravated by sitting but is usually relieved upon sitting on a toilet seat. The increase in pain is related to the increased pressure on the perineum with sitting, which can be minimized by sitting on a wide "donut" cushion or some improvised sitting pad that avoids pressure on the perineum.

Pharmacological Measures

Although no controlled trial has been conducted on the pharmacological management of pudendal neuralgia, the choice of neuropathic pain medication should be similar to other neuropathic pain syndromes. Tricyclic antidepressants and gabapentinoids (gabapentin, pregabalin) are generally considered first-line agents because of their efficacy and low side effect profile [39, 40]. Selective norepinephrine reuptake inhibitors (SNRIs) have also recently been shown to be effective for the treatment of neuropathy [39]. A thorough discussion of oral medication used for neuropathic pain can be found in Chapter 17.

Physical Therapy

The impairments from pudendal neuralgia can extend to include structural, muscular, and connective tissue dysfunctions, resulting in functional limitations and disability. The physical therapist can help this group of patients to minimize the impairment and functional limitation with various techniques [41] as discussed in Chapter 13.

Pudendal Nerve Block

Considering the diagnostic and therapeutic purposes of the pudendal nerve block, we suggest a protocol of three blocks, two at the ischial spine level and one at Alcock's canal, performed on a monthly basis. The block can last for hours, days, weeks, or months. Unfortunately, the long-term response rate is unknown. Most studies to date have not excluded nonresponders in the long-term evaluation of pudendal injections. It is likely that initial nonresponders had an incorrect diagnosis of pudendal neuralgia. Despite this, Amarenco suggested a 15% response rate at 1 year [7]. In the authors' institution (Peng and Gordon), the 3-month response rate was 66%, which drops to 33%

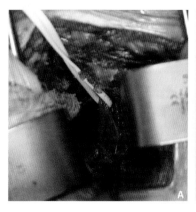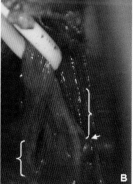

Figure 17.3 (a) The right pudendal nerve has been decompressed. A small inferior rectal nerve is narrow and flattened (left) similar to the main trunk (right). Normal volume and shape of nerve is evident in the vessel loop. (b) Enlarged picture of the nerve with the vessel loop.

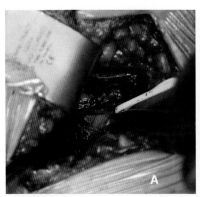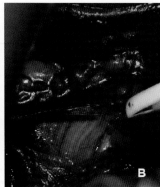

Figure 17.4 (a) Exposure of the left ischiorectal fossa via an oblique incision between sacrum (superiorly) to ischial tuberosity (inferiorly). The pudendal nerve is identified after opening the fascia over the obturator muscle (the pudendal canal). The nerve is flattened, its fibers splayed, and fascicles are apparent. The changes are caused by repetitive flexion of the muscle forcing the nerve against the fascia, which in this case is thicker than usual. Pallor of the nerve suggests vascular impairment. Perineurium is not seen. Anatomic evidence of compression in the pudendal canal occurs in fewer than 10% of our surgeries. (b) Enlarged picture of the nerve with pickups holding fascia open.

at 6 months for those who initially reported temporary relief from the block.

The pudendal nerve block can be repeated. There is no general consensus on the maximum number of nerve blocks that may be given, but we consider it advisable to avoid more than six injections per year to minimize the systemic effects of steroid.

Pudendal Nerve Decompression Surgery

Pudendal neuropathy is a "tunnel syndrome" that may require decompression surgery in over one-third of patients. The "clamp" between the sacrotuberous and sacrospinous ligaments must be released by transecting the sacrospinous ligament (90%) or decompressing the pudendal canal (<10%). The pathophysiology and effectiveness of a transgluteal approach were described by Robert et al. [3]. This incision permits visualization of the nerve from above the ischial spine to the urogenital diaphragm. Anomalies of the nerve and ligaments are common; therefore, the procedure requires meticulous dissection (Figures 17.3 and 17.4). Other decompression techniques include a pararectal incision, a transperineal approach, and a laparoscopic approach [42–44].

Surgical success rates range from 60% to 70%, but pain-free status may require 4–5 years. Bladder, bowel, and sexual dysfunctions show variable improvement

[45]. Neurophysiological tests may improve after surgery [45]. Surgical complications are typically of short duration and may include neuropraxia with patchy areas of numbness, occasional aggravation of pain, and urinary hesitancy. Persistent symptoms beyond 4–6 months require re-evaluation for concurrent neuropathies (ilioinguinal, middle cluneal) and attention to spinal cord wind-up (sensitization).

Conclusion

Pudendal neuralgia can be debilitating and is associated with significant functional limitations and disability. The diagnosis is based on clinical presentation, neurophysiologic testing, and nerve blockade. Pudendal neuralgia is managed with a multimodal approach including modification of activities, pharmacological treatment, physical therapy, pudendal nerve block and, in refractory cases, surgery.

References

1 Beco J, Mouchel J. (2002) Understanding the concept of perineology. *International Urogynecology Journal and Pelvic Floor Dysfunction* **13**, 275–77.
2 Beco J. Pudendal neuropathy: one of the main "defects" in perineology. Available at: http://www.perineology.com/files/beco-athens2006.pdf.

3 Robert R, Prat-Pradal D, Labat JJ, *et al.* (1998) Anatomic basis of chronic perineal pain: role of the pudendal nerve. *Surgical and Radiologic Anatomy* **20**, 93–8.

4 Benson JT, Griffis K. (2005) Pudendal neuralgia, a severe pain syndrome. *Amercan Journal of Obstetrics and Gynecology* **192**, 1663–68.

5 Lefaucheur J-P, Labat J-J, Amarenco G, *et al.* (2007) What is the place of electroneuromyographic studies in the diagnosis and management of pudendal neuralgia related to entrapment syndrome? *Neurophysiologie Clinique* **37**, 223–28.

6 Graham B, Regehr G, Naglie G, *et al.* (2006) Development and validation of diagnostic criteria for carpal tunnel syndrome. *Journal of Hand Surgery* **31A**, 919.e1–919.e7.

7 Amarenco G, Kerdraon J, Bouju P, *et al.* (1997) Treatments of perineal neuralgia caused by involvement of the pudendal nerve. *Revue Neurologique* **153**, 331–34.

8 Robert R, Labat JJ, Bensignor M, *et al.* (2005) Decompression and transposition of the pudendal nerve in pudendal neuralgia: a randomized controlled trial and long-term evaluation. *European Urology* **47**, 403–8.

9 Mahakkanukrauh P, Surin P, Vaidhayakarn P. (2005) Anatomical study of the pudendal nerve adjacent to the sacrospinous ligament. *Clinical Anatomy* **18**, 200–35.

10 Hough DM, Wittenberg KH, Pawlina W, *et al.* (2003) Chronic perineal pain caused by pudendal nerve entrapment: anatomy and CT-guided perineural injection technique. *AJR American Journal of Roentgenology* **181**, 561–67.

11 Shafik A, Doss SH. (1999) Pudendal canal: surgical anatomy and clinical implications. *American Surgery* **65**, 176–80.

12 Shafik A, el-Sherif M, Youssef A, *et al.* (1995) Surgical anatomy of the pudendal nerve and its clinical implications. *Clinical Anatomy* **8**, 110–15.

13 Schraffordt SE, Tjandra JJ, Eizenberg N (2004) Anatomy of the pudendal nerve and its terminal branches: a cadaver study. *ANZ Journal of Surgery* **74**, 23–26.

14 Sedy J, Nanka O, Belisova M, Walro JM, *et al.* (2006) Sulcus nervi dorsalis penis/clitoridis: anatomic structure and clinical significance. *European Urology* **50**, 1079–85.

15 Ashton-Miller JA, Delancey JOL. (2007) Functional anatomy of the female pelvic floor. *Annals of the New York Academy of Sciences* **1101**, 266–96.

16 Leibovitcha I, Morb Y. (2005) The vicious cycling: bicycling related urogenital disorders. *European Urology* **47**, 277–87.

17 Schrader SM, Breitenstein MJ, Clark JC, *et al.* (2002) Nocturnal penile tumescence and rigidity testing in bicycling patrol officers. *Journal of Andrology* **23**, 927–34.

18 Allen RE, Hosker GL, Smith AR, *et al.* (1990) Pelvic floor damage and childbirth: a neurophysiological study. *BJOG* **97**, 770–79.

19 Lien KC, Morgan DM, Delancey JOL, *et al.* (2005) Pudendal nerve stretch during vaginal birth: a 3D computer simulation. *American Journal of Obstetrics and Gynecology* **192**, 1669–76.

20 Soulie M, Vazzoler N, Seguin P, *et al.* (2002) Urological consequences of pudendal nerve trauma during orthopedic surgery: review and practical advice. *Progrés en Urologie* **12**, 504–9.

21 Amarenco G, Ismael SS, Bayle A, *et al.* (2001) Electrophysiological anlaysis of pudendal neuropathy following traction. *Muscle and Nerve* **24**, 116–19.

22 Alevizon SJ, Finan MA. (1996) Sacrospinous colpopexy: management of postoperative pudendal nerve entrapment. *Obstetrics and Gynecology* **88**, 713–15.

23 Antolak SJ, Hough DM, Pawlina W. (2002) The chronic pelvic pain syndrome after brachytherapy for carcinoma of the prostate. *Journal of Urology* **167**, 2525.

24 Antolak S, Hough D, Pawlina W, *et al.* (2002) Anatomical basis of chronic pelvic pain syndrome: the ischial spine and pudendal nerve entrapment. *Medical Hypotheses* **59**, 349–53.

25 Amarenco G, Ismael SS, Bayle B, *et al.* (2001) Electrophysiological analysis of pudendal neuropathy following traction. *Muscle and Nerve* **24**, 116–19.

26 Ricchiutu VS, Haas CA, Seftel AD, *et al.* (2000) Pudendal nerve injury associated with avid bicycling. *Journal of Urology* **162**, 2099–2100.

27 Benson JT. Neurophysiology of the female pelvic floor. (1994) *Current Opinion in Obstetrics and Gynecology* **6**, 320–23.

28 Bleustein CB, Eckholdt E, Arezzo JC, *et al.* (2003) Quantitative somatosensory testing of the penis: optimizing the clinical neurological examination. *Journal of Urology* **169**, 2266–69.

29 Dyck PJ, O'Brien PC, Kosanke JL, *et al.* (1993) A 4, 2, and 1 stepping algorithm for quick and accurate estimation of cutaneous sensation threshold. *Neurology* **43**, 1508–12.

30 Snooks SJ, Swash M. (1984) Abnormalities of the innervation of the urethral striated sphincter musculature in incontinence. *British Journal of Urology* **56**, 410–15.

31 Hogan QH, Abram SE. (1997) Neural blockade for diagnosis and prognosis: a review. *Anesthesiology* **86**, 216–41.

32 Bowes WA. (1989) Clinical aspects of normal and abnormal labor. In: Creasy RK, Resnik R. (eds.) *Maternal–Fetal Medicine: Principles and Practice*, 2nd ed. WB Saunders, Philadelphia, pp. 510–46.

33 Naja Z, Ziade MF, Lonnqvist PA. (2005) Nerve stimulator–guided pudendal nerve block decreases posthemorrhoidectomy pain. *Canadian Journal of Anesthesiology* **52**, 62–68.

34 Imbelloni LE, Vieira EM, Gouveia MA, *et al.* (2007) Pudendal block with bupivacaine for postoperative pain relief. *Diseases of the Colon and Rectum* **50**, 1656–61.

35 Shafik A. (1998) Pudendal canal syndrome as a cause of vul-
    vodynia and its treatment by pudendal nerve decompression.
    European Journal of Obstetrics and Gynecology **80**, 215–20.

36 Calvillo O, Skaribas IM, Rockett C. (2000) Computed
    tomography–guided pudendal nerve block: a new diagnos-
    tic approach to long-term anoperineal pain: a report of two
    cases. *Regional Anesthesia and Pain Medicine* **25**, 420–23.

37 Rofaeel A, Peng PWH, Chan VWS. (2008) Feasibility of real-
    time ultrasound for pudendal nerve block inpatients with
    chronic perineal pain. *Regional Anesthesia and Pain Medicine*
    33, 139–45.

38 Peng PWH, Tumber PS. (2008) Ultrasound-guided interven-
    tional procedures for patients with chronic pelvic pain: a
    description of techniques and review of the literature. *Pain
    Physician* **11**, 215–24.

39 Dworkin RH, O'Connor AB, Backonja M, *et al.* (2007) Phar-
    macologic management of neuropathic pain: evidence-based
    recommendations. *Pain* **132**, 237–51.

40 Moulin DE, Clark AJ, Gilron I, *et al.* (2007) Pharmacologic
    management of chronic neuropathic pain: consensus state-
    ment and guidelines from the Canadian Pain Society. *Pain
    Management Research* **12**, 13–21.

41 Prendergast, SA, Rummer, EH. (2007) The role of physical
    therapy in the treatment of pudendal neuralgia. *Vision* **15**,
    1–2.

42 Shafik A. (1992). The posterior approach in the treatment of
    pudendal canal syndrome. *Coloproctology* **14**, 310–15.

43 Beco J, Climov D, Bex M. (2004) Pudendal nerve decompres-
    sion in perineology: a case series. *BMC Surgery* **4**, 15.

44 Bautrant E, de Bisschop E, Vaini-Elies V, *et al.* (2003) Modern
    algorithms for treating pudendal neuralgia; 2122 cases and
    104 decompressions. *Journal de Gynécologie, Obstétrique et
    Biologie de la Reproduction* **32**, 705–12.

45 Shafik A. (1998) Pudendal canal syndrome. A new etiological
    factor in prostadynia and its treatment by pudendal canal
    decompression. *Pain Digest* **8**, 32–36.

CHAPTER 18

Congenital Anomalies of the Female Genital Tract

Lara J. Burrows

The Center for Vulvovaginal Disorders, Washington, DC, USA

Introduction

Congenital anomalies of the female genital tract are uncommon and may be challenging to diagnose. While the evaluation of these conditions is not typically performed in a sexual pain center, women with these conditions may present for evaluation of sexual dysfunction which may include dyspareunia. This chapter will review the embryology of the lower female genital tract and the more common congenital anomalies. Management of these patients should entail a multidisciplinary approach led by a compassionate provider who is experienced in managing women with sexual pain.

Early Development of the Female Genital Tract

The prevalence of Müllerian anomalies is 2–3% [1]. Although the genitalia of the developing embryo may be affected at any time during development, the gonads do not acquire their male or female phenotype until the seventh week of development [2]. Most anomalies result from the arrest of development of the uterovaginal primordium during the eighth week; usually there is a failure of the Müllerian ducts to fuse properly, resulting in structural abnormalities of the uterus, fallopian tubes, and upper vagina [3].

It is beyond the scope of this book to discuss in detail human female genital embryology, but a few key concepts

Female Sexual Pain Disorders 1st edition. Edited by A. Goldstein, C. Pukall & I. Goldstein. © 2009 Blackwell Publishing, ISBN: 9781405183987.

should be noted. In the absence of Müllerian-inhibiting substance, the Müllerian (paramesonephric) ducts develop into the uterus, fallopian tubes, and upper third of the vagina. The Wolffian (mesonephric) ducts regress and differentiate into the labia majora, labia minora, and clitoris. The caudal tip of the Müllerian duct fuses with the urogenital sinus to form the vaginal plate and by the fifth month, the vagina is entirely canalized [3]. Interestingly, the vulva is unique in that it is the only place in the human body where all three embryologic layers (ectoderm, mesoderm, and endoderm) may be visualized together. The vulvar vestibule itself is mesodermal in origin, whereas the tissues distal to it are derived from ectoderm, and those proximal to it are from the endoderm.

Lastly, anomalies of the urinary tract appear in approximately 23% of patients with malformations of the genital tract. Therefore, when a congenital anomaly is found in the lower genital tract, the upper genital and tract and urologic system should be evaluated.

Dyspareunia and Specific Congenital Anomalies of the Female Genital Tract

Given that female sexual pain has only recently become a topic of scientific study and given that congenital anomalies of the female genital tract are uncommon, it is not surprising that there is a paucity of data on the subject of dyspareunia in women with congenital malformations. Nevertheless, congenital anomalies may be associated with female sexual dysfunction and sexual pain. Therefore, they should be considered when evaluating a patient with dyspareunia. Congenital anomalies of the vulva and vagina may be classified as (1) developmental abnormalities of external genitalia; (2) genetic and chromosomal abnormalities; and (3) anomalies associated with uterovaginal and vulvovaginal abnormalities. Although many conditions may be associated with anomalies of the lower female genital tract, this chapter will discuss the more commonly described conditions.

The Clitoris

Clitoral hypertrophy is most commonly seen in association with congenital adrenal hyperplasia (discussed below). While it is quite possible that adult women with clitoral hypertrophy might have discomfort with intercourse, the vast majority of females with this condition are diagnosed and managed in early childhood. The treatment for clitoral hypertrophy is surgical correction by means of a reduction clitoroplasty, and more recently, a nerve-sparing clitoroplasty has been described [4].

Periclitoral abscesses, a rare cause of dyspareunia, are uncommon in women who have not undergone female genital cutting (see Chapter 36). However, noncircumcised females who develop a periclitoral abscess caused by a pilonidal sinus tract have been reported [5]. This condition may be diagnosed with history and physical examination and treated with marsupialization and antibiotic therapy if needed.

The Vulva

Congenital labia fusion is typically seen in female infants with female pseudohermaphroditism (an individual who is genetically XX, and phenotypically male or has ambiguous genitalia; see below). Acquired labial agglutination, as its name implies, is not a congenital disorder, yet it may be misdiagnosed as labioscrotal fusion (implying a genetic or chromosomal etiology) in young children. Labial agglutination has also been observed in postmenopausal women [6]. Although it is uncommon, it is likely that this condition would be associated with dyspareunia.

Approximately 43% of women with hypertrophic (enlarged) labia minora complain of discomfort with intercourse [7]. This condition may be congenital or acquired, and it is managed with a surgical repair called a "labiaplasty." There has recently been increasing public awareness of this procedure with some associated controversy, as some women are requesting it for cosmetic purposes.

Prolapsed urethral mucosa typically presents in premenarchal girls and postmenopausal women. The common-

ality among these two populations is estrogen deficiency, and treatment involves estrogen replacement. Typically, these patients are asymptomatic and the prolapsed urethral mucosa is commonly seen on physical examination especially in a postmenopausal woman. When symptomatic, the most common associated symptom is spotting. Although the association between prolapsed urethral mucosa and dyspareunia has not been rigorously studied, it is possible that this condition may be associated with coital discomfort.

It is becoming increasingly clear that a subset of patients with provoked vestibulodynia (PVD) actually suffer from a congenital defect. It has been shown that women with primary PVD (they have always had dyspareunia) have a markedly increased number of C-afferent nociceptive nerve fibers in the vulvar vestibule [8]. Subsequent studies have demonstrated that these women also have umbilical hypersensitivity [9]. As both the vulvar vestibule and the umbilicus are of the same embryologic origin (the urogenital sinus), this association implies that this subset of PVD patients actually have a congenital disorder. It is the author's opinion that women who suffer from primary congenital PVD are best managed with a vestibulectomy.

The Vagina

Imperforate hymen is the most common obstructive lesion of the female reproductive tract, but it is still a rare anomaly with an incidence of less than 1% [10, 11]. This anomaly is typically diagnosed at birth or in infancy with a bulging introitus due to mucocolpos from vaginal secretions. Sometimes the individual is not symptomatic until menarche, at which time she usually presents with a bulging hymen and hematocolpos.

While it is possible that an imperforate hymen may be associated with pain upon attempted intercourse, this entity is typically diagnosed before the patient becomes sexually active. These patients are readily managed at any age with a surgical procedure that involves incising the membrane near the hymeneal ring and evacuation of accumulated blood and debris. It is important to note, however, that post-traumatic scarring that may be associated with dyspareunia can mimic an imperforate hymen [12]. This overlap underscores the importance of a careful history and physical examination in all patients suspected of having a congenital anomaly.

When there is incomplete union of the urogenital sinus and Müllerian ducts or failed canalization of the vaginal plate, a *transverse* vaginal septum may result. The septum may be located in the upper, middle, or lower third of the vagina. This condition occurs in approximately one in every 18,000–30,000 women [13, 14]. Typically, there is a single septum, although multiple septae may be present. These patients may present with a variety of symptoms depending on the severity of the anomaly, including mucocolpos (in children), hematocolpos (in adolescents), spotting, dysmenorrhea, lower abdominal pain, and urinary symptoms.

Joki-Erkkila et al. found that 19% of women with a transverse vaginal septum had dyspareunia as a presenting symptom [15]. The diagnosis is made by a careful physical examination as well as ultrasound or magnetic resonance imaging (MRI) to define the location, thickness, and number of septae. Treatment involves surgical resection of the septum with end-to-end anastomosis of the upper and lower edges of the vaginal wall [10]. These patients typically go on to have normal sexual function but have decreased reproductive capacity.

It is also possible to have a *longitudinal* vaginal septum (also called a double vagina). This may also be associated with a septate uterus (the uterus has a normal external appearance, but has two endometrial cavities). A longitudinal vaginal septum is caused by a defect in the fusion or reabsorption of the midline septum between the Müllerian ducts. Approximately 10% of women with a longitudinal vaginal septum present with dyspareunia [15]. Individuals with a longitudinal vaginal septum have an increased incidence of uterine anomalies while those with a transverse vaginal septum and hymeneal malformations do not. Patients with a longitudinal vaginal septum may be diagnosed and managed in a similar fashion to those with a transverse vaginal septum. They may go on to have normal sexual relations, but have decreased reproductive capacity.

Mayer–Roikitansky–Kuster–Hauser syndrome (MRKH), or uterovaginal agenesis, refers to absence of the vagina with varying degrees of uterine development. It occurs in one in every 5,000 females and is caused by failure of the Müllerian system to develop [16]. In these females, the external genitalia appear normal, although a blind vaginal pouch is present. These patients typically present with amenorrhea, although lack of normal sexual intercourse may also precipitate an evaluation. In a study by Mizia et al., 21% of patients with MRKH in their case series had attempted sexual intercourse and all reported severe dyspareunia [17].

MRKH is diagnosed by a careful history, physical examination, and imaging studies. Sometimes a karyotype is obtained to differentiate between gonadal dysgenesis or male pseudohermaphoditism (see below). In addition, approximately one third of these patients have urological abnormalities (such as unilateral renal agenesis or a horseshoe kidney), congenital cardiac defects, and skeletal anomalies. Therefore, further evaluation in these areas is warranted [10, 16]. Patients with MRKH have normal ovarian function; thus, they do not require hormone replacement therapy and may have genetic children.

A number of management options are available to patients with MRKH. Nonsurgical options include vaginal dilators (the Frank method) which are used for 20 minutes daily with progressively larger dilators [18]. This method may create a functional vaginal in several months. Other options include the Vecchieti operation which applies a transvaginal or laparoscopic traction device for 7–9 days [19]. For patients who cannot tolerate or who have not been successful with these conservative treatment options, numerous methods for the surgical creation of a neovagina have been described [20]. Some patients with MRKH or vaginal agenesis of another etiology who have had a vagina created surgically may have subsequent dyspareunia [21]. Sometimes the dyspareunia has been associated with stenosis or strictures of the neovagina, but deep dyspareunia has been described as well. In patients who have a neovagina, postoperative care with dilators and eventually vaginal intercourse is key in order to maintain vaginal patency.

Another rare congenital anomaly of the female genital tract is a unicornuate uterus. This occurs when the Müllerian ducts do not fuse properly. One side typically produces a normal uterine cavity with a fallopian tube and cervix, but the affected side may fail to develop altogether or may develop partially as a horn that may be either connected to or separate from the uterus. A unicornuate uterus with a rudimentary horn is the rarest congenital anatomic anomaly of the female genital system and it may be associated with dyspareunia [22]. Depending on the patient's symptoms, surgical treatment may be necessary.

During embryologic development, the distal mesonephric ducts in the female are absorbed, but occasionally they may persist as vestigial remnants in the anterolateral vaginal wall, extending to the hymen. Gartner's duct cysts arise from these embryonic remnants. These cysts usually develop along the lateral walls of the vagina or fornix. Sometimes, they can cause dyspareunia, although they are usually asymptomatic unless they are large [10]. Gartner's duct cysts are usually diagnosed by physical examination, but should the diagnosis be in question, ultrasound is of value. Gartner's duct cysts typically do not require intervention unless they are symptomatic, in which case they may be marsupialized. Infrequently, Gartner's duct cysts are associated with other urologic abnormalities such as ectopic ureters and renal agenesis [23, 24].

Genetic and Chromosomal Abnormalities

There are several genetic or chromosomal abnormalities that are associated with abnormalities of the female genitalia. For the purposes of this chapter, female pseudohermaphroditism, androgen insensitivity syndrome, and gonadal dysgenesis are most clinically relevant.

A female pseudohermaphrodite has ovaries, but genital development displays masculine characteristics [16]. Most infants affected by this disorder have congenital adrenal hyperplasia (CAH). This autosomal recessive disorder is caused by a deficiency in one of the enzymes required for adrenal synthesis of corticosteroids and leads to androgen excess in the female fetus, resulting in masculinized external genitalia. This condition is usually diagnosed and treated in infancy; however, if left untreated, females with CAH will progressively become virilized, sometimes as early as 2 years of age.

Gastaud et al. [25] reported on sexual function in a series of women with CAH. Although these women had all been diagnosed and treated early in life, 56% reported various degrees of pain with intercourse. Thirty-seven percent of women in this series also said that they had never had vaginal intercourse with their partner, and about half of these women cited abnormal genitalia or fear of pain as the reason for their abstinence.

A male pseudohermaphrodite refers to an individual who is genetically a male (XY) but exhibits abnormal virilization (or no virilization) of the external genitalia. One of the most common causes of male pseudohermaphroditism is androgen insensitivity syndrome (previously called testicular feminization). Gynecologists are frequently involved in the care of these individuals as they are phenotypically female and have been raised as such. In this X-linked recessive disorder, early in fetal de-

velopment, male external genitalia do not develop due to defective androgen receptors, resulting in the birth of a phenotypically female infant. In these patients, the vagina ends in a shallow, blind pouch; however, elongation of the vagina with intercourse has been reported [26]. Alternatively, dilator therapy or the surgical creation of a neovagina may be necessary.

When gonads fail to develop as in gonadal dysgenesis, the individual is a phenotypic female. In Turner syndrome, which is characterized by a loss of one X chromosome, or an abnormality of an X chromosome, these females have sexual infantilism. However, studies on sexual function in women with Turner syndrome found that women who were in an intimate relationship appeared to have normal sexual function [27].

Conclusion

Female sexual pain is a topic of scientific study and includes female sexual pain secondary to congenital abnormalities. Congenital anomalies of the female reproductive tract are uncommon and may be part of a syndrome with systemic manifestations or represent an isolated defect. While most anomalies are diagnosed and managed in childhood before coitarche, this is not always the case. Additionally, despite optimal medical and/or surgical management, these individuals may still have sexual pain. Optimal management of an individual with dyspareunia in the setting of a congenital anomaly requires an empathetic clinician who can make an accurate diagnosis and ensure adequate treatment, and who can provide appropriate emotional support.

References

1 Sanfilippo JS, Wakim NG, Schikler KN, et al. (1986) Endometriosis in association with uterine anomaly. *American Journal of Obstetric Gynecology* **154**, 39–43.
2 Sadler TW. (1990) *Langman's Medical Embryology*, 6th ed. Williams & Wilkins, Baltimore.
3 Lin PC, Bhatnagar KP, Nettleton GS, et al. (2002) Female genital anomalies affecting reproduction. *Fertility and Sterility* **78**, 899–915.
4 Poppas DP, Hochsztein AA, Baergen RN, et al. (2007) Nerve-sparing ventral clitoroplasty preserves dorsal nerves in congenital adrenal hyperplasia. *Journal of Urology* **178**, 1802–6.

5 Mendilcioglu I. (2007) Recurrent periclitoral abscess: treatment of a rare cause of vulvar pain. *European Journal of Obstetrics and Gynecology and Reproductive Biology* **131**, 101–2.

6 Julia J, Yacoub M, Levy G. (2003) Labial fusion causing urinary incontinence in a postmenopausal female: a case report. *International Urogynecological Journal of Pelvic Floor Dysfunction* **14**, 360–61.

7 Rouzier R, Louis-Sylvestre C, Paniel BJ, *et al.* (2000) Hypertrophy of labia minora: experience with 163 reductions. *American Journal of Obstetrics and Gynecology* **182**, 35-40.

8 Bohm-Starke N, Hilliges M, Falconer C, *et al.* (1998) Increased intraepithelial innervation in women with vulvar vestibulitis syndrome. *Gynecological and Obstetric Investigation* **46**, 256–60.

9 Burrows LJ, Klingman D, Pukall CF, *et al.* (2008) Umbilical hypersensitivity in women with primary vestibulodynia. *The Journal of Reproductive Medicine* **53**, 413–16.

10 Goldstein D. (2008) How to diagnose and repair congenital uterovaginal malformations. *OBG Management* **20**.

11 Attaran M, Gidwani G. (1999) Obstructive Müllerian anomalies. In: Gidwani G, Falcone T. (eds.) *Congenital Malformations of the Female Reproductive Tract. Diagnosis and Management,* Lippincott Williams & Wilkins, Philadelphia, pp. 145–68.

12 Berkowitz CD, Elvik SL, Logan M. (1987) A simulated "acquired" imperforate hymen following the genital trauma of sexual abuse. *Clinical Pediatrics* **26**, 307–9.

13 Acien P. (1997) Incidence of Müllerian defects in fertile and infertile women. *Human Reproduction* **12**, 1372–76.

14 Emans SJ, Goldstein DP. (1983) *Pediatric and Adolescent Gynecology.* Lippincott Williams & Wilkins, Philadelphia.

15 Joki-Erkkila MM, Heinonen PK. (2003) Presenting and long-term clinical implications and fecundity in females with obstructing vaginal malformations. *Journal of Pediatric and Adolescent Gynecology* **16**, 307–12.

16 Speroff L, Fritz MA. (2005) *Clinical Gynecologic Endocrinology and Infertility,* 7th ed. Lippincott Williams & Wilkins, Philadelphia.

17 Mizia K, Bennett MJ, Dudley J, *et al.* (2006) Müllerian dysgenesis: a review of recent outcomes at Royal Hospital for Women. *Australian and New Zealand Journal of Obstetrics and Gynaecology* **46**, 29–31.

18 Frank RT. (1935) Formation of artificial vagina without operation. *American Journal of Obstetrics and Gynecology* **35**, 1053–55.

19 Veronikis DK, McClure GB, Nichols DH. (1997) The Vecchietti operation for constructing a neovagina: indications, instrumentation, and techniques. *Obstetrics and Gynecology* **90**, 301–4.

20 Davies MC, Creighton SM. (2007) Vaginoplasty. *Current Opinion in Urology* **17**, 415–18.

21 Communal PH, Chevret-Measson M, Golfier F, *et al.* (2003) Sexuality after sigmoid colpopoiesis in patients with Mayer–Rokitansky–Kuster–Hauser syndrome. *Fertility and Sterility* **80**, 600–6.

22 Atmaca R, Germen AT, Burak F, *et al.* (2005) Acute abdomen in a case with noncommunicating rudimentary horn and unicornuate uterus. *Journal of the Society of Laparoendoscopic Surgeons* **9**, 235–37.

23 Dwyer PL, Rosamilia A. (2006) Congenital urogenital anomalies that are associated with the persistence of Gartner's duct: a review. *American Journal of Obstetrics and Gynecology* **195**, 354–59.

24 Lee MJ, Yoder IC, Papanicolaou N, *et al.* (1991) Large Gartner duct cyst associated with a solitary crossed ectopic kidney: imaging features. *Journal of Computer-Assisted Tomography* **15**, 149–51.

25 Gastaud F, Bouvattier C, Duranteau L, *et al.* (2007) Impaired sexual and reproductive outcomes in women with classical forms of congenital adrenal hyperplasia. *Journal of Clinical Endocrinology and Metabolism* **92**, 1391–96.

26 Moen MH. (2000) Creation of a vagina by repeated coital dilatation in four teenagers with vaginal agenesis. *Acta Obstetricia et Gynecologica Scandinavica* **79**, 149–50.

27 Sheaffer AT, Lange E, Bondy CA. (2008) Sexual function in women with Turner syndrome. *Journal of Womens Health* **17**, 27–33.

CHAPTER 19
Endometriosis

Jennifer Droz,[1] *Fred M. Howard*[2]

[1] University of Rochester Medical Center, Rochester, NY, USA
[2] University of Rochester School of Medicine and Dentistry, Rochester, NY, USA

Introduction

Endometriosis is the presence of endometrial glands or stroma outside of the endometrial cavity. It affects 1–7% of the general population [1]. Endometriosis encompasses a wide spectrum of presentations ranging from disease found incidentally during laparoscopy to extensive, seemingly malignant disease that can spread outside of the pelvis and into the upper abdomen. The severity of symptoms also varies greatly and does not always correlate with the amount of endometriosis.

Classically, endometriosis presents with one or more of the following: an adnexal mass, infertility, or pelvic pain. Up to 70% of women with endometriosis have some type of pain symptoms, most commonly dysmenorrhea, noncyclic pelvic pain, or deep dyspareunia [2, 3]. A total of 60–79% of patients undergoing surgery for endometriosis have been affected by deep dyspareunia, resulting in a negative attitude toward sexuality, anxiety toward and avoidance of intercourse, lower levels of desire and arousal, and fewer orgasms [4, 5]. Women with uterosacral ligament endometriosis in particular have the most severe impairment of sexual function, higher intensity of pain, and less satisfying orgasms [6].

Etiology

The two etiological aspects of endometriosis of clinical importance are the cause of the disease and the cause of

symptoms of endometriosis (pelvic pain and infertility). Neither is completely understood.

The etiology of endometriosis is complex. Both genetic and environmental factors are important. There are several general theories regarding the etiology of endometriosis (Table 19.1). None of these theories is sufficient to explain the protean manifestations and locations of endometriosis, or the predilection of some women, but not others, to develop endometriosis. The theory of retrograde menstruation leading to the implantation of endometrial cells in the peritoneal cavity (also known as Sampson's theory) is supported by observational data [7, 8].

Adolescents with obstructive reproductive tract malformations [9, 10] and adult women with cervical stenosis both have high rates of endometriosis [11]. However, most, if not all, women experience some form of retrograde menstruation, so retrograde menstruation is not the sole source of endometriosis [12]. There must be other factors that allow implantation, invasion, and proliferation of ectopic endometrium in some, but not all, women. Other theories include immune system defects [13–15], genetic predisposition [16], metaplasia of coelomic epithelium into endometrial cells [17], and lymphatic spread of disease [18].

Recently, research has focused on environmental factors and on the unique attributes of the endometrial cells of endometriosis. Environmental pollutants such as polychlorinated biphenyls (PCBs) and dioxin have been associated with an increased risk of confirmed endometriosis among women undergoing laparoscopy [19–21]. This effect has also been shown experimentally in primates [22]. Endometriotic cells have the ability to produce enzymes such as aromatase, an enzyme that is not present in normal endometrium and is integral to the conversion of

Female Sexual Pain Disorders 1st edition. Edited by A. Goldstein, C. Pukall & I. Goldstein. © 2009 Blackwell Publishing, ISBN: 9781405183987.

Table 19.1 Theories of etiology of endometriosis.

Retrograde menstruation (Sampson's theory)
Metaplasia
Lymphatic and vascular metastases
Immunologic defect
Genetic predisposition
Abnormal endometrium in endometriosis

androstenedione and testosterone to estrogen, a conversion usually done only in the ovary [23]. The ability to produce estrogen locally may lead to auto-stimulation of endometriotic lesions. Not only do endometriotic lesions show high levels of estradiol biosynthesis, they also show low estradiol inactivation compared to normal endometrium. Additionally, there is some evidence that alterations in progesterone receptors in endometriosis may play a role in the development or progression of endometriotic lesions.

The etiology of pain symptoms with endometriosis is less well understood, although there is ample epidemiological evidence of the relationship of endometriosis and pelvic pain symptoms. Because endometriosis is most commonly a disease of the pelvic viscera and visceral peritoneum, endometriosis pain is usually visceral in origin. Visceral pain has a number of characteristics that are important to any understanding of endometriosis-associated pain: (1) not all viscera are sources of visceral pain, possibly due to lack of sensory receptors or the lack of an appropriate nociceptive stimulus; (2) visceral pain is not always linked to injury and thus may be functional; (3) visceral pain frequently results in somatic referral of pain, possibly due to central convergence of visceral and somatic afferents; and (4) visceral pain tends to be diffuse or poorly localized, probably due to the low concentration of nociceptive afferents within viscera [24]. Visceral nociception and pain are generated in response to distention, ischemia, inflammation, and traction on mesentery. In the case of endometriosis, inflammation may be the primary nociceptive stimulus. A number of studies have shown that endometriotic lesions produce and release inflammatory mediators, particularly prostaglandins $F_{2\alpha}$ and E_2, potent mediators of the inflammatory response [25–27].

In addition to directly causing visceral pain, inflammation induced by endometriosis may also enhance pain sensitivity. The presence of inflammation tends to significantly enhance both the sensitivity and the severity of visceral pain. This characteristic of visceral pain may be relevant in patients with endometriosis, because in the presence of local inflammation, visceral afferents may develop peripheral hypersensitization and start to respond to previously innocuous physiological stimuli.

In addition to nociceptive pain, neuropathic pain may also be a significant factor in endometriosis-associated pelvic pain. For example, there are significant differences in the uterine innervation of women with endometriosis and chronic pelvic pain compared to those without pelvic pain. Women with endometriosis and chronic pelvic pain have an increase in nerve fibers, microneuroma formation, and perivascular nerve proliferation in their uteri [28]. These neural changes may be a cause of both dysmenorrhea and chronic pelvic pain.

Finally, referred visceral pain with hyperalgesia may be an important mechanism in endometriosis-associated pain. Referral of pain with hyperalgesia of somatic tissue is a well-known characteristic of visceral pain. In the case of endometriosis, there are both animal experimental and human clinical evidence of hyperalgesia of the vagina, abdominal wall, and lumbosacral back. Referred pain with hyperalgesia may be an important mechanism in the generation of dyspareunia in women with endometriosis [29–32].

Epidemiology

Endometriosis is estimated to be present in 1–7% of the general population, although the true prevalence is unknown. In women undergoing laparoscopy for pelvic pain and infertility, endometriosis lesions are present 33% and 40% of the time, respectively [33].

Seventy percent of women with endometriosis diagnosed by laparoscopy experience pelvic pain of some type [34]. There is not a direct relationship between severity of pelvic pain and the extent of disease: A patient with large, bilateral endometriomas and stage IV endometriosis obliterating the posterior cul-de-sac can experience little or no pain, whereas a woman with only a few lesions identified laparoscopically can have debilitating pain symptoms. This is not inconsistent with modern theories of pain, especially chronic pain, but can make clinical management perplexing. There is, however, a relationship between pain relief with surgical treatment and extent of disease [35].

Diagnosis

History

Endometriosis occurs in women of reproductive age, so it is rarely a cause of pelvic pain or dyspareunia in post-menopausal women. About 60% of women with endometriosis have the onset of their symptoms before 20 years of age [2]. Ninety percent or more of women with pelvic pain and endometriosis classically present with a history of dysmenorrhea [2, 36]. A common complaint, dyspareunia occurs with deep penetration and not with initial entry. Dyspareunia occurs in up to 60% of patients with pain symptoms [2]. Rarely is dyspareunia an isolated pain symptom of endometriosis. Deep dyspareunia is often associated with uterosacral and/or rectovaginal endometriosis lesions; 60–78% of women with deep dyspareunia had positive uterosacral ligament pathology during laparoscopy [37].

Physical Examination

Physical examination findings in women with endometriosis are often negative. Many women only have tenderness during menses, and sometimes repeating the exam at this time can be useful [38]. Other women with endometriosis have persistent areas of tenderness that coincide with areas of endometriosis, whether or not they are menstruating [39]. In particular, a fixed retroverted uterus with posterior tenderness and tender nodularity of the uterosacral ligaments or cul-de-sac are suggestive of endometriosis. Narrowing of the posterior vaginal fornix may rarely be present. There may be lateral displacement or deviation of the cervix [40]. Asymmetrically enlarged, tender ovaries that are fixed to the broad ligaments or pelvic sidewalls are sometimes found. In patients with endometriomas, a tender adnexal mass may be noted. In women whose primary complaint is deep dyspareunia, localized tenderness of the cervix, cul-de-sac, or a fixed, retroverted uterus may be found at the time of examination.

Imaging Studies

Radiologic studies can be useful in the preoperative evaluation and surgical planning in a patient with suspected endometriosis, but are not sensitive or specific for diagnostic purposes. Pelvic ultrasound findings of a hypoechoic adnexal mass with diffuse low-level internal echoes consistent with an endometrioma can guide the operative plan, particularly when ovarian endometriomas are small and do not result in an enlarged ovary visible laparoscopically. Magnetic resonance imaging has also been described to identify endometriosis lesions, particularly in unusual locations, such as with rectal, nervous system, or thoracic involvement.

Laparoscopy

The diagnosis of endometriosis is based on positive histology, and should not be based solely on a visual diagnosis made at the time of laparoscopy. Histologic diagnosis is important because endometriosis lesions can have many different appearances, from the "classic" powder burn lesions (black, brown, or gray) to the "atypical" lesions which can be clear, red, yellow, or white [41]. Also, many other lesions can look like endometriosis, such as hemangiomas, old suture, ovarian carcinoma, residual carbon deposits from prior surgery, and even normal peritoneum. When the diagnosis is based only on the visual appearance, the diagnosis is incorrect 50–55% of the time [42]. Conversely, relying only on visual diagnosis can lead to underdiagnosis or understaging, as many atypical lesions are actually endometriosis.

Endometriosis most commonly involves the pelvic organs. In one study of 716 women with endometriosis diagnosed at the time of laparoscopy, lesions were found at the following locations: posterior cul-de-sac and uterosacral ligaments, 69%; ovary, 45%; ovarian fossa, 33%; vesicouterine fold, 24% [43]. Appendiceal involvement has been found in 10–20% of cases of pelvic endometriosis [44]. Extraperitoneal disease is much less common, but can involve the gastrointestinal and urinary tracts, the thorax, and even the nervous system [45]. Adhesions are a common operative finding and endometriosis can be found in half of adhesions, so adhesion tissue should be excised and sent for histologic evaluation in women with endometriosis.

Laparoscopy is the ideal diagnostic tool, with histologic sampling for reasons outlined above. Compared with laparotomy, laparoscopy allows for magnification of lesions and results in easier identification of microscopic endometriosis, particularly in the setting of "atypical" lesions. Many women with endometriosis will likely undergo more than one operation, and laparoscopy results in less adhesive disease, shorter hospital stay, and a better cosmetic result.

Treatment

Treatment of endometriosis may be surgical, medical, or both. Many factors must be considered in planning treatment and the patient needs to be actively involved in treatment decisions. Her understanding of the disease and her unique needs and problems will influence her decisions about treatment. From the physician's perspective, the location and extent of endometriosis, the severity of symptoms, and any other pelvic pathology will influence recommendations. The patient's age, reproductive plans, duration of pain or infertility, and attitude toward surgery or toward hormonal medications may be vital components of treatment planning. Treatment may need to be modified, based on the tolerance of the therapy or the persistence or worsening of symptoms.

Medical Treatment

Most medical therapies for endometriosis work by decreasing estrogen levels. For the majority of the commonly used medical treatments there is good evidence supporting their efficacy for symptomatic relief of pain.

Danazol, a 17-ethinyl-testosterone derivative, is an oral medication that induces amenorrhea and lowers estrogen levels by directly inhibiting steroidogenesis at the ovarian and adrenal levels. This induces atrophic changes in the endometrium and endometriosis. It was the first drug approved by the U.S. Food and Drug Administration (FDA) for the treatment of endometriosis, and at one time was considered the gold standard in medical treatment of endometriosis. However, the extensive side effects profile which includes acne, edema, weight gain, hirsutism, voice changes, hot flushes, abnormal uterine bleeding, decreased breast size, decreased libido, vaginal dryness, nausea, weakness, and muscle cramps [46], makes it difficult for many patients to tolerate and limits its effectiveness as a treatment option. An early uncontrolled study showed that about 75% of patients had relief of either pelvic pain or dysmenorrhea, and about 60% had relief of dyspareunia [47].

Gonadotropin-releasing hormone agonists (GnRHa) are analogues of naturally occurring gonadotropin-releasing hormone that shut down production and release LH and FSH, thereby dramatically reducing estradiol levels. This induces a pseudomenopausal state. Clinical trials show that efficacy is comparable to danazol. The hypoestrogenic state results in hot flushes, vaginal dryness, decreased libido, emotional lability, and decreased bone

density. Loss of lumbar spinal bone density averages 3.2% at 6 months and 6.3% at 12 months. Add-back therapy with the progestin norethindrone acetate, with or without estrogen, reduces the loss of bone density and decreases other side effects without loss of efficacy [48]. The GnRH agonists currently available for use in the United States are nafarelin, leuprolide, and goserelin.

Progestins are synthetic steroids with progesterone-like activity. Those that have been shown to have efficacy in clinical trials include medroxyprogesterone acetate (MPA) [49], norethindrone acetate [50, 51], and gestrinone (not available in the United States) [52].

Combined oral contraceptives (COCs) are widely used to treat endometriosis-associated pelvic pain. COCs inhibit ovulation, decrease gonadotropin levels, and decrease menstrual flow. At least one randomized clinical trial suggests that COCs are almost as effective as GnRH agonists for the treatment of pelvic pain and dyspareunia [53]. Both COCs and GnRH agonists decreased pelvic pain, but the GnRH agonist was somewhat more effective in relief of dysmenorrhea and dyspareunia. Side effects of COCs include nausea, headache, abnormal uterine bleeding, thrombophlebitis, and thromboembolism.

Surgical Treatment

Although many patients with suspected endometriosis based upon history and physical exam findings are treated presumptively and successfully with medical therapy, diagnostic laparoscopy is still recommended for diagnosis. Treatment can be combined with diagnosis in this setting [54]. Excision, coagulation, and vaporization with various energy sources have been described as appropriate treatment options for the conservative surgical management of endometriosis, both for pelvic pain and for infertility. Regardless of energy source, care should be taken to treat all lesions identified and to remove or ablate each lesion in its entirety. This is especially important for deeply infiltrating lesions such as those commonly present in the uterosacral ligaments or in the rectovaginal septum. Any lesion greater than 5 mm in diameter should be excised in order to be sure that the entire lesion is removed.

There are two randomized clinical trials validating the efficacy of laparoscopic surgical treatment of endometriosis. The first used laser energy to destroy the lesions [54]. At six months postoperatively, 23% of the placebo group showed decreased pain and 62% of the surgically treated group showed decreased pain. Over the subsequent 6–12 months, 16% of the surgically treated patients required repeat surgery compared to 52% of the control group. In a study of excision of endometriotic lesions, there was improvement of symptoms in 80% of the treated group versus 32% of the control group [55]. Additionally, observational studies suggest that dyspareunia improves in 70–80% after conservative surgical treatment.

In addition to conservative surgical management with excision or ablation of endometriosis, procedures such as presacral neurectomy and uterosacral neurectomy (transection of the uterosacral ligament) are frequently performed to further improve pelvic pain in a patient who requests conservative, fertility-sparing management. Two randomized clinical trials have shown that presacral neurectomy combined with endometriosis surgery improves midline dysmenorrhea more than endometriosis surgery without presacral neurectomy [56, 57]. The second study also showed slight improvements in dyspareunia and nonmenstrual pelvic pain with presacral neurectomy. Long-term complications of presacral neurectomy include constipation and urinary urgency. Two randomized clinical trials with endometriosis surgery have shown that uteroscral neurectomy does not improve dysmenorrhea, dyspareunia, or nonmenstrual pelvic pain over that obtained solely with excision or ablation of endometriosis [58, 59].

For women who are not interested in future childbearing, hysterectomy with or without bilateral salpingo-oophorectomy is also an option for treatment. There is no consensus regarding the necessity of removal of ovaries with endometriosis, although one study reported 62% recurrence of pain when one or both ovaries were retained, compared to 10% after both were removed [60].

Conclusion

The etiology of endometriosis and its associated symptoms are complex and poorly understood. The diagnosis can be implied by history, physical exam, and radiologic studies, but histologic documentation of endometriosis cells is required to confirm the diagnosis. Endometriosis can be managed both medically and surgically. The primary purpose of surgical treatment is the removal or destruction of all endometriotic lesions. Surgery for en-

dometriosis can be very challenging, and should be done by a skilled surgeon who is well versed in pelvic surgery, especially retroperitoneal dissection.

References

1 Barbieri RL. (1990) Etiology and epidemiology of endometriosis. *American Journal of Obstetrics and Gynecology* **162**, 565–67.

2 Ballweg ML. (2004) Impact of endometriosis on women's health: comparative historical data show that the earlier the onset, the more severe the disease. *Best Practice and Research Clinical Obstetrics and Gynaecology* **18**, 201–18.

3 Fedele L, Bianchi S, Bocciolone L, *et al.* (1992) Pain symptoms associated with endometriosis. *Obstetrics and Gynecology* **79**, 767–69.

4 Ferrero S, Abbamonte LH, Giordano M, *et al.* (2007) Deep dyspareunia and sex life after laparoscopic excision of endometriosis. *Human Reproduction* **22**, 1142–48.

5 Ferrero S, Abbamonte LH, Parisi M, *et al.* (2007) Dyspareunia and quality of sex life after laparoscopic excision of endometriosis and postoperative administration of triptorelin. *Fertility and Sterility* **87**, 227–29.

6 Ferrero S, Esposito F, Abbamonte LH, *et al.* (2005) Quality of sex life in women with endometriosis and deep dyspareunia. *Fertility and Sterility* **83**, 573–79.

7 Halme J, Hammond MG, Hulka JF, *et al.* (1984) Retrograde menstruation in healthy women and in patients with endometriosis. *Obstetrics and Gynecology* **64**, 151–54.

8 Geist SH. The viability of fragments of menstrual endometrium. (1933) *American Journal of Obstetrics and Gynecology* **25**, 751.

9 Goldstein DP, De Cholnoky C, Emans SJ. (1980) Adolescent endometriosis. *Journal of Adolescent Health Care* **1**, 37–41.

10 Olive DL, Henderson DY. (1987) Endometriosis and Mullerian anomalies. *Obstetrics and Gynecology* **69**, 412–15.

11 Barbieri RL. (1998) Stenosis of the external cervical os: an association with endometriosis in women with chronic pelvic pain. *Fertility and Sterility* **70**, 571–73.

12 Koninckx PR, Ide P, Vandenbroucke W, *et al.* (1980) New aspects of the pathophysiology of endometriosis and associated infertility. *The Journal of Reproductive Medicine* **24**, 257–60.

13 Giudice LC, Tazuke SI, Swiersz L. (1998) Status of current research on endometriosis. *The Journal of Reproductive Medicine* **43**, 252–62.

14 Dmowski WP, Steele RW, Baker GF. (1981) Deficient cellular immunity in endometriosis. *American Journal of Obstetrics and Gynecology* **141**, 377–83.

15 Antsiferova YS, Sotnikova NY, Posiseeva LV, *et al.* (2005) Changes in the T-helper cytokine profile and in lymphocyte

activation at the systemic and local levels in women with endometriosis. *Fertility and Sterility* **84**, 1705–11.

16 Kennedy S, Mardon H, Barlow D. (1995) Familial endometriosis. *Journal of Assisted Reproductive Genetics* **12**, 32–34.

17 El-Mahgoub S, Yaseen S. (1980) A positive proof for the theory of coelomic metaplasia. *American Journal of Obstetrics and Gynecology* **137**, 137–40.

18 Javert CT. (1951) Observations on the pathology and spread of endometriosis based on the theory of benign metastasis. *American Journal of Obstetrics and Gynecology* **62**, 477–87.

19 Cervone P, Boso CF, Painvain E, *et al.* (1999) [Peritoneal cyst. A case report]. *Minerva Ginecologica* **51**, 449–51.

20 Mechsner S, Schwarz J, Thode J, *et al.* (2007) Growth-associated protein 43-positive sensory nerve fibers accompanied by immature vessels are located in or near peritoneal endometriotic lesions. *Fertility and Sterility* **88**, 581–87.

21 Eskenazi B, Mocarelli P, Warner M, *et al.* (2002) Serum dioxin concentrations and endometriosis: a cohort study in Seveso, Italy. *Environmental Health Perspectives* **110**, 629–34.

22 Rier SE, Martin DC, Bowman RE, *et al.* (1993) Endometriosis in rhesus monkeys (*Macaca mulatta*) following chronic exposure to 2,3,7,8-tetrachlorodibenzo-*p*-dioxin. *Fundamentals of Applied Toxicology* **21**, 433–41.

23 Letterie GS, Yon JL. (1995) Use of a long-acting GnRH agonist for benign cystic mesothelioma. *Obstetrics and Gynecology* **85**, 901–03.

24 Cervero F, Laird JM. (1999) Visceral pain. *Lancet* **353**, 2145–48.

25 Lessey BA, Metzger DA, Haney AF, *et al.* (1989) Immunohistochemical analysis of estrogen and progesterone receptors in endometriosis: comparison with normal endometrium during the menstrual cycle and the effect of medical therapy. *Fertility and Sterility* **51**, 409–15.

26 Muzii L, Marana R, Brunetti L, *et al.* (2000) Atypical endometriosis revisited: clinical and biochemical evaluation of the different forms of superficial implants. *Fertility and Sterility* **74**, 739–42.

27 Vernon MW, Beard JS, Graves K, *et al.* (1986) Classification of endometriotic implants by morphologic appearance and capacity to synthesize prostaglandin F. *Fertility and Sterility* **46**, 801–6.

28 Atwal G, du PD, Armstrong G, *et al.* (2005) Uterine innervation after hysterectomy for chronic pelvic pain with, and without, endometriosis. *American Journal of Obstetrics and Gynecology* **193**, 1650–55.

29 Giamberardino MA, Berkley KJ, Affaitati G, *et al.* (2002) Influence of endometriosis on pain behaviors and muscle hyperalgesia induced by a urethral calculosis in female rats. *Pain* **95**, 247–57.

30 Giamberardino MA, Vecchiet L. (1995) Visceral pain, referred hyperalgesia and outcome: new concepts. *European Journal of Anaesthesiology Supplement* **10**, 61–66.

31 Giamberardino MA, De Laurentis S, Affaitati G, *et al.* (2001) Modulation of pain and hyperalgesia from the urinary tract by algogenic conditions of the reproductive organs in women. *Neuroscience Letters* **304**, 61–64.

32 Yoon SM, Jung JK, Lee SB, *et al.* (2002) Treatment of female urethral syndrome refractory to antibiotics. *Yonsei Medical Journal* **43**, 644–51.

33 Howard FM. (1993) The role of laparoscopy in chronic pelvic pain: promise and pitfalls. *Obstetric and Gynecological Survey* **48**, 357–87.

34 Mahmood TA, Templeton AA, Thomson L, *et al.* (1991) Menstrual symptoms in women with pelvic endometriosis. *British Journal of Obstetrics and Gynaecology* **98**, 558–63.

35 Sutton CJ, Ewen SP, Whitelaw N, *et al.* (1994) Prospective, randomized, double-blind, controlled trial of laser laparoscopy in the treatment of pelvic pain associated with minimal, mild, and moderate endometriosis. *Fertility and Sterility* **62**, 696–700.

36 Forman RG, Robinson JN, Mehta Z, *et al.* (1993) Patient history as a simple predictor of pelvic pathology in subfertile women. *Human Reproduction* **8**, 53–55.

37 Chapron C, Dubuisson JB. (1996) Laparoscopic treatment of deep endometriosis located on the uterosacral ligaments. *Human Reproduction* **11**, 868–73.

38 Koninckx PR, Meuleman C, Oosterlynck D, *et al.* (1996) Diagnosis of deep endometriosis by clinical examination during menstruation and plasma CA-125 concentration. *Fertility and Sterility* **65**, 280–87.

39 Ripps BA, Martin DC. (1991) Focal pelvic tenderness, pelvic pain, and dysmenorrhea in endometriosis. *The Journal of Reproductive Medicine* **36**, 470–72.

40 Propst AM, Storti K, Barbieri RL. (1998) Lateral cervical displacement is associated with endometriosis. *Fertility and Sterility* **70**, 568–70.

41 Stripling MC, Martin DC, Chatman DL, *et al.* (1988) Subtle appearance of pelvic endometriosis. *Fertility and Sterility* **49**, 427–31.

42 Walter AJ, Hentz JG, Magtibay PM, *et al.* (2001) Endometriosis: correlation between histologic and visual findings at laparoscopy. *American Journal of Obstetrics and Gynecology* **184**, 1407–11.

43 Koninckx PR, D'Hooghe TD, Oosterlynck D. (1991) Response to letter to the editor. *Fertility and Sterility* **56**, 590.

44 Pittaway DE. (1983) Appendectomy in the surgical treatment of endometriosis. *Obstetrics and Gynecology* **61**, 421–24.

45 Batt RE, Yeh J, Koninckx PR. (2004) Asymmetric distribution of sciatic nerve endometriosis. *Obstetrics and Gynecology* **103**, 400–1.

46 Telimaa S, Ronnberg L, Kauppila A. (1987) Placebo-controlled comparison of danazol and high-dose medroxyprogesterone acetate in the treatment of endometriosis after conservative surgery. *Gynecological Endocrinology* **1**, 363–71.

47 Barbieri RL, Evans S, Kistner RW. (1982) Danazol in the treatment of endometriosis: analysis of 100 cases with a 4-year follow-up. *Fertility and Sterility* **37**, 737–46.

48 Hornstein MD, Surrey ES, Weisberg GW, *et al.* (1998) Leuprolide acetate depot and hormonal add-back in endometriosis: a 12-month study. *Lupron Add-Back Study Group. Obstetrics and Gynecology* **91**, 16–24.

49 Schlaff WD, Carson SA, Luciano A, *et al.* (2006) Subcutaneous injection of depot medroxyprogesterone acetate compared with leuprolide acetate in the treatment of endometriosis-associated pain. *Fertility and Sterility* **85**, 314–25.

50 Muneyyirci-Delale O, Karacan M. (1998) Effect of norethindrone acetate in the treatment of symptomatic endometriosis. *International Journal of Fertility and Womens Medicine* **43**, 24–27.

51 Vercellini P, Pietropaolo G, De Giorgi O, *et al.* (2005) Treatment of symptomatic rectovaginal endometriosis with an estrogen–progestogen combination versus low-dose norethindrone acetate. *Fertility and Sterility* **84**, 1375–87.

52 Gestrinone Italian Study Group. (1996) Gestrinone versus a gonadotropin-releasing hormone agonist for the treatment of pelvic pain associated with endometriosis: a multicenter, randomized, double-blind study. *Fertility and Sterility* **66**, 911–19.

53 Vercellini P, Trespidi L, Colombo A, *et al.* (1993) A gonadotropin-releasing hormone agonist versus a low-dose oral contraceptive for pelvic pain associated with endometriosis. *Fertility and Sterility* **60**, 75–79.

54 Howard FM. (1994) Laparoscopic evaluation and treatment of women with chronic pelvic pain. *Journal of the American Association of Gynecologic Laparoscopists* **1**, 325–31.

55 Abbott J, Hawe J, Hunter D, *et al.* (2004) Laparoscopic excision of endometriosis: a randomized, placebo-controlled trial. *Fertility and Sterility* **82**, 878–84.

56 Candiani GB, Fedele L, Vercellini P, *et al.* (1992) Presacral neurectomy for the treatment of pelvic pain associated with endometriosis: a controlled study. *American Journal of Obstetrics and Gynecolgy* **167**, 100–3.

57 Zullo F, Palomba S, Zupi E, *et al.* (2003) Effectiveness of presacral neurectomy in women with severe dysmenorrhea caused by endometriosis who were treated with laparoscopic conservative surgery: a 1-year prospective randomized double-blind controlled trial. *American Journal of Obstetrics and Gynecology* **189**, 5–10.

58 Vercellini P, Aimi G, Busacca M, *et al.* (2003) Laparoscopic uterosacral ligament resection for dysmenorrhea associated with endometriosis: results of a randomized, controlled trial. *Fertility and Sterility* **80**, 310–19.

59 Sutton C, Pooley AS, Jones KD, *et al.* (2001) A prospective, randomized, double-blind controlled trial of laparoscopic uterine nerve ablation in the treatment of pelvic pain associated with endometriosis. *Gynaecological Endoscopy* **10**, 217–22.

60 Namnoum AB, Hickman TN, Goodman SB, *et al.* (1995) Incidence of symptom recurrence after hysterectomy for endometriosis. *Fertility and Sterility* **64**, 898–902.

CHAPTER 20
Pelvic Inflammatory Disease

Nancy D. Gaba

The George Washington University Medical Center, Washington, DC, USA

Introduction

Pelvic inflammatory disease (PID) is a highly prevalent disorder that affects one million American women each year [1]. PID is caused by sexually transmitted infections (STIs) (see Chapter 11) which have ascended to the upper genital tract (uterus, fallopian tubes) and intraperitoneal cavity. PID is a polymicrobial infectious process; commonly isolated organisms include *Chlamydia trachomatis, Neisseria gonorrheae, Escheria coli,* and *Enterococcus* species. The major sequelae of this disorder include infertility, ectopic pregnancies, bowel obstructions, pelvic pain, and deep dyspareunia. This chapter reviews the relationship between PID, pelvic adhesions, and pelvic pain, and discusses how diagnosis and management can impact the long-term complications of PID.

The Link Between Pelvic Adhesions, Pelvic Pain, and Dyspareunia

Pelvic adhesions are abnormal attachments between organs and other tissues that form after any intraperitoneal insult. Adhesions form because the normal peritoneal healing process is either altered or disrupted. Adhesions form from tissue trauma that may result from infections such as PID, as well as injury, surgery, radiation, ischemia, or foreign-body reactions. Any of these triggers can then lead to activation of stromal mast cells, the first and most important trigger in the cascade of events that lead to adhesion formation.

Mast cells release vasoactive substances, such as histamine and kinins, which increase vascular permeability (see Chapter 27). In addition, mast cells induce fibrin deposition. These fibrin deposits are made up of cellular exudate, leukocytes, and macrophages. A fibrinous exudate usually forms within 3 hr of injury. The invasion of fibroblasts and blood vessels soon follows. Under normal circumstances, healing occurs by a combination of fibrosis (scarring) and mesothelial regeneration. Normally, most fibrinous exudates are transient and break down within 72 hr, but trauma-induced local suppression of peritoneal fibrinolysis predisposes to the formation of adhesions [2].

A postmortem study of motor vehicle accident victims showed that 93% of subjects who underwent prior surgery had adhesions. Only 10% of those who never had surgery had adhesions [3]. Other studies have shown that up to 20% of clinically significant pelvic adhesions are caused by inflammatory conditions, including PID. The presence of adhesions in patients who have never had intra-abdominal surgery suggests that other etiologies, including PID, may be responsible. As PID is highly prevalent, it is possible that PID can be a common cause of adhesions. The American Fertility Society has developed criteria to describe the severity of adhesions [4, 5].

Significant basic science and clinical research has been directed toward the prevention of adhesions to preserve fertility. Less attention has been paid to adhesion prevention and its effects on chronic pelvic pain (CPP) or dyspareunia. In addition, research has focused on suppressing the formation of adhesions after general and gynecologic surgery, but little effort has been spent on reducing adhesions after PID.

Studies of adhesion prevention were initiated in the 1980s and 1990s, often utilizing elaborate animal models.

Female Sexual Pain Disorders 1st edition. Edited by A. Goldstein, C. Pukall & I. Goldstein. © 2009 Blackwell Publishing, ISBN: 9781405183987.

For example, one group of investigators found that injured rat peritoneal cells contained an increased amount of transforming growth factor beta (TGF-β) [6]. This protein was not expressed as strongly in tissues without adhesions. TGF-β has been found in human adhesions as well, suggesting that it plays a role in fibrosis and adhesion formation. If it is possible to prevent the expression of TGF-β, or suppress its action, adhesion formation may be prevented.

Although several mechanisms for this possible suppression have been suggested, one involves the omega-3 fatty acid docosahexaenoic acid (DHA). This acid is known for its ability to act as an antagonist to peroxisome proliferator activated receptors which are nuclear receptors that activate the inflammatory cascade involving lipid metabolism, fatty acid oxidation, cytokine production, and others mediators involved in adhesion formation. When DHA is applied directly to cell cultures, it has been shown to substantially decrease levels of adhesion related markers in peritoneal adhesions and fibroblasts [7].

Landmark studies on PID were conducted in Scandinavia during the 1970s and 1980s when long-term outcomes in patients with PID were analyzed for the first time. These outcomes included pelvic pain and pelvic adhesions but neglected to study important concerns such as pelvic pain and dyspareunia. In fact, because these studies were conducted using laparoscopic evidence of PID as an inclusion criterion, many women were discovered to have Fitz–Hugh–Curtis syndrome (perihepatic adhesions), at the time of diagnosis [8]. Since that time, analyses of screening plans, antibiotic treatment regimens, outpatient versus inpatient management options, and assessments of cost-effectiveness of management have often included data on chronic pelvic pain, adhesions, quality of life, sexual function, and cost. The most notable of these studies was the large, multicenter, randomized controlled trial known as the PID Evaluation and Clinical Health (PEACH) study, in which patients with PID were followed for up to 7 years postdiagnosis. Important data regarding long-term outcomes including CPP, infertility, and quality-of-life measures were gained from these studies [9].

The U.S. Centers for Disease Control list three major criteria and five associated criteria for the diagnosis of PID (Table 20.1) [1]. Most patients with PID have fever, adnexal tenderness, and an elevated white blood cell count. However, up to two-thirds of women do not

Table 20.1 Centers for Disease Control criteria for PID.

Minimal criteria
- Lower abdominal tenderness
- Uterine/adnexal tenderness
- Cervical motion tenderness

Additional criteria
- Oral temperature >38.3°C (101°F)
- Abnormal cervical or vaginal mucopurulent discharge
- Presence of white blood cells (WBCs) on saline microscopy of vaginal secretions
- Elevated erythrocyte sedimentation rate
- Elevated C-reactive protein level
- Laboratory documentation of cervical infection with *Neisseria gonorrhoeae* or *Chlamydia trachomatis*

Definitive criteria
- Histopathologic evidence of endometritis on endometrial biopsy Transvaginal sonography or magnetic resonance imaging techniques showing thickened, fluid-filled tubes with or without free pelvic fluid or tubo-ovarian complex
- Laparoscopic abnormalities consistent with PID

have these hallmark findings, and in many cases the PID goes unrecognized [1]. In some women, the only evidence of PID is laparoscopic findings of acute or chronic salpingitis.

Although it is not necessary to perform laparoscopy to make the diagnosis of PID, the PEACH trial demonstrated that laparoscopy can reveal many findings suggestive of acute infection [9]. These include erythematous, swollen fallopian tubes with or without purulent discharge, or a peritubal abscess in severe cases. In general, there are no adhesions in the early stages of PID. Subacute cases can demonstrate gelatinous red adhesions, yellow liquid in the cul-de-sac, and yellow pseudocysts around the tubes and ovaries. In longstanding cases or in patients with recurrent PID, dense and fibrous adhesions, occluded fallopian tubes, and hydro/pyosalpinges may be seen. On second-look laparoscopy 3–6 months after an episode of PID, the duration of the PID was found to be strongly associated with the presence of pelvic adhesions and obstruction of the fallopian tubes [10]. These investigators also observed a 22% incidence of CPP, especially in patients who had chronic abscesses. Not surprisingly, more extensive adhesions were associated with a higher incidence of infertility and CPP.

Pelvic adhesions are often associated with pain because the peritoneum is rich in pain fibers that conduct pain stimuli to the central nervous system. Sulaiman and colleagues developed a mouse model that confirmed that both myelinated and nonmyelinated nerve fibers are present within four weeks of adhesion formation [11]. Immunohistochemistry also demonstrated nerve fibers within the adhesions. The nerve fibers, which were both myelinated and unmyelinated, expressed both calcitonin gene related protein and substance P [12].

Other markers of pain have been found in pelvic adhesions. In a small study of patients with pelvic pain and pelvic adhesions, cyclooxygenase-2 (COX-2) mRNA and its protein were present in adhesion fibroblasts [13]. The authors of this study suggested that the regulation of COX-2 could help reduce adhesion formation. The heterogeneity of the type of cells that exist within adhesions is indicative of the complexity of adhesive disease and its multifactorial origins.

PID has a polymicrobial etiology. Up to 50% of cases of PID are associated with *C. trachomatis* and/or *N. gonorrheae* [9]. The PEACH trial showed that lower genital tract inflammation was highly associated with upper genital tract infection and a positive test for *N. gonorrheae* and *C. trachomatis* in patients with mild to moderate PID. In the young (age ≤ 25), mostly black (65%) population described in the PEACH trial, a high titer of immunoglobulin G (IgG) antibodies to *C. trachomatis* was associated with significantly lower pregnancy rates, presumably from tubal disease caused by pelvic adhesions [14]. Treating and preventing chlamydia could potentially lower the incidence of tubal factor infertility, adhesion formation, CPP, and dyspareunia in patients with PID.

Prevention of PID

The Centers for Disease Control and Prevention (CDC) recommends chlamydia screening at least annually for young women and adolescents who are sexually active, or more frequently if symptoms such as abnormal discharge and bleeding develop [15]. However, a recent analysis showed that it was cost-effective to screen women every 5 months instead of every year, and this may indeed lead to improved diagnosis and treatment of PID and its associated side effects [16]. In addition, it has been shown in a study of almost 6000 patients that safe-sex counseling can increase condom use and decrease transmission

of chlamydia and other sexually transmitted infections including HIV [17].

Diagnosis, Management, and Prevention of Adhesions

While the gold standard method for the diagnosis of pelvic adhesions is surgery, it would be preferable if the diagnosis could be made less invasively. Advances in imaging technologies such as ultrasound, computed tomography (CT scan), and magnetic resonance imaging (MRI) have led to the investigation of these modalities to diagnose adhesions. A prospective study of 120 women with CPP examined both "soft" and "hard" markers in predicting pelvic pathology [18]. Soft markers included site-specific pelvic tenderness, ovarian mobility, and the presence of loculated peritoneal fluid in the pelvis. Only 6 of 37 (16%) patients with soft markers actually had pelvic adhesions, indicating that ultrasound is a poor way to diagnose adhesions in patients with CPP. MRI has also shown some promise in the diagnosis of pelvic adhesions with a sensitivity of 73% and specificity of 87% [19, 20].

There have been many in vivo studies of adhesion prevention. Recently, many commercially available products have been marketed as adhesion blockers. These include dextran, hyaluronic acid, hydrogel, fibrin, cellulose, and combinations of these which are sold under different brand names. Although there are no data on the prevention of adhesion formation after an episode of PID, animal models have been used to demonstrate that adhesion barriers can be helpful in adhesion prevention during sepsis. A group of Turkish investigators developed a rat model for a polymicrobial infection using cecal puncture. They demonstrated that the incidence of adhesions as well as the tensile strength of adhesions was significantly reduced in rats treated with a hyaluron-based agent when compared to placebo [21]. As PID is a similar infection to the one induced in this study, it is possible that such a barrier could be used in patients with PID to reduce the risk of long-term sequelae.

Recent Cochrane reviews have evaluated the role of fluid and pharmacological agents as well as barrier agents for adhesion prevention after gynecologic and fertility preserving pelvic surgery [22, 23]. Individual pharmacological and fluid agents, such as steroids, antihistamines, dextran, and hyaluronic acid were compared with no treatment or placebo. Also studied were synthetic barriers including oxidized regenerated cellulose, polytetrafluoroethylene, and fibrin sheets. It was found that there is insufficient evidence that steroids, icodextrin, and dextran prevent adhesion formation. There was some indication that fluids containing hyaluronic acid may help reduce adhesion formation. Limited data are available with respect to long-term outcomes such as pregnancy and fertility rates. With respect to adhesion barriers, both oxidized regenerated cellulose and polytetrafluoroethylene were found to reduce adhesion formation, although the polytetrafluoroethylene must be removed and is therefore of limited value [22, 23]. This suggests that there is likely no benefit for the prevention of pelvic pain or dyspareunia.

Women with a history of PID are more likely to suffer from sexual dysfunction, although a large study in the United States did not find that history of STIs was associated with a higher risk of sexual pain [24]. Data from the PEACH trial show that CPP is prevalent in women with a history of PID [25]. The rates of CPP were highest in patients who used condoms the least, suggesting that PID and other STIs are responsible [26]. Specifically, these patients also had a diminished quality of life, especially in their reported physical functioning, bodily pain, vitality, social functioning, and mental health [27]. In addition, Steege and Stoute [28] showed that laproscopic lysis of adhesions improves both pain during daily activities and dyspareunia.

Conclusion

PID and its sequelae affect millions of women in the United States at substantial costs. It has been estimated that 4.2 billion dollars a year are spent in medical care for PID [29]. Overall, private insurance covered the largest portion of the costs of PID (41%), followed by public payment sources. Prevention of PID is needed both to reduce human suffering and to contain rising costs [29]. Because the association between PID, pelvic adhesions, and dyspareunia is strong [30], further research is necessary to help reduce the impact of PID and subsequent adhesive disease on dyspareunia and sexual function.

References

1 Centers for Disease Control Website, http://www.cdc.gov/std/PID/STDFact-PID.htm

2 Practice Committee of the American Society for Reproductive Medicine, Society of Reproductive Surgeons. (2007) Pathogenesis, consequences, and control of peritoneal adhesions in gynecologic surgery. *Fertility and Sterility* **88**, 21–26.

3 Weibel, MA, Majno G. (1973) Peritoneal adhesions and their relation to abdominal surgery, a postmortem study. *American Journal of Surgery* **126**, 345–53.

4 American Fertility Society. (1988) The AFS classification of adnexal adhesions. *Fertility and Sterility* **49**, 944–55.

5 Adhesions Scoring Group. (1994) Improvement of the interobserver reproducibility of the adhesion scoring system. *Fertility and Sterility* **62**, 984–88.

6 Chegini N, Gold LI, Williams S, *et al.* (1994) Localization of transforming growth factor beta isoforms TGFB1, TGFB-2, and TGFB-3 in surgically induced pelvic adhesions in the rat. *Obstetrics and Gynecology* **83**, 449–54.

7 Victory R, Saed GM, Diamon MP. (2007) Antiadhesion effects of docosahexaenoic acid on normal human peritoneal adhesion fibroblasts. *Fertility and Sterility* **88**, 1657–62.

8 Westrom L, Joesoef R, Reynolds G, *et al.* (1992) Pelvic inflammatory disease and fertility: a cohort study of 1,844 women with laparoscopically verified disease and 657 control women with normal laparoscopic findings. *Sexually Transmitted Diseases* **19**, 185–92.

9 Haggerty SL, Hillier, Bass DC, Ness RB. (2004) Bacterial vaginosis and anaerobic bacteria are associated with endometritis. *Clinical Infectious Diseases* **39**, 990–95.

10 Henry-Suchet, J. (2000) PID: Clinical and laparoscopic aspects. *Annals of the New York Academy of Sciences.* **900**, 301–8.

11 Sulaiman H, Gabells G, Davis C, *et al.* (2000) Growth of nerve fibers into murine peritoneal adhesions. *Journal of Pathology* **192**, 396–403.

12 Sulaiman H, Gabella G, Davis C, *et al.* (2001) Presence and distribution of sensory nerve fibers in human peritoneal adhesions. *Annals of Surgery* **234**, 256–61.

13 Saed GM, Munkarah AR, Diamond MP. (2003) Cyclooxygenase-2 is expressed in human fibroblasts isolated from intraperitoneal adhesions but not from normal peritoneal tissues. *Fertility and Sterility* **79**, 1404–08.

14 Ness RB, Soper DE, Richter HE, *et al.* (2008) Chlamydia antibodies, chlamydia heat shock protein, and adverse sequelae after pelvic inflammatory disease: the PID evalauation and clinical health (PEACH) study. *Sexually Transmitted Diseases* **35**, 129–35.

15 CDC Guidelines for Treating STIs. (2006) www.cdc.gov/std/treatment/

16 Smith KJ, Cook RL, Roberts MS. (2007) Time from sexually transmitted infection acquisition to pelvic inflammatory disease development, influence of cost-effectiveness of different screening intervals. *Value in Health* **10**, 358–66.

17 Project RESPECT Study Group: Kamb ML, Fishbein M, Douglas JM, Jr., *et al.* (1998) Efficacy of risk-reduction counseling to prevent human immunodeficiency virus and sexually transmitted diseases: a randomized controlled trial. *Journal of the American Medical Association* **280**, 1161–67.

18 Okaro E, Condous G, Khalid A, *et al.* (2006) The use of ultrasound-based "soft markers" for the prediction of pelvic pathology in women with chronic pelvic pain: can we reduce the need for laparoscopy? *Obstetrical and Gynaecological Survey* **61**, 379–80.

19 Byrne H, Ball E, Davis C. (2006) The role of magnetic resonance imaging in minimal access surgery. *Current Opinion on Obstetrics and Gynecology* **18**, 369–73.

20 Katayama M, Masui T, Kobayashi S, *et al.* (2001) Evaluation of pelvic adhesions using multiphase and multislice MR imaging with kinematic display. *American Journal of Roentgenology* **177**, 107–110.

21 Tuzuner A, Kuzu MA, Akin B, *et al.* (2004) The effect of hyaluronan-based agents on adhesion formation in an intra-abdominal sepsis model. *Digestive Diseases and Sciences* **49**, 1054–62.

22 Metwally M, Watson A, Lilford R, *et al.* (2006) Fluid and pharmacological agents for adhesion prevention after gynaecological surgery. *The Cochrane Database of Systematic Reviews* **2**.

23 Ahmad G, Duffy JMN, Farquhar C, *et al.* (2008) Barrier agents for adhesion prevention after gynaecological surgery. *The Cochrane Database of Systematic Reviews* **3**.

24 Laumann EO, Paik A, Rosen RC. (1999) Sexual dysfuction in the United States: prevalence and predictors. *Journal of the American Medical Association* **281**, 537–44.

25 Haggerty CL, Peipert J, Weitzen S, *et al.* (2005) Predictors of chronic pelvic pain in an urban population of women with symptoms and signs of pelvic inflammatory disease. *Sexually Transmitted Diseases* **32**, 293–99.

26 Ness RB, Randall H, Richter HE, *et al.* (2004) Condom use and the risk of recurrent pelvic inflammatory disease, chronic pelvic pain, or infertility following an episode of pelvic inflammatory disease. *American Journal of Public Health* **94**, 1327–29.

27 Haggerty CL, Schulz R, Ness RB. (2003) Lower quality of life among women with chronic pelvic pain after pelvic inflammatory disease. *Obstetrics and Gynecology* **102**, 934–39.

28 Steege JF, Stout AL. (1991) Resolution of chronic pelvic pain after laparoscopic lysis of adhesions. *American Journal of Obstetrics and Gynecolpgy* **165**, 278–83.

29 Washington AE, Katz P. (1991) Cost of and payment source for pelvic inflammatory disease: trends and projections, 1983 through 2000. *Journal of the American Medical Association* **266**, 2565–69.

30 Marks C, Tideman RL, Estcourt CS, *et al.* (2000) Diagnosing PID: getting the balance right. *International Journal of STD and AIDS* **11**, 545–47.

CHAPTER 21

Dyspareunia and Irritable Bowel Syndrome (IBS)

Ami D. Sperber,[1] *Douglas A. Drossman*[2]

[1] Ben-Gurion University of the Negev, Beer-Sheva, Israel
[2] University of North Carolina, Chapel Hill, NC, USA

Introduction

In this chapter, we assess available data on associations between irritable bowel syndrome (IBS) and dyspareunia. IBS will be defined and a short summary of its characteristics provided. Sexual dysfunction (including dyspareunia) and chronic pelvic pain (CPP) will be discussed in the context of the well-recognized phenomenon of comorbidity between IBS and extra-intestinal unexplained symptoms and functional disorders. The chapter will conclude with a conceptual and mechanistic model and discussion of these associations.

Irritable Bowel Syndrome

Irritable bowel syndrome (IBS) is the best known of the functional gastrointestinal (GI) tract disorders, all characterized by chronic or recurrent GI tract symptoms that are not explained by structural abnormalities, infection, or metabolic changes on routine testing [1, 2]. Patients with IBS suffer from chronic abdominal pain, usually in the lower abdomen, with an impaired bowel pattern. The latter can be constipation, diarrhea, or mixed constipation and diarrhea. Although the range of prevalence rates for IBS in studies conducted throughout the world is broad (from 2% to 25%), in the Western world, it is generally agreed that 10–20% of adults meet diagnostic criteria for IBS [1, 3, 4].

Female Sexual Pain Disorders 1st edition. Edited by A. Goldstein, C. Pukall & I. Goldstein. © 2009 Blackwell Publishing, ISBN: 9781405183987.

The burden of IBS on the health care services is substantial. As many as 28% of referrals for gastroenterology consultations are for IBS [5]. Absenteeism rates from work or school are significantly higher among patients with IBS than nonaffected individuals [6]. The cost of health services for patients with IBS is very high [7, 8].

Approximately 60–70% of IBS patients are women [6], making it a serious women's health concern. The results of studies have shown that a greater awareness of IBS on the part of gynecologists could reduce the rate of unnecessary diagnostic tests and procedures in women complaining of pelvic/lower abdominal pain. Because of the similarity in pain of bowel and gynecological origin, the cause of women's symptoms may be difficult to determine [9] and women with unrecognized IBS may undergo unnecessary pelvic laparoscopy or even surgery.

For many years IBS was considered a "diagnosis of exclusion." However, over the past 20 years expert working groups have developed symptom-based, consensus-diagnostic criteria for IBS and the other functional GI disorders [1]. Known as the Rome criteria (Rome III in its latest version) (Table 21.1), these criteria have contributed to positive developments in the field of functional GI disorders. IBS can now be confidently diagnosed on the basis of a cluster of symptoms with a minimal diagnostic workup [10].

IBS is a complex, multifactorial disorder. Research on the pathophysiology of IBS has focused on the bidirectional signaling pathways and information processing centers between the GI system and the central nervous system, known as the brain–gut axis [11–14]. The experience of abdominal pain and/or altered motility and bowel

Table 21.1 Rome III diagnostic criteria for IBS.*

Recurrent abdominal pain or discomfort** at least 3 days/month in the last 3 months associated with *two or more* of the following:
1. Improvement with defecation;
2. Onset associated with a change in frequency of stool;
3. Onset associated with a change in form (appearance) of stool.

* Criterion fulfilled for the last 3 months with symptom onset at least 6 months prior to diagnosis.
** "Discomfort" means an uncomfortable sensation not described as pain.

habits can be caused by impaired activity in the intestinal lumen, the intestinal mucosa, or the enteric nervous system [15–17].

Brain–gut activity is mediated by biochemical factors incorporating input from the neuroendocrine and neuroimmunological systems [18]. Peripheral stressors and/or changes to the intestinal mucosa (e.g., following acute gastroenteritis [19, 20], transient mucosal inflammation, and/or prior abdominal or pelvic surgery [21–23] may affect afferent stimuli from the gut. A major factor in the experience of symptoms is abnormal central processing of peripheral afferent visceral signals, leading to a lowered threshold for pain (hypersensitivity) and increased selective attention to gut-related stimuli (hypervigilance) [24].

Similar processes have been implicated in "functional" gynecological disorders related to CPP and dyspareunia, including vestibulodynia. Pukall et al. reported that women with vestibulodynia have augmented sensory genital processing similar to other "hypersensitivity syndromes" such as IBS [25, 26].

Comorbid Conditions and Symptoms in IBS

In a systematic review of the literature, Whitehead et al. [27] reported that 50% of IBS patients complain of at least one other unexplained somatic symptom and that a significant number of IBS patients meet diagnostic criteria for other functional somatic syndromes [28] including CPP and dyspareunia.

When patients with IBS also suffer from other chronic unexplained symptoms (such as dyspareunia) and/or other non-GI functional disorders (such as CPP),

there is a significant increase in symptom severity and comorbid psychopathology with a corresponding reduction in quality of life as compared to IBS patients without chronic comorbid conditions [27–29].

Prevalence of Sexual Dysfunction Among IBS Patients

Some studies examine the link between IBS and dyspareunia (Table 21.2), although there are more studies investigating the association between IBS and CPP. These studies have reported an increased prevalence of sexual dysfunction among IBS patients, including reduced sexual drive [30], increased dyspareunia [31, 32] and more severe IBS symptoms following intercourse. IBS patients report a high rate of intercourse avoidance [33]. The presence of sexual dysfunction in IBS may be affected by factors such as a history of sexual abuse and disorders of the pelvic floor.

Whorwell et al. [31] assessed 100 consecutive IBS patients (90 women and 10 men) in the UK for noncolonic comorbid conditions in comparison with 100 controls matched to the patients by age, sex, and social class. Among the IBS patients, 42% reported dyspareunia compared to 5% of the controls (P < 0.0001). This significant association was not affected by the presence or absence of psychological comorbidity. In contrast, there was no significant difference between the groups in the percentage reporting premenstrual tension (63% and 55%, respectively).

Prior et al. [34] evaluated 798 patients referred by general practitioners to a gynecological clinic over a 6-year period. Of these, 63 were referred for dyspareunia of whom 52.4% were found to meet diagnostic criteria for IBS (40.8–59.2, 95% CI, P < 0.001). This strong association was not related to overlap with other indications for referral to the gynecology clinic. Interestingly, the prevalence of IBS was particularly high among women complaining of dyspareunia and dysmenorrhea, but was similar to rates for controls in women who came to the gynecology clinic for other indications such as termination of sterilization, for cervical abnormalities, and because of prolapse, cysts, or vulvar warts.

Longstreth et al. [9] assessed 86 women undergoing gynecological laparoscopy for CPP. IBS was diagnosed in 47.7% of these women. Those with IBS were compared

Table 21.2 Reported rates of dyspareunia and sexual dysfunction in women with IBS, with and without CPP.

Study	Dyspareunia	Decreased libido	After intercourse IBS worsens	Increased IBS symptoms leads to reduced sexual activity	Avoid intercourse
Whorwell [31] (90% women)	42%	–	–	–	–
Guthrie [49]	17%	–	69%	–	–
Walker [50]	52%	28%	16%	–	–
Prior [34]*	52.4	–	–	–	–
Longstreth [9]†	78.4%	–	–	–	–
Corney [33]		–	–	–	48.3%
Nyhlin [51]	8%	–	–	–	–
Walker [52]	42%	–	–	–	–
Fass [30]‡	32%	36%	–	15%	32%
Zondervan [35] (IBS and CPP)	79.3%	–	–	53%§	32.6%
Williams [53] (IBS + CPP)	12.7–37.5§§	–	–	–	–

*Women with dyspareunia who were diagnosed with IBS.
†Women with CPP and IBS referred for diagnostic pelvic laparoscopy.
‡Women with IBS and a sexual problem over previous 6 months.
§IBS, CPP, and genitourinary symptoms.
§§Mixed dyspareunia = 12.7%; functional = 11.8%; organic, 37.5%.

with those without IBS on a series of demographic and clinical variables as well as findings at laparoscopy. No significant difference was found between the two groups in terms of age, symptoms (pain duration, abnormal menstrual bleeding, depression, chronic headache or backache), or findings on laparoscopy (adhesions, endometriosis, functional ovarian cyst, uterine fibroid, chronic PID, neoplastic ovarian cyst, or other findings). However, there was a significant difference between the groups in rates of dyspareunia. Among women with IBS, 78.4% complained of dyspareunia compared with 53.8% among those without IBS ($P < 0.05$).

Zondervan et al. [35] conducted a community-based survey of a representative sample of women in a district of England examining the overlap among CPP, dysmenorrhea, dyspareunia, and IBS. Among women with CPP without IBS, 41% reported dyspareunia over the previous three months (compared with 13.8% among women without either CPP or IBS). The percentage of women reporting dyspareunia increased to 79.3% among women who reported CPP and IBS. Another finding of interest was that among women with CPP without IBS, 22% reported having sexual intercourse less frequently because of the pain compared with 53% among women with CPP, IBS, and genitourinary symptoms ($P < 0.01$).

Fass et al. [30] surveyed 683 consecutive patients with IBS or functional dyspepsia for sexual dysfunction and compared them with a comparison group of 247 controls. Any participant who reported interference with sexual functioning over the previous 6 months was asked to characterize the problem in terms of decreased sexual drive, pain during intercourse, symptoms that directly prevent intercourse, and exacerbation of sexual problems at the time of exacerbation of bowel problems.

The prevalence of any reported sexual dysfunction among patients was 40.6% (males and females), which was significantly higher than among controls (OR 4.33, $P < 0.001$). Among women with IBS with a sexual problem over the previous 6 months, 36% reported a decreased sexual drive, 32% reported dyspareunia, 32% reported that bowel symptoms directly prevented them from engaging in intercourse, and 15% reported that sexual dysfunction worsened directly in relation to the severity of their bowel problems. However, in all, only 14% of women with IBS reported dyspareunia.

CPP Among Female IBS Patients

Another related problem is the high rate of CPP in IBS patients. Many IBS patients undergo gynecological work-ups, including pelvic laparoscopy for pelvic pain, without any pathological findings. The prevalence of CPP in IBS was reported to be 14% [32]. The rates of IBS in women with CPP are even higher, ranging from 29% to 79% [32, 36]. Williams et al. [37] studied 987 new patients to a CPP clinic and reported that 35% met the Rome I criteria for IBS, although IBS was not diagnosed previously in 40% of these patients. In contrast to the studies depicted above, this study failed to demonstrate a relationship between IBS and dyspareunia among women with CPP for any type of deep dyspareunia (organic, functional, or mixed). Similar percentages of women with and without IBS reported this problem.

History of Abuse and Possible Association with Sexual Dysfunction in IBS

Studies have demonstrated that IBS patients have higher rates of sexual abuse, including threatened sex, incest, forced intercourse, lifetime sexual victimization, severe lifetime sexual trauma, and severe child sexual abuse than patients with structural GI diseases [38–41], an association that appears to hold true for many of the functional somatic disorders.

There is also a documented association between sexual abuse and CPP. Walker et al. [42] conducted an in-depth study of CPP, psychiatric diagnoses and childhood sexual abuse among 55 women scheduled to undergo diagnostic laparoscopy either with CPP (study group) or without it (controls). Compared with the controls, the women with CPP had a significantly higher prevalence of depression and somatization disorder, a significantly higher percentage of childhood sexual abuse and more sexual dysfunction, in particular, significantly more functional dyspareunia and more inhibited sexual desire. Among women with previous sexual abuse, there was a statistically significant association between depression and pelvic pain, which was not found among women without a history of sexual abuse.

Latthe et al. published a systematic review of CPP, including dyspareunia, and looked at its association with predisposing factors, including abuse history [43]. Of the studies identified, 19 evaluated dyspareunia and 68% of these met the review's quality criteria. The authors reported, on the basis of seven studies, that a history of sexual abuse was associated with dyspareunia with an OR of 2.67 (99% CI 2.16 to 3.29; $P < 0.001$).

Toward a Unifying Model of Brain–Gut Interactions and Dyspareunia: The Relationship of Psychosocial Distress to Functional GI Symptoms

Dyspareunia and CPP are recognized as comorbid conditions in women with IBS. As reviewed above, the more comorbid conditions IBS patients have, the greater the psychosocial difficulties they manifest and the worse their quality of life [27]. There are peripheral contributions to the initiation of sensory signals and central contributions to the perception and overall experience of these signals as symptoms and behaviors. Thus, the central effects refer to central nervous system (CNS) processing of peripheral sensory information, including facilitation of ascending pain signals and descending inhibition of these signals [44]. This central processing can be modulated by psychosocial factors such as stressful life events, a history of abuse, poor coping skills, nonsupportive social networks, and maladaptive ("catastrophic") cognitions [11, 45]. Patients with more comorbid somatic conditions tend to have more central effects and greater symptom severity. The following studies illustrate the capability of psychosocial factors to regulate GI symptoms via the CNS.

We recently reported that significantly more women undergoing elective gynecological surgery reported abdominal pain both 3 and 12 months after surgery than nonsurgical controls [23]. The only presurgery variables that predicted this development were psychosocial ones, implying that pain development was associated with central registration and amplification of the afferent signal (via cognitive and emotional input). Pukall et al. used functional MRI to show that women with vestibulodynia have augmented sensory processing [25]. Women with both IBS and dyspareunia would be expected, based on the conceptual model presented here (Figure 21.1), to have more psychological difficulties, more central effects, hypervigilance to gut and pelvic-related sensory stimuli, and lower quality of life than women with either entity alone.

Other brain imaging studies have demonstrated an association between sexual abuse and disinhibition of afferent pain signals that was modulated by changes in

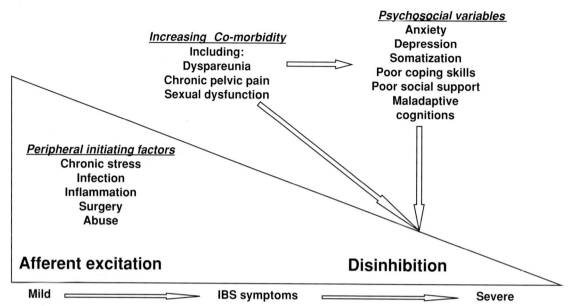

Figure 21.1 A conceptual model showing IBS symptom severity as a function of the interaction between peripheral sensory initiating factors and central processing variables. Central processing of the afferent signals leads to disinhibition and more severe IBS symptoms. It is increased by the presence of chronic comorbid conditions (including dyspareunia), which also have a negative effect on psychosocial variables, another factor that increases central signal processing and disinhibition. The triangle shape demonstrates that most patients have mild or moderate symptoms while a minority has more severe symptoms.

psychological distress [46]. A brain imaging study was performed on a young woman who had been the victim of childhood and adult sexual abuse. When she exhibited increased psychological distress, there was activation of the cingulate cortex leading to decreased inhibition of afferent sensory signals generated by rectal distension. In contrast, after successful psychological treatment there was less activation of this brain center and reduced sensitivity to peripheral pain. More recently, we have shown that groups of patients with a history of abuse and IBS have greater activation of the anterior mid-cingulate cortex which correlated with the patients' reports of pain [47].

Figure 21.1 presents a conceptual model in which afferent excitation (e.g., infection, inflammation, surgery, abuse) causes a level of distress with mild IBS symptom severity. However, with an increasing number of comorbid conditions (including dyspareunia, chronic pelvic pain, and sexual dysfunction), IBS symptoms become moderate to severe. This is modulated by psychosocial factors (anxiety, depression, somatization, poor coping skills, poor social support, and maladaptive cognitions) by means of

CNS disinhibition. The psychosocial factors are themselves affected negatively by the presence of chronic co-morbidity.

Future research might focus on the effect of comorbid IBS and dyspareunia on central processing, as assessed for example by brain imaging techniques, and the modulating effect of psychosocial variables. The results of such studies could have implications for centrally targeted treatments in IBS and in CPP and dyspareunia [48].

References

1 Longstreth GF, Thompson WG, Chey WD, *et al.* (2006) Functional bowel disorders. In: Drossman SA, Corazzari E, Delvaux M, *et al.* (eds.). Rome III. *The Functional Gastrointestinal Disorders.* Degnon Associates, Inc., McLean, VA, pp. 487–555.

2 Drossman DA, Camilleri M, Mayer EA, *et al.* (2002) AGA technical review on irritable bowel syndrome. *Gastroenterology* **23**, 2108–31.

3 Cremonini F, Talley NJ. (2005) Irritable bowel syndrome: epidemiology, natural history, health care seeking and emerging

risk factors. *Gastroenterology Clinics of North America* **34**, 189–204.

4 Hungin AP, Whorwell PJ, Tack J, *et al.* (2003) The prevalence, patterns, and impact of irritable bowel syndrome: an international survey of 40,000 subjects. *Alimentary Pharmacology and Therapeutics* **17**, 643–50.

5 Mitchell CM, Drossman DA. (1987) Survey of the AGA membership relating to patients with functional gastrointestinal disorders. *Gastroenterology* **92**, 1282–84.

6 Drossman DA, Li Z, Andruzzi E, *et al.* (1993) U.S. householder survey of functional GI disorders: prevalence, sociodemography, and health impact. *Digestive Disease and Sciences* **38**, 1569–80.

7 Talley NJ, Gabriel SE, Hamsen WS, *et al.* (1995) Medical costs in community subjects with irritable bowel syndrome. *Gastroenterology* **109**, 1736–41.

8 Sandler RS, Everhart JE, Donowitz M, *et al.* (2002) The burden of selected digestive diseases in the United States. *Gastroenterology* **122**, 1500–11.

9 Longstreth G, Preskill DB, Youkeles L. (1990). Irritable bowel syndrome in women having diagnostic laparoscopy or hysterectomy: relation to gynecologic features and outcome. *Digestive Disease and Sciences* **35**, 1285–90.

10 Cash BD, Schoenfeld P, Chey WD. (2002) The utility of diagnostic tests in irritable bowel syndrome patients: a systematic review. *American Journal of Gastroenterology* **97**, 2812–19.

11 Drossman DA. (2006) The functional gastrointestinal disorders and the Rome III process. In: Drossman DA, Corazziari E, Delvaux M, *et al.* (eds.). *Rome III. The Functional Gastrointestinal Disorders.* 2nd. ed. Degnon Associates, Inc., McLean, VA, pp. 1–29.

12 Hobson AR, Aziz Q. (2004) Brain imaging and functional gastrointestinal disorders: has it helped our understanding? *Gut* **53**, 1198–1206.

13 Mayer EA, Naliboff BD, Chang L, *et al.* (2001) Stress and irritable bowel syndrome. *American Journal of Physiology—Gastrointestinal and Liver Physiology* **280**, G519–24.

14 Wood JD, Grundy D, Al-Chaer ED, *et al.* (2006) Fundamentals of neurogastroenterology: basic science. In: Drossman SA, Corazziari E, Delvaux M, *et al.* (eds.). *Rome III: The Functional Gastrointestinal Disorders.* 3rd ed. Degnon Associates, Inc., McLean, VA.

15 Spiller RC. (2003) Postinfectious irritable bowel syndrome. *Gastroenterology* **124**, 1662–71.

16 Mertz H, Naliboff B, Munakata J, *et al.* (1995) Altered rectal perception is a biological marker of patients with irritable bowel syndrome. *Gastroenterology* **109**, 40–52.

17 Munakata J, Naliboff B, Harraf F, *et al.* (1997) Repetitive sigmoid stimulation induces rectal hyperalgesia in patients with irritable bowel syndrome. *Gastroenterology* **112**, 55–63.

18 Chadwick VS, Chen W, Shu D, *et al.* (2002) Activation of the mucosal immune system in irritable bowel syndrome. *Gastroenterology* **122**, 1778–83.

19 Gwee KA, Leong YL, Graham C, *et al.* (1999) The role of psychological and biological factors in postinfective gut dysfunction. *Gut* **44**, 400–6.

20 Neal KR, Barker L, Spiller RC. (2002) Prognosis in postinfective irritable bowel syndrome: a six-year follow-up study. *Gut* **51**, 410–13.

21 Longstreth GF, Yao JF. (2004) Irritable bowel syndrome and surgery: a multivariable analysis. *Gastroenterology* **126**, 1665–73.

22 Hasler WL, Schoenfeld P. (2003) Systematic review: abdominal and pelvic surgery in patients with irritable bowel syndrome. *Alimentary Pharmacology and Therapeutics* **17**, 997–1005.

23 Sperber AD, Blank Morris C, Greemberg L, *et al.* (2008) Development of abdominal pain and IBS following gynecological surgery: a prospective, controlled study. *Gastroenterology* **134**, 75–84.

24 Chang L, Mayer EA, Johnson T, *et al.* (2000) Differences in somatic perception in female patients with irritable bowel syndrome with and without fibromyalgia. *Pain* **84**, 297–307.

25 Pukall CF, Strigo IA, Binik YM, *et al.* (2005) Neural correlates of painful genital touch in women with vulvar vestibulitis syndrome. *Pain* **115**, 118–27.

26 Pukall CF, Binik YM, Khalife S, *et al.* (2002) Vestibular tactile and pain thresholds in women with vulvar vestibulitis syndrome. *Pain* **96**, 163–75.

27 Whitehead WE, Palsson O, Jones KR. (2002) Systematic review of the comorbidity of irritable bowel syndrome with other disorders: what are the causes and implications? *Gastroenterology* **122**, 1140–56.

28 Sperber AD, Atzmon Y, Neumann L, *et al.* (1999) Fibromyalgia in the irritable bowel syndrome: studies of prevalence and clinical implications. *American Journal of Gastroenterology* **94**, 3541–46.

29 Markowitz M, Harris W, Ricci JF, *et al.* (2001) Comorbid conditions in patients with irritable bowel syndrome: data from a national IBS awareness registry. *Gastroenterology* **120**, 105.

30 Fass R, Fullerton S, Naliboff B, *et al.* (1998) Sexual dysfunction in patients with irritable bowel syndrome and nonulcer dyspepsia. *Digestion* **59**, 79–85.

31 Whorwell PJ, McCallum M, Creed FH. (1986) Noncolonic features of irritable bowel syndrome. *Gut* **27**, 37–40.

32 Walker EA, Katon WJ, Jemelka R, *et al.* (1991) The prevalence of chronic pelvic pain and irritable bowel syndrome in two university clinics. *Journal of Psychosomatic Obstetrics and Gynaecology* **12**, 65–75.

33 Corney RH, Stanton R. (1990) Physical symptom severity, psychological and social dysfunction in a series of outpatients with irritable bowel syndrome. *Journal of Psychosomatic Research* **34**, 483–91.

34 Prior A, Wilson K, Whorwell PJ, *et al.* (1989) Irritable bowel syndrome in the gynecological clinic: survey of 798 new referrals. *Digestive Diseases and Sciences* **34**, 1820–24.

35 Zondervan KT, Yudkin PL, Vessey MP, *et al.* (2001) Chronic pelvic pain in the community: symptoms, investigations, and diagnoses. *American Journal of Obstetrics and Gynecology* **184**, 1149–55.

36 Longstreth GF. (1994) Irritable bowel syndrome and chronic pelvic pain. *Obstetrical and Gynecological Survey* **49**, 505–7.

37 Williams RE, Hartmann KE, Sandler RS, *et al.* (2005) Recognition and treatment of irritable bowel syndrome among women with chronic pelvic pain. *American Journal of Obstetrics and Gynecology* **192**, 761–67.

38 Drossman SA, Leserman J, Nachman N, *et al.* Sexual and physical abuse in women with functional or organic gastrointestinal disorders. *Annals of Internal Medicine* **113**, 828–33.

39 Walker EA, Katon WJ, Roy-Byrne PP, *et al.* (1993) Histories of sexual victimization in patients with irritable bowel syndrome or inflammatory bowel disease. *American Journal of Psychiatry* **150**, 1502–6.

40 Drossman DA, Talley NJ, Olden KW, *et al.* (1995) Sexual and physical abuse and gastrointestinal illness: review and recommendations. *Annals of Internal Medicine* **123**, 782–74.

41 Drossman SA, Li Z, Leserman J, *et al.* (1996) Health status by gastrointestinal diagnosis and abuse history. *Gastroenterology* **110**, 999–1007.

42 Walker EA, Katon WJ, Harrop-Griffiths J, *et al.* (1988) Relationship of chronic pelvic pain to psychiatric diagnoses and childhood sexual abuse. *American Journal of Psychiatry* **145**, 75–80.

43 Latthe P, Mignini L, Gray R, *et al.* (2006) Factors predisposing women to chronic pelvic pain: systematic review. *BMJ* **332**, 749–55.

44 Naliboff BD, Derbyshire SW, Munakata J, *et al.* (2001) Cerebral activation in patients with irritable bowel syndrome and control subjects during rectosigmoid stimulation. *Psychosomatic Medicine* **63**, 365–75.

45 Creed F, Levy R, Bradley L, *et al.* (2006) Psychosocial aspects of functional gastrointestinal disorders. In: Drossman SA, Corazziari E, Delvaux M. (eds). *Rome III. The Functional Gastrointestinal Disorders.* Degnon Associates, Inc., McLean, VA, pp. 295–368.

46 Drossman DA, Ringel Y, Vogt BA, *et al.* (2003). Alterations of brain activity associated with resolution of emotional distress and pain in a case of severe irritable bowel syndrome. *Gastroenterology* **124**, 754–61.

47 Ringel Y, Drossman DA, Leserman JL, *et al.* (2008) Effect of abuse history on pain reports and brain responses to aversive visceral stimulation: an fMRI study. *Gastroenterology* **134**, 396–404.

48 Drossman DA. (2005) Brain imaging and its implications for studying centrally targeted treatments in irritable bowel syndrome: a primer for gastroenterologists. *Gut* **54**, 569–73.

49 Guthrie E, Creed FH, Whorwell PJ. (1987) Severe sexual dysfunction in women with the irritable bowel syndrome: comparison with inflammatory bowel disease and duodenal ulceration. *BMJ (Clinical Research Ed)* **295**, 577–78.

50 Walker E, Katon W, Harrop-Griffiths J, *et al.* (1988) Relationship of chronic pelvic pain to psychiatric diagnoses and childhood sexual abuse. *American Journal of Psychiatry* **145**, 75–80.

51 Nyhlin H, Ford MJ, Eastwood J, *et al.* (1993) Nonalimentary aspects of the irritable bowel syndrome. *Journal of Psychosomatic Research* **37**, 155–62.

52 Walker EA, Gelfand AN, Gelfand MD, *et al.* (1996) Chronic pelvic pain and gynecological symptom symptoms in women with irritable bowel syndrome. *Journal of Psychosomatic Obstetrics and Gynaecology* **17**. 39–46.

53 Williams RE, Hartmann KE, Sandler RS, *et al.* (2004) Prevalence and characteristics of irritable bowel syndrome among women with chronic pelvic pain. *Obstetrics and Gynecology* **104**, 452–58.

CHAPTER 22

Pelvic Organ Prolapse and Sexual Pain

Gordon Davis,[1] *Joe Brooks*[2]

[1] The University of Arizona School of Medicine, Tucson, AZ, USA
[2] The Arizona Vulva Clinic, Phoenix, AZ, USA

Introduction

The integrity of the supportive structures of the lower genital tract is not given its due consideration as causative factors of sexual pain. Pelvic organ prolapse (POP) can be a significant cause of vaginal and rectal pressure and pain. In addition, women with POP frequently complain that they have the sensation of "bulging" or that "something is falling out." POP can also cause incontinence of urine or stool. Because of these symptoms, POP presents significant barriers to sexual function. It has been demonstrated that women with POP suffer from sexual dysfunction.

In addition, POP may exacerbate other vulvar diseases that may in themselves cause sexual dysfunction. For example, urinary incontinence may worsen the symptoms of lichen sclerosus. In addition, as the symptoms of POP overlap with other vulvar pain syndromes, it is possible that the diagnosis of POP may be overlooked and incorrectly diagnosed as provoked vestibulodynia (PVD) or generalized vulvodynia (GVD). Therefore, an understanding of anatomic distortions that may be found in women with POP is necessary when addressing a patient who presents with sexual complaints. The goal of this chapter is to review POP and its effects on dyspareunia.

Female Sexual Pain Disorders 1st edition. Edited by A. Goldstein, C. Pukall & I. Goldstein. © 2009 Blackwell Publishing, ISBN: 9781405183987.

Diagnosing Pelvic Organ Prolapse

The initial evaluation of POP begins with a visual inspection of the perineum. Patients with high degrees of prolapse manifest a bulge or protrusion of the most dependent part of the prolapse at the introitus when the labia minora are separated. The examiner should realize, however, that the supine position is associated with a spontaneous reduction of prolapse. This is a clinical correlate to the relief of symptoms women with POP often obtain when they are resting in the supine position. Therefore, we recommend that the examination of the internal structures be conducted with the patient both supine and standing [1]. Examination in the supine position allows for visual inspection, whereas examination in the erect position provides thorough palpation of sites of endopelvic fascial defects and their associated organs.

The authors advocate the "semi-squat" standing position (Figure 22.1). When the patient is standing erect, the examiner and the patient can often palpate the bulge associated with POP. Cystocele, rectocele, and enterocele are diagnosed entirely on physical examination by observation and palpation. Magnetic resonance imaging (MRI) and other imaging techniques can confirm the clinical impression of prolapse, but they are rarely indicated.

POP is described in levels of degree or extent. Sexual complaints are believed to be related to stage. The preferred staging system for POP is the Pelvic Organ Prolapse Quantification system (POP-Q) [2]. This staging system defines the hymen as the key anatomic landmark.

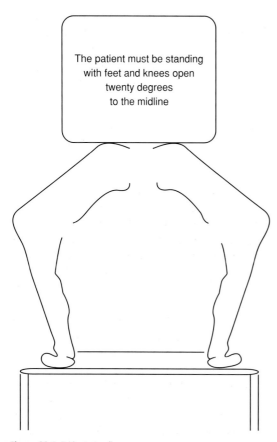

The patient must be standing with feet and knees open twenty degrees to the midline

Figure 22.1 Patient standing.

Descent beyond the hymen is usually symptomatic and may manifest as sexual pain. Further, with descent beyond the hymen, the degree of prolapse is considered more severe [3]. Irritative symptoms increase as the prolapsing organ (i.e., bladder, cervix, uterus) descends to the level of the vulvar vestibule, because the vestibule has a higher density of nociceptors than the prolapsing organ.

Evaluation of Anterior Defects

Anterior separation is defined as hypermobility of the urethra, including cystocele and anterior enterocele. Anterior separation may produce vulvar pain referable to the urogenital triangle of the vulva. The patient may describe her pain as "vaginal." The patient may gesture with her hand, pushing downward on her mons pubis, as if to indicate that her symptoms are arising in the anterior vulvar triangle.

Following initial inspection, two fingers are inserted into the introitus, with the examiner's palm facing downwards. The integrity of the posterior pelvic floor structures is evaluated and the patient's ability to contract and relax the pelvic floor muscles is assessed. The examiner then rotates his or her hand 180° to palpate the urethra. The urethra is then between the examiner's two fingers. The patient is asked to valsalva, and the urethra can be felt to descend and move outward, especially when urethral hypermobility is present. The pubic symphysis and the arcus tendineus fasciae pelvis attachments are then palpable superior and lateral to the urethra. Palpation of Cooper's ligament should be performed in patients with a history of a prior retropubic surgery (e.g., Burch procedure). The examiner may then palpate a bulge superior to the urethra (cystocele). The examination continues with a single speculum blade examination that allows visualization of the complete vaginal canal and the anterior bulge. Excessive tenderness in this region may suggest that further evaluation of the bladder mucosa is indicated. However, cystoscopy is not routinely performed in the evaluation of anterior defects.

Suburethral and paraurethral prolapse are referred to as cystourethroceles. Forceful separation of the endopelvic fascia from its attachment at the pubic rami or attenuation of the midline fascial fibers is responsible for the findings of an anterior "bulge." Hypermobility of the urethra can be associated with stress urinary incontinence, which may cause inflammation at the vestibule, contributing to introital dyspareunia.

A Q-tip® test (not to be confused with the cotton swab test performed in the evaluation of PVD) is then performed by placing a cotton-tip applicator into the urethra to measure the arc of movement greater than 30° as the patient strains. If positive, this test may be suggestive of an anterior urethral separation. While the Q-tip test may be useful, it is not considered diagnostic of a distinct pathology. In addition, it may not be necessary in patients with higher stages of prolapse as it has been shown that virtually all these patients will have urethral hypermobility [4]. Neither urodynamic studies nor closing urethral pressure profiles are required if urethral hypermobility is found on physical examination. These tests are only necessary when evaluating a woman with urinary incontinence.

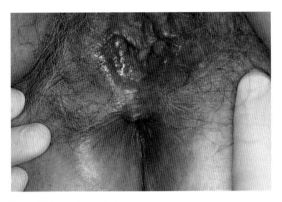

Figure 22.2 The dove-tail sign.

Evaluation of Posterior Defects

Examination of the posterior compartment is the next step in the evaluation and may provide clues to the severity of POP. An inspection of an intact perineal body will demonstrate skin creases arranged radially around the anus. In the event of perineal body disruption, the normal posterior corrugated peri-anal skin is accentuated and the anterior perineal skin exhibits an "ironed out" appearance. This finding is highly suggestive of both prolapse and anal sphincter disruption, and is referred to as the dove-tail sign [5] (Figure 22.2). Digital rectal examination is performed to assess the degree of attenuation of the perineal body and rectovaginal septum. This is accomplished by palpating the rectovaginal tissue between the thumb and forefinger.

Parturition and the Perineum

Vaginal birth has a substantial impact on the perineum (see Chapter 34). The most significant risk factor for POP is vaginal delivery. The relative risk for hospital admission due to POP rises to 4 with one vaginal delivery and to 8.4 with two [6]. Vaginal birth is also associated with direct injury to the anal sphincter and fecal incontinence. Despite adequate primary repair at time of parturition, approximately 30–50% of patients who have a third- or fourth-degree sphincter disruption will suffer from chronic anal incontinence, dyspareunia, fecal urgency, and perineal pain [7, 8]. Incontinence, particularly fecal, is associated with a delay in the postpartum resumption of sexual activity [9].

Cardinal movements of the fetus during birth including descent and rotation may tear or avulse any of the supportive structures that comprise the perineal body. A prolonged second stage or vaginal operative delivery separates these musculotendinous structures even further and increases the risk of anal incontinence. Six months after delivery, 20% of women report dyspareunia and approximately 18% have resumed sexual activity [10, 11]. Laceration and extensive separation of these tissues may result in POP in any compartment as well as compromise of the perineal body.

The perineal laceration staging system describes a spectrum of lacerations and avulsions, not descent of pelvic organs. Repairs performed at the time of delivery are variable and often incomplete in that they may not address the re-approximation of the individual constituents that make up the perineal body. After childbirth, long-term follow-up studies indicate that separation of supportive tissues allows for protrusion of the vaginal mucosa over the healed, but separated, perineal structures. As prolapse develops, which may occur years after intrapartum injury, there is a saccular protrusion of the rectovaginal wall [12]. Over time, this may cause a cystocele or rectocele.

Significant intrapartum fascial disruption progresses under ordinary forces that increase intra-abdominal pressures such as lifting, pulling, straining, and gravity [13]. Additional risk factors for POP include activities or conditions that cause an increase in intra-abdominal pressure including chronic coughing, chronic constipation, obesity, ascites, abdominal tumors, connective tissue disorders, aging, and possibly pudendal nerve disorders (see Chapter 17) [14].

Mucosal Factors

Irritative symptoms may present as the mucosa extends to or beyond the hymen [15]. The authors believe that the supporting connective tissues may stretch or break causing a "mucosal prolapse." The organ and mucosal surfaces in patients with POP can suffer from compromised blood supply due to the elongation of the adjunctive supportive tissues such as the blood vessels, nerves, and connective tissue of the prolapsed organ. Though largely unstudied, the authors believe that this mucosal prolapse is a significant cause of sexual pain in women with POP.

With advanced degrees of POP (e.g., procedentia), severe irritative signs appear on the mucosa and ischemic "pressure" ulcers are common. The mucosa of the prolapsed organ may become keratinized. In premenopausal women, or in postmenopausal women on hormonal therapy, cervical mucous may contribute to vulvovaginal irritation. In women with an active cervical transformation zone, the cervix is easily traumatized and may become infected by flora from the vagina, skin, or bowel [16].

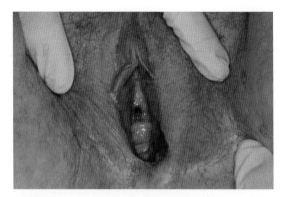

Figure 22.3 Lichen planus complicated by prolapse.

Vulvar Effects of POP That May Exacerbate Sexual Pain

The support of the vaginal introitus is provided by the superficial and deep perineal pouches. These pouches contain three thin muscles and bulbous erectile tissue [17]. The superficial perineal pouch lies between the Colles' fascia and inferior fascia of the urogenital diaphragm. Frequently, fascial defects in the anterior pouch lead to POP. Anteriorly, this pouch extends to the potential space between the superficial fascia and the anterior abdominal muscles where the origins of ischiocavernosis and bulbocavernosis muscles are found. These muscles undergo rhythmic contraction during orgasm and work in concert with the larger supportive structures found in the anal triangle of the perineum. The bulbospongiosis, ischicavernosis, and the external anal sphincter muscles unite to form the central tendon of the perineum which is often referred to as the "perineal body" [18]. Defects in the perineal body are a frequent cause of POP.

Painful symptoms may occur during sexual activity due to the malposition of the cervix or vaginal cuff. Sexual pain may also occur from tears in the four fornices of the vagina, the urethrovesical junction, and the levator hiatus (including the lower one-third of the vagina as well as the perineal body and associated anorectal canal) [19].

Vulvar Consequences of Perineal Disruption and Incontinence

Persistent rubbing at the introitus by the prolapsing organ will affect the vulvar mucosa, causing an irritant reaction. This irritation can exacerbate other disorders of the vulva such as lichen sclerosus, lichen simplex chronicus, or lichen planus, which further complicates management of

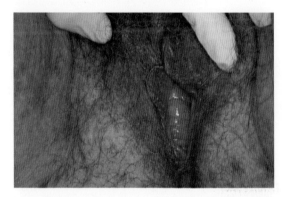

Figure 22.4 Lichen simplex chronicus complicated by prolapse.

these conditions (see Chapter 9) (Figures 22.3 and 22.4). In fact, these dermatoses may be refractory to treatment until such anatomic conditions are corrected. In addition, lesions caused by the erosive effects of POP on the tissue of the introitus may mimic erosive lichen planus. Furthermore, the changes produced by POP, or incontinence of urine or stool, may mimic PVD or GVD. Treatment of urinary incontinence has been shown to improve the patient's related sexual symptoms and to improve her overall quality of life [20].

Prolapse and Cervical Discharge

A functioning cervix is the source of discharge/mucous that is usually absorbed by the vaginal fornices. The non-water components [including sugars and immunoglobulin A (IgA)] and other proteins are broken down and reabsorbed into the circulatory system. This discharge can be very irritating to the mucosa and epithelium of the vulva.

With uterine descent, the anatomy of the fornices is distorted and this mucous absorption function is disrupted. This causes an increase in the amount of irritating mucous in contact with the vulvar skin.

Uterine Prolapse

A prolapsed uterus is graded by the position the cervix occupies within the vagina with regard to the hymen [21]. Painful symptoms tend to be minimal with first-degree uterine prolapse. However, patients may note an increase in vaginal discharge after their first childbirth. In second- or third-degree uterine prolapse, fullness, pressure, vaginal discharge, and a sensation of organs "falling out" are common reports. This may follow the birth of only one child, but it is more common in multiparous woman [22]. With advanced prolapse, the descending part may be a source of friction to the vestibule. This may cause erosion, infection, or exacerbation of preexisting disease. Therefore, the treatment of uterine prolapse may be necessary to treat vulvar diseases and dyspareunia.

Surgical Repair of Uterine Prolapse

Surgical repair of uterine prolapse includes hysterectomy or uterine suspension techniques. Uterine suspension techniques have been described since the early 1880s [23]. As a result of surgery with unclear indications, such surgeries decreased in popularity in the 1950s, and they were rarely performed prior to the last decade. Lately, however, uterine suspension surgeries have enjoyed a resurgence in popularity as less invasive techniques have emerged. There are approximately 200 published techniques for performing suspension of the uterus and cervix [23–25].

Surgical repair of the posterior musculature is often employed in combination with other repairs of POP. The sole aim of surgical repair is to re-establish normal pelvic anatomy and maintain sexual function. Identification of the rectum follows the usual gynecological principles for posterior colporrhaphy. Careful dissection minimizes blood loss and reveals an areolar space (rectocele space) where muscle separation or fascial tears have occurred. The authors believe in the traditional approach to rectocele repair and do not use Richardson's "site-specific" technique [26]. Although this may be a contrarian view to

the state-of-the-art approach [25], we believe in the Harvard technique advocated by Parsons and Ulfelder in the older surgical literature [27].

We feel, as experienced surgeons in this area, that there are three cardinal sutures for the re-establishment of the perineum. These sutures re-approximate fascia and the levator ani muscles, thereby re-establishing the perineal body's prior association with the distal levator musculature. This is accomplished within the first 3–4 cm of the rectocele space. We make no attempt to plicate the levator musculature beyond the perineal body or across the rectocele.

These sutures are placed in succession until the space created by the separation of the levators has been closed. As each suture is placed laterally, the rectum is held posteriorly with the index finger. Traction is applied to the first suture to allow the fascial margins to be seen for placement of the subsequent sutures. This technique of suture placement ensures proper repair of the perineal defect contiguous to the rectocele defect. We repair the fascia to complete our rectocele repair. It does not create a simple "nonanatomic barrier," but re-approximates vital perineal supportive musculature and torn or attenuated rectovaginal fascia. Perineorrhaphy plays a key role in lasting endurance of an appropriate colporrhaphy. We concur that an inadequately restored, or worse, ignored perineal body defect presents a major bottleneck to the success of not only a posterior repair but also any of the restorative repairs, both anteriorly and posteriorly, no matter how well executed [28].

The paramount importance of the perineal body repair is exemplified by Grody, a very well respected vaginal reconstructive surgeon who stated, "If significant defects in the perineal body are ignored and not completely repaired to natural configuration in this commonly coexistent lesion in pelvic floor anatomical failure, then no matter how wonderful the surgeon feels about his or her effort in correcting the other defects, the operation is almost certainly doomed to fail in time" [29, 30].

Summary

A clear understanding of the relationship between POP and sexual pain is essential to effective treatment of patients with dyspareunia. A systematic, anatomical approach to POP and the lower genital tract will help the practitioner in decision-making when treating patients with sexual pain. There is a strong association between parturition and POP although other risk factors exist. Urine and/or feces, as seen with urinary and anal incontinence, can be an irritant to the introitus and surrounding tissues. Cervical discharge in estrogenized women is also a common irritant that may be seen as the cervix descends toward the hymen. Further, our belief is that the anatomical support defects should be considered as possible complicating factors to sexual function in vulvar dermatoses. Surgical repairs should be performed as indicated for effective relief for patients who suffer from POP.

References

1 Barber MD, Lambers AR, Visco AG, *et al.* (2000) Effect of patient position on clinical evaluation of pelvic organ prolapse. *Journal of Obstetrics and Gynecology*, **96**, 18–22.

2 Bump RC, Mattiasson A, Bo K, *et al.* (1996) The standardization of terminology of female pelvic organ prolapse and pelvic floor dysfunction. *American Journal of Obstetrics and Gynecology* **175**, 10.

3 The American Geriatric Society. (2002–2004) *Geriatric Review Syllabus*, 5th ed. Blackwell, Oxford, pp. 139–142.

4 Cogan SL, Webber AM, Hammel JP. (2002) *Journal of Obstetrics and Gynecology*, **99**, 473–76.

5 Haslam J, Laycock J. (2007) Therapeutic management of incontinence and pelvic pain: pelvic organ disorders, 2nd ed. Springer, London, pp. 259–62.

6 Mant J, Painter R, Vessey M. (1997) Epidemiology of genital prolapse: observation from the Oxford Family Planning Association Study. *British Journal of Obstetrics and Gynaecology* **104**, 579–85.

7 Donnelly V, Fynes M, Campbell D, *et al.* (1998) Obstetric events leading to anal sphincter damage. *Obstetrics and Gynecology* **92**, 955–61.

8 Fornell EK, Berg G, Hallböök Matthiesen LS, Sjodahl R. (1996) Clinical consequences of anal sphincter rupture during vaginal delivery. *Journal of the American College of Surgeons* **183**, 553–58.

9 Handa VL, Cundiff F, Chang H, *et al.* (2008) Female sexual function and pelvic floor disorders. *American Journal of Obstetrics and Gynecology* **111**, 1045–52.

10 Glazener C. (1997) Sexual function after childbirth: women's experiences, persistent morbidity and lack of professional recognition. *British Journal of Obstetrics and Gynaecology* **104**, 330–35.

11 Barrett G, Pendry E, Peacock J, *et al.* (2000) Women's sexual health after childbirth. *British Journal of Obstetrics and Gynaecology* **107**, 186–95.

12 Hall AF, Theofrastous JP, Cundiff GW. (1996) Interobserver and intraobserver reliability of the proposed International Incontinence Society, Society of Gynecological Surgeons, and American Urogynecologic Society, Pelvic Organ Prolapse classification system. *American Journal of Obstetrics and Gyecology* **175**, 1467.

13 Gerten KA, Richter HE, Wheeler TL, *et al.* (2008) Intraabdominal pressure changes associated with lifting: implications for postoperative activity restrictions. *American Journal of Obstetrics and Gynecology* **53**, 306–7.

14 Bent A, Ostergard D, Cundiff G, *et al.* (2003) *Ostergard's Urogynecology and Pelvic Floor Dysfunction*, 5th ed. Lippincott, Williams & Wilkins, Philadelphia, pp. 40–41.

15 Walters MD, Karram MN. (1999) *Urogynecology and Reconstructive Pelvic Surgery*, 2nd ed. Mosby, St. Louis.

16 Neimark M, Davila GW, Kopka SL. (2003) Le Fort colpocleisis: a fesable treatment for pelvic organ prolapse in the elderly woman. *Journal of Pelvic Surgery* **9**, 83–89.

17 Dally AF (1991) Perineum. In: Agur A. (ed.) *Grant's Atlas of Human Anatomy*, 9th ed. Lippincott, Williams & Wilkins.

18 Standring S. (2004) *Gray's Anatomy: The Anatomical Basis of Clinical Practice*, 39th ed. Churchill Livingstone.

19 Bent AE, Ostergard DR, Cundiff G. (eds.) (2003) *Ostergard's Urogynecology and Pelvic Floor Dysfunction*, 5th ed. Lipppincott, Williams & Wikins, Philadelphia.

20 Pace G, Vicentini C. (2008) Female sexual function evaluation of the tension-free vaginal tape (TVT) and transobturator suburethral tape (TOT) incontinence surgery: results of a prospective study. *The Journal of Sexual Medicine* **5**, 387–93.

21 Bump RC, Mattiasson A, Bo K, *et al.* (1996) The standardization of terminology of female pelvic organ prolapse and pelvic floor dysfunction. *American Journal of Obstetrics and Gynecology* **175**, 10–17.

22 Beers MH, Porter RS, Jones TV. (2005) *The Merck Manual*, Merck, Whitehouse Station, NJ.

23 Fluhmann CF. (1955) The rise and fall of suspension operations for uterine retrodisplacement. *Bulletin of the John Hopkins Hospital* **96**, 59–70.

24 Narayanan S. (2008) Laparoscopic uterine sling suspension: a new technique of uterine suspension in women desiring surgical management of uterine prolapse with uterine conservation. *British Journal of Obstetrics and Gynaecology* **115**, 128–28.

25 Rock J, Jones HW. (2003) *TeLinde's Operative Gynecology*, 9th ed. Lippincott, Williams & Wilkins, Philadelphia, pp. 620–21.

26 Richardson AC, Lyon JB, Williams NL. (1976) A new look at pelvic relaxation. *American Journal of Gynecology* **126**, 568–73.

27 Parsons L, Ulfelder H. (1968) *An Atlas of Pelvic Operations*, 2nd ed. WB Saunders, Philadelphia, pp. 256–57.

28 Rock J, Jones HW. (2003) *TeLinde's Operative Gynecology*, 9th ed. Lippincott, Williams & Wilkins, Philadelphia, pp. 978–79.

29 Miller CE. (2005) Surgeons respond to pelvic reconstruction column. *OB/GYN News,* March 1.

30 Grody MHT. (2003) Posterior compartment defects. In: Rock J, Jones HW. (eds.) *TeLinde's Operative Gynecology*, 9th ed. Lippincott, Williams & Wilkins, Philadelphia, pp. 966–71.

CHAPTER 23

Cognitive-Behavioral, Physical Therapy, and Alternative Treatments for Dyspareunia

Sophie Bergeron, Tina Landry, Bianca Leclerc
Université du Québec à Montréal, Montréal, Québec, Canada

Introduction

Cognitive-behavioral sex therapy/pain management and physical therapy (PT) are the main nonmedical interventions available to women with vulvodynia, while more recent options include hypnosis and acupuncture. Although these four modalities are widely used in the multidisciplinary treatment of musculoskeletal chronic pain problems [1] with success rates comparable to that of other medical interventions [2], they remain under-recommended in the treatment of vulvodynia.

This chapter describes cognitive-behavioral therapy (CBT), PT, and alternative treatments for vulvodynia from both clinical and scientific perspectives. Specifically, we (1) explain the rationale underlying the use of psychological and pelvic floor rehabilitation interventions; (2) detail the main strategies and techniques that comprise each of these two interventions; (3) summarize the empirical evidence concerning the effectiveness of CBT, PT, acupuncture, and hypnosis; and (4) emphasize the need to approach the treatment of vulvodynia from a multimodal, multidisciplinary perspective.

Why Manage Vulvodynia with Psychotherapy and Pelvic Floor Rehabilitation?

Because psychological and PT interventions are less mainstream in comparison to medical management of vul-

Female Sexual Pain Disorders 1st edition. Edited by A. Goldstein, C. Pukall & I. Goldstein. © 2009 Blackwell Publishing, ISBN: 9781405183987.

vodynia, they are often less obvious treatment choices. Nonetheless, there are compelling reasons for their use in the treatment of vulvar pain. First, CBT is the only treatment that directly targets distressing sexual and couple issues. Second, CBT provides psychological support to women and couples grappling with a misunderstood condition that may generate feelings of shame, anger, inadequacy, and hopelessness. Third, individual and dyadic psychological factors have been shown to contribute to the experience of vulvar pain [3]. Fourth, psychological approaches to pain management have been shown to be successful in terms of diminished pain intensity and frequency of pain behaviours, and improved coping [4]. Fifth, CBT leads to reduced pain intensity and catastrophizing, improved sexual functioning, and treatment satisfaction in women with provoked vestibulodynia (PVD) [2]. Lastly, it is a great complement to another nonmedical intervention, pelvic floor rehabilitation.

In terms of pelvic floor PT and its rationale, a controlled study conducted by Reissing et al. [5] showed that women with PVD present with significantly more pelvic floor muscle hypertonicity than pain-free controls. These findings suggest that pelvic floor dysfunction may contribute to the development and maintenance of vulvar pain and should be targeted via pelvic floor rehabilitation in PT. Furthermore, retrospective and prospective studies have shown that PT and biofeedback help women with PVD reduce their pain and improve their sexual functioning [6].

It can become even more worthwhile to combine CBT and PT into an integrated form of care that may allow women to avoid the negative sexual side effects of certain pain medications and the invasiveness of vestibulectomy [7]. Indeed, both interventions share similar goals and strategies (e.g., the use of systematic desensitization to decrease the fear of pain and penetration), and they can possibly potentiate each other's effectiveness via a simultaneous focus on mind and body [8].

Intervention Strategies

Psychological Interventions

Psychological interventions range from pain education and exposure-type exercises such as vaginal dilation, to more sophisticated, in-depth psychotherapy focusing on issues related to relationship discord or psychosexual development. We have developed a CBT group treatment for women with PVD [9]. For some patients, these ten group sessions will be enough to bring about satisfactory improvements in pain and sexual functioning. Others will shy away from such a format and prefer individual and/or couple therapy sessions tailored specifically to their clinical presentation. With parsimony guiding our clinical approach, we prefer to begin with CBT strategies and work our way toward more intensive psychotherapy when necessary; that is, when the patient expresses this need or when too many roadblocks impede progress via short-term treatment.

Keeping this framework in mind, the goals of CBT are to enable patients to: reconceptualize vulvodynia as a multidimensional pain problem influenced by cognitive, emotional, behavioral, and couple factors; modify such factors to help increase adaptive coping (e.g., reduce pain catastrophizing) and decrease pain intensity; improve the quality of women and/or couples' sexual functioning, and steer the focus away from intercourse with a view toward developing more positive attitudes about other pleasurable sexual activities; reduce avoidance of physical intimacy and nonpenetrative sex; facilitate adherence to other treatment regimens (e.g., medical management) and assessment and intervention procedures (e.g., gynaecological examinations); and consolidate skills and maintain gains.

The treatment generally includes the following:
1 information about the nature of CBT;
2 education and information about vulvodynia and how it impacts negatively on desire, arousal, and orgasm;

3 education concerning a multifactorial view of pain and the interdependent roles of cognitive, affective, behavioral, relationship, and biomedical factors in the maintenance of persistent pain;
4 use of a pain diary;
5 relaxation techniques;
6 exposure exercises such as vaginal dilation (i.e., inserting increasingly larger fingers into the vagina while in a relaxed state);
7 cognitive restructuring exercises (i.e., replacing distorted or irrational beliefs about pain and sexuality with realistic ones);
8 distraction techniques focusing on sexual imagery;
9 rehearsal of coping self-statements; and
10 communication skills training related to romantic relationships, in particular, the expression of emotional needs and sexual preferences.

Because more substantial work concerning sexual desire, intimacy, or other systemic issues may be warranted, the partner should be included in the process as much as possible, although this need not be via formal couple therapy. This may allow the partner to receive needed support, and may develop both partners' awareness of, and empathy for what each is experiencing.

In our clinical experience, we have found that patients do not always fit into our neatly elaborated treatment programs. It is thus necessary to develop a flexible attitude and tailor the treatment to the needs of each patient, while making pain and sexual impairment the central focus of therapy. This has the benefit of validating the woman's suffering, strengthening the therapeutic alliance between patient and health professional, and facilitating parsimony and cost-effectiveness.

Pelvic Floor Rehabilitation

Some patients notice their hypertonic pelvic floor, especially during attempted penetration, and know intuitively that this tension may be contributing to their pain experience. Pelvic floor PT has the advantage of being short term (6–10 sessions) and may be seen as less threatening than CBT because the focus of PT is not on talking about intimate aspects of their sex lives.

The main goal of PT is to rehabilitate the pelvic floor musculature by increasing awareness and proprioception; increasing strength, speed, endurance, and muscle discrimination; decreasing hypertonicity; increasing elasticity of the tissues at the vaginal opening; and decreasing fear of vaginal penetration. These goals are achieved through education about the role of the pelvic floor musculature in the maintenance of vulvodynia, electromyographic (EMG) biofeedback, electrical stimulation, and manual techniques (e.g., stretching). Patients are instructed to complete home exercises (e.g., vaginal dilation/stretching), and to eventually incorporate larger accommodators or dildos, including a male partner's penis, when relevant [8, 10].

As is the case with psychological interventions, the involvement of the significant other in treatment is important because he/she often does not understand exactly where it hurts and may inadvertently be contributing to the maintenance of the pain. The PT sessions present the partner with an opportunity to actually feel the muscle hypertonicity and to observe the patient's protective reactions against pain. The partner can be trained to practice some of the exercises with the patient and to be actively involved in the rehabilitation process.

In short, pelvic floor rehabilitation is a modality that patients usually enjoy taking part in, although it can be anxiety-provoking and involve some degree of pain in the beginning. Patients often progress relatively quickly, which is empowering and may have a positive ripple effect on other aspects of vulvodynia, including sexuality.

Do Psychological and PT Interventions Help? An Overview of Empirical Findings

CBT

Prior to 2000, only two published studies focused on the effectiveness of a combination of sex therapy and behavioral pain management. Weijmar Schultz et al. [11] were the first to investigate this intervention approach with a partially randomized trial in which 14 women with PVD were either assigned to a behavioral treatment or to this same treatment preceded by surgery. Results revealed no significant difference between treatments, with 86% of women in both groups reporting symptom resolution or reduction at follow-up. In a similar prospective study involving seven women with PVD and vaginismus, 43% improved to the point of being able to resume intercourse following treatment [12]. While the findings from these first studies were encouraging, their interpretation was

complicated by unstandardized treatment protocols and small sample sizes.

Since then, more methodologically sound studies assessing CBT have been conducted. First, ter Kuile and Weijenborg [13] prospectively evaluated the efficacy of 12 two-hour sessions of group CBT with 76 women with PVD. At posttreatment, participants reported a significant reduction of dyspareunia and vaginal muscle tension, in addition to significant improvement of sexual satisfaction and perceived pain control. However, no significant difference was reported with regards to relationship satisfaction and psychological distress, likely because these variables did not reach clinical thresholds at pretreatment.

Bergeron et al. [14] conducted a randomized study comparing group CBT (8 two-hour sessions), biofeedback, and vestibulectomy. At the 6-month follow-up, women in all three groups reported significant pain reduction, with overall success rates of 68% for vestibulectomy, 39% for CBT, and 35% for biofeedback. While vestibulectomy resulted in significantly more pain reduction, all three interventions resulted in equally significant psychosexual functioning improvements. Whereas 9% of the vestibulectomy participants reported a worsening of their pain at posttreatment, no such deterioration was reported by participants of the two behavioral treatments. A 2.5-year follow-up indicated that vestibulectomy participants still had significantly lower pain levels than biofeedback and CBT participants overall. Pain reduction and sexual functioning gains were maintained at follow-up in all three treatment modalities [15]. Moreover, with regard to pain during intercourse, vestibulectomy did not prove superior to CBT, suggesting that the long-term effects of both treatments may be equivalent.

In a recently completed study [2], 97 women with PVD were randomly assigned to a 13-week trial of either corticosteroid cream or group CBT. Although both groups reported significant pain reduction at posttreatment and 6-month follow-up, women in the CBT group reported significantly less pain than those assigned to the topical treatment condition. In addition, the CBT intervention yielded significantly more improvements in sexual functioning, reduced pain catastrophizing, and higher satisfaction with treatment.

Overall, results indicate that CBT leads to significant improvements in pain and psychosexual functioning, even when delivered in a research context with short-term treatment duration and group format. It seems reasonable to hypothesize that CBT delivered in actual clinical practice may be more effective as it is specifically tailored to patients' and couples' needs. Additionally, by targeting multiple factors associated with pain, it seems that this type of intervention may help break the negative cycle of pain and contribute to maintenance of gains over time.

Pelvic Floor PT/Biofeedback

Glazer et al. [16] were the first to retrospectively study the effectiveness of biofeedback with a group of 33 women experiencing PVD. At 6-month follow-up, destabilization of pelvic floor muscles greatly improved, 52% of women were pain-free, and 79% of women who had been abstaining from intercourse were able to resume regular activity. In their later retrospective, longer-term study involving 43 women with generalized vulvodynia (GVD), Glazer et al. [6] showed that treatment gains resulting from biofeedback were maintained 3–5 years posttreatment. Similar results were reported in another retrospective study investigating the effectiveness of PT, including biofeedback, with 35 women experiencing PVD [17]. Results not only showed a 52% success rate with regards to pain reduction, but also a significant improvement in women's sexual functioning.

Two remaining studies investigated biofeedback using more rigorous study designs. First, a prospective study involving 29 women with PVD revealed that pain significantly decreased as pelvic floor musculature contractile strength increased [18]. Moreover, among 24 women reporting negligible or mild dyspareunia, 69% reported resuming sexual activity posttreatment. Finally, in a randomized clinical trial involving 46 women with PVD, Danielsson et al. [19] compared the efficacy of biofeedback to that of a nonsurgical medical treatment (i.e., topical lidocaine). Results showed no significant difference between treatments, with both modalities significantly improving pain, quality of life, and psychosexual functioning. At the 12-month follow-up, 78% of the women in the biofeedback group considered themselves cured or improved compared to 63% in the lidocaine group.

Taken together, these five studies suggest that interventions specifically targeted toward the pelvic floor musculature not only yield satisfactory pain reduction, but also help women regain a healthier sex life. Although more randomized controlled trials are warranted to further corroborate results, patients can benefit from being more routinely informed of this treatment modality.

Acupuncture and Hypnosis

In addition to CBT and interventions targeting the pelvic floor musculature, two acupuncture and two hypnosis studies have been published thus far. First, Powell and Wojnarowska [20] prospectively investigated five weekly sessions of acupuncture in 12 women with GVD. At a 5-week follow-up, 17% of the women reported being completely cured, 25% reported short-term symptom control with relapse after treatment cessation, and the remaining 58% felt no improvement. The other prospective study involved 14 women with PVD who received ten weekly or biweekly acupuncture sessions [21]. Although pain outcome was not published, participants reported a significant improvement in their quality of life following treatment.

The efficacy of hypnosis was first assessed in a case study involving one woman with PVD who reported complete pain relief and nearly complete anticipatory anxiety reduction at a 12-month follow-up [22]. More recently, Pukall et al.'s [23] prospective hypnotherapy study involving eight women with PVD showed both significant pain reduction and improvement in sexual satisfaction.

In sum, while hypnotherapy may offer encouraging treatment gains that appear to be maintained over time, acupuncture seems to provide limited, short-term pain relief. Nonetheless, the small sample sizes of these studies indicate that the evaluation of alternative treatments is preliminary. Large-scale, controlled studies are needed to further investigate their effectiveness.

Conclusions

Based on the growing scientific evidence supporting their effectiveness, we believe that psychological and pelvic floor rehabilitation interventions are beneficial for the treatment of vulvodynia. They target pain reduction and psychosexual consequences; they provide long-term maintenance of treatment gains; they have success rates similar or superior to some medical treatments [2, 19]; and they result in no documented adverse effects. Considering these advantages, CBT and PT should be recommended as first-line interventions for vulvodynia. Acupuncture and hypnosis require further empirical validation. However, because women afflicted with vulvodynia do not benefit equally from treatment, future research should examine predictors of therapeutic success to guide health professionals' treatment decision process and to identify women at risk of developing problematic outcomes.

Optimal treatment of pain ultimately involves an integrated approach to care. Based on an exhaustive meta-analytic review of empirical evidence, Wampold [24] outlined the common factors that make psychotherapy successful: the healing context; the therapeutic alliance (the fact that therapist and patient are aligned regarding goals, tasks, and their overall collaborative relationship); and the belief in the rationale for treatment and in the treatment itself. These may well be factors that are the pillars of any high-quality health care, in particular, when the medical condition is as complex and challenging as vulvodynia.

What guidelines may help health care providers work in synergy to offer a multidisciplinary, multimodal treatment approach for women with vulvodynia? First, the patient has to trust that the health professional believes that her pain is real, and is knowledgeable and competent to alleviate the pain to some degree. An initial step is often to provide patient education concerning the specific vulvodynia condition with which she is afflicted, in addition to education about pain and its biopsychosocial nature. This subsequently serves as a platform from which to explain the rationale of each intervention. Finally, a multimodal, integrated approach involves keeping informed about what other health professionals are doing and developing a collaborative relationship with one's interdisciplinary colleagues in an effort to convey hope and encouragement to women grappling with a distressing pain condition.

References

1 Flor H, Fydrich T, Turk DC. (1992) Efficacy of multidisciplinary pain treatment centers: a meta-analytic review. *Pain* **49**, 221–30.

2 Bergeron S. (2008) Provoked vestibulodynia: A randomized comparison of cognitive-behavioral therapy and medical management. Paper presented at the meeting of the *International Society for the Study of Women's Sexual Health*, San Diego, CA.

3 Desrochers G, Bergeron S, Landry T, *et al.* (2008) Do psychosexual factors play a role in the etiology of provoked vestibulodynia? A critical review. *Journal of Sex and Marital Therapy* **34**, 198–226.

4 Morley S, Eccleston C, Williams A. (1999) Systematic review and meta-analysis of randomized controlled trials of cognitive behaviour therapy and behaviour therapy for chronic pain in adults, excluding headache. *Pain* **80**, 1–13.

5 Reissing ED, Binik YM, Khalifé S, *et al.* (2003) Etiological correlates of vaginismus: sexual and physical abuse, sexual knowledge, sexual self-schema, and relationship adjustment. *Journal of Sex and Marital Therapy* **29**, 47–59.

6 Glazer HI. (2000) Dysesthetic vulvodynia: long-term follow-up after treatment with surface electromyography-assisted pelvic floor muscle rehabilitation. *The Journal of Reproductive Medicine* **45**, 798–802.

7 Weijmar Schultz WC, van de Wiel HB. (2002) Vulvar vestibulitis syndrome: care made to measure. *Journal of Psychosomatic Obstetrics and Gynaecology* **23**, 5–6.

8 Bergeron S, Lord MJ. (2003) The integration of pelvi-perineal re-education and cognitive-behavioural therapy in the multidisciplinary treatment of the sexual pain disorders. *Sexual and Relationship Therapy* **18**, 135–41.

9 Bergeron S, Binik YM, Larouche J. (2001) *Treatment Manual for Cognitive-Behavioral Group Therapy with Women Suffering from Vulvar Vestibulitis Syndrome.* Unpublished treatment manual, McGill University, Montreal.

10 Rosenbaum TY. (2007) Physical therapy management and treatment of sexual pain disorders. In: Leiblum SR (ed.) *Principles and Practice of Sex Therapy*, 4th ed. The Guilford Press, New York, pp. 157–180.

11 Weijmar Schultz WC, Gianotten WL, van der Meijden WI, *et al.* (1996) Behavioral approach with or without surgical intervention to the vulvar vestibulitis syndrome: a prospective randomized and nonrandomized study. *Journal of Psychosomatic Obstetrics and Gynecology* **17**, 143–48.

12 Abramov L, Wolman I, David MP. (1994) Vaginismus: an important factor in the evaluation and management of vulvar vestibulitis syndrome. *Gynecologic and Obstetric Investigation* **38**, 194–97.

13 ter Kuile MM, Weijenborg PT. (2006) A cognitive-behavioral group program for women with vulvar vestibulitis syndrome (VVS): factors associated with treatment success. *Journal of Sexual and Marital Therapy* **32**, 199–213.

14 Bergeron S, Binik YM, Khalifé S, *et al.* (2001) A randomized comparison of group cognitive-behavioral therapy, surface electromyographic biofeedback, and vestibulectomy in the treatment of dyspareunia resulting from vulvar vestibulitis. *Pain* **91**, 297–306.

15 Bergeron S, Khalifé S, Glazer HI, *et al.* (2008) Surgical and behavioral treatments for vestibulodynia: two-and-one-half-year follow-up and predictors of outcome. *Obstetrics and Gynecology* **111**, 159–66.

16 Glazer HI, Rodke G, Swencionis C, *et al.* (1995) Treatment of vulvar vestibulitis syndrome with electromyographic

biofeedback of pelvic floor musculature. *The Journal of Reproductive Medicine* **40**, 283–90.

17 Bergeron S, Brown C, Lord MJ, *et al.* (2002) Physical therapy for vulvar vestibulitis syndrome: a retrospective study. *Journal of Sex and Marital Therapy* **28**, 183–92.

18 McKay E, Kaufman RH, Doctor U, *et al.* (2001) Treating vulvar vestibulitis with electromyographic biofeedback of pelvic floor musculature. *The Journal of Reproductive Medicine* **46**, 337–42.

19 Danielsson I, Torstensson T, Brodda-Jansen G, *et al.* (2006) EMG biofeedback versus topical lidocaine gel: a randomized study for the treatment of women with vulvar vestibulitis. *Acta Obstetricia et Gynecologica Scandinavica* **85**, 1360–67.

20 Powell J, Wojnarowska F. (1999) Acupuncture for vulvodynia. *Journal of the Royal Society of Medicine* **92**, 579–81.

21 Danielsson I, Sjoberg I, Ostman C. (2001) Acupuncture for the treatment of vulvar vestibulitis: a pilot study. *Acta Obstetricia et Gynecologica Scandinavica* **80**, 437–41.

22 Kandyba K, Binik YM. (2003) Hypnotherapy as a treatment for vulvar vestibulitis syndrome: a case report. *Journal of Sex and Marital Therapy* **29**, 237–42.

23 Pukall CF, Kandyba K, Amsel R, *et al.* (2007) Effectiveness of hypnosis for the treatment of vulvar vestibulitis syndrome: a preliminary investigation. *Journal of Sexual Medicine* **4**, 417–25.

24 Wampold BE. (2001) *The Great Psychotherapy Debate: Models, Methods and Findings.* Lawrence Erlbaum, Mahwah. NJ.

24

CHAPTER 24

Topical and Injectable Therapies for Vulvar Pain

Colleen M. Kennedy,[1] *Catherine M. Leclair,*[2] *Lori A. Boardman*[3]

[1] University of Iowa, Iowa City, IA, USA
[2] Oregon Health & Science University, Portland, OR, USA
[3] University of Central Florida College of Medicine, Orlando, FL, USA

Introduction

The study of vulvar disease is a relatively new science. Some conditions such as lichen sclerosus have been fairly well defined clinically and histopathologically, and treatments are based on well-designed, placebo-controlled trials. However, when women suffer from other types of vulvar pain disorders such as generalized vulvodynia (GVD), provoked vestibulodynia (PVD), and pelvic floor dysfunction (PFD), the treatments are frequently based solely on anecdotal evidence. This chapter examines topical and injectable treatments for these conditions.

Benefit of Topical and Injectable Therapy

Despite limited evidence to support the use of tricyclic antidepressants (TCAs) and anticonvulsants for the treatment of vulvodynia, these medications have become mainstays of therapy for GVD and PVD (see Chapter 26). However, the common side effects of these medications, particularly the anticholinergic effects of the TCAs (e.g., dry mouth, constipation) and the sedation and dizziness associated with gabapentin (an anticonvulsant), limit their clinical applicability.

For example, one placebo-controlled trial of the TCA amitriptyline, found that 92% of interstitial cystitis pa-

tients taking 100 mg or less experienced significant side effects, especially dry mouth [1]. Some vulvodynia experts believe that compounding amitriptyline and gabapentin into topical formulations has significant potential in the treatment of vulvar pain syndromes. Although optimal dosing and product stability have yet to be determined, trials to investigate and resolve these issues are planned.

Topical therapy can circumvent systemic side effects in at least two ways. First, the topical route of delivery reduces systemic absorption of the medication; second, the amount of active drug in topical preparations is significantly less than in oral medications. Although data on using topical agents with vulvar pain patients is sparse, studies of topical preparations in the treatment of other forms of chronic neuropathic pain suggest beneficial outcomes with minimal side effects. For example, in a trial of two commercially available topical medications, 5% doxepin and 0.025% capsaicin, overall pain scores were significantly reduced and side effects were minor, with only 15% of patients using topical doxepin experiencing drowsiness [2].

Many local therapies have shown promise in the treatment of vulvar pain disorders. In a number of case series and small uncontrolled trials, injectable interferon, injectable steroids and lidocaine, topical nitroglycerin, topical lidocaine, and topical capsaicin have shown some efficacy. Of the topical preparations, lidocaine, capsaicin, and nitroglycerin have all demonstrated promise as treatments for PVD.

Female Sexual Pain Disorders 1st edition. Edited by A. Goldstein, C. Pukall & I. Goldstein. © 2009 Blackwell Publishing, ISBN: 9781405183987.

Side Effects and Limitations of Topical and Injectable Therapy

Skin reactions to topical medications are not uncommon, and it is often the base of the cream, ointment, or gel that is to blame rather than the active ingredient. Thus, it is imperative to choose the proper vehicle when employing topical therapy, especially when it is to be applied to the sensitive vulvar skin/mucosa. Many topical formulations include well-known irritants, such as propylene glycol, or allergens, such as dibucaine. For patients with sensitivities to any of these ingredients, the use of a compounding pharmacy can be invaluable. The authors have found that acid mantle base and methylcellulose gel are generally very well tolerated. In addition, glycerin can replace propylene glycol as an emollient for women who are sensitive to the former. In general, ointments are better tolerated and often provide a protective barrier, whereas creams contain more preservatives and may cause burning on application.

Common reactions associated with topical anesthetics include stinging, erythema, and edema. Benzocaine, an anesthetic frequently found in over-the-counter topical preparations such as Vagisil™, should be avoided due to its association with allergic contact dermatitis. Patients should also realize that if an anesthetic is present on the skin during intercourse, their partners may experience numbness or side effects. Although the occurrence of serious reactions to topical formulations has not been well studied, they can occur with both lidocaine (e.g., double vision) and the tricyclic antidepressants (e.g., seizures, stroke, and myocardial infarction) [3].

Topical Therapy for Treatment of PVD and GVD

At present, there are no FDA-approved medications (systemic, topical, or injectable) for the treatment of vulvar pain symptoms. Many local therapies have shown promise in the reduction of vulvar pain symptoms in small case series and reports; however, placebo-controlled trials are lacking. When physicians on a referral list from the National Vulvodynia Association were surveyed regarding practice patterns, topical lidocaine was the most common first-line therapy for the treatment of PVD [4]. Based on its treatment efficacy (see below), this is certainly a reasonable and easily obtainable first choice of therapy.

To date, there are only two published randomized placebo-controlled trials on topical therapy for the treatment of PVD. In the first study, Nyirjesy et al. used 4% cromolyn sulfate cream to treat 26 recalcitrant PVD patients and found that placebo users were as likely to experience resolution of their pain as patients who used cromolyn [5]. In a second, small trial, Zycynski et al. randomly assigned 14 vestibulitis patients to use either 0.025% capsaicin or placebo five times a day for six weeks [6]. Of the nine women who completed the protocol, capsaicin users demonstrated a significant reduction in pain scores, as compared to those on placebo. Over the next 6 weeks, all patients were treated with capsaicin, and at the 12-week period, all reported similar pain relief, regardless of initial exposure.

Topical Anesthetics

Topical anesthetics, including lidocaine (2% jelly or 5% ointment; AstraZeneca Pharmaceuticals LP, Wilmington, DE), are the most commonly prescribed topical medications for the treatment of vulvar pain [3, 4]. Other topical anesthetics commonly employed include the following: EMLA (eutectic mixture of lidocaine and prilocaine, AstraZeneca, Wilmington, DE) and LMX-4 (4% liposomal lidocaine, Ferndale Laboratories, Ferndale, MI). Benzocaine, a potent sensitizer found in several over-the-counter agents including Vagisil (Combe, Inc., White Plains, NY) should not be used to treat vulvar pain.

In Zolnoun et al.'s trial of 5% lidocaine ointment in the treatment of 61 women with PVD, a significant increase in patients' ability to have intercourse (76% vs. 36% at baseline) and a decrease in intercourse-related pain was found [7]. In this study, patients applied copious amounts of the ointment to a cotton-ball, which was then placed in the vestibule at bedtime. Patients performed this regimen nightly for an average of 7 weeks, although many continued to use the ointment at least sporadically in the following months. In another report, Danielsson et al. compared biofeedback and topical lidocaine gel in 46 women with PVD and found improved sexual functioning in both groups at 12 months [8].

Topical Capsaicin

Capsaicin is the purified extracted alkaloid from red chili peppers. Capsaicin selectively binds to TRPV1, a calcium channel in peripheral sensory nerve endings [9]. Prolonged activation of TRPV1 by capsaicin results in the depletion of substance P in the peripheral neurons leading to hypoathesia. Pain relief is not instantaneous, and repetitive application of capsaicin is required over weeks or months to cause depletion of substance P.

Topical capsaicin is available to treat neuropathic pain, and has shown efficacy in small studies, such as those conducted by Friedrich in 1988 [10] and Zyczynski in 1997 [6]. In a recent trial involving 52 women with PVD, Steinberg and colleagues instructed patients to use 0.025% capsaicin cream for 20 minutes each day [11]. After 12 weeks of treatment, women reported a significant decrease in discomfort and an increase in ability to have sexual intercourse (from 62% pretreatment to 95% following therapy). In this trial, however, some patients also needed topical lidocaine for pain control. Murina and colleagues also evaluated capsaicin 0.05% cream in 19 women, and while 59% noted improvement of symptoms, no complete remission was observed. Furthermore, severe burning was reported by all the women studied, and symptoms recurred after the use of capsaicin cream was discontinued [12]. Thus, Murina concluded that the use of capsaicin should be considered only as a "last-choice" medical approach. It should be noted that the concentration in the Murina study was twice the concentration used in the Steinberg study.

Topical Nitroglycerin

Walsh et al. evaluated topical 0.2% nitroglycerin cream in a pilot study of 34 women with vulvodynia [13]. Patients were instructed to use the cream for 5–10 minutes prior to intercourse and to apply the cream at least three times a week for 4–6 weeks. Although all patients tolerated the initial dose applied in the clinic, ten discontinued the cream after one or two applications at home. Six patients noted headache as the primary reason for discontinuing the medication. Of the 21 women who completed both the pre- and postpain scale questionnaire, all noted a decrease in pain during sexual activity. Although such results are encouraging, the subject population was heterogeneous and included women with both PVD and GVD. Furthermore, the majority of women who completed therapy experienced headaches, leading the researchers to conclude that a larger placebo-controlled study is necessary to establish the optimal dose with minimal side effects [13].

Topical Estrogen and Testosterone

Many practitioners advocate the use of topical estrogen with or without topical testosterone in women with vulvodynia. Compared to women without pain, decreased estrogen receptor expression in women with PVD may explain, in part, the efficacy of topical estrogen in this population [14]. See Chapter 28 for a discussion of the rationale for the use of topical testosterone in women with PVD.

Compounded TCA and Gabapentin

The use of topical (compounded) tricyclics and antiepileptics has been described, largely to avoid the dose-limiting systemic effects these medications can cause. Except for topical 5% Doxepin (Bradley Pharmaceuticals, Fairfield, NJ), these agents are not commercially available for topical use and must be compounded by a qualified pharmacist. The Vulvodynia Guideline by Haefner et al. notes the use of topical amitriptyline 2% (Elavil; AstaZeneca Pharmaceuticals, Wilmington, DE) and baclofen 2% (Novartis Pharmaceuticals, East Hanover, NJ) in water washable base for PVD and vaginismus [3]. However, such use is not based on clinical studies. Gabapentin has also been compounded as a topical therapy (usually dosed in the range 2–6%) and utilized with promising results. Boardman and colleagues reported that following a minimum of eight weeks of therapy, the mean pain score among 35 evaluable women with vulvodynia was significantly reduced from 7.26 to 2.49. Overall, 28/35 (80%) demonstrated ≥ 50% improvement in pain scores [15].

Evidence Supporting Injectable Therapy in the Treatment of Vulvar Pain

The use of injectable therapy in the management of vulvar pain has been limited by patient acceptance and inconsistent results. Local injection has been most commonly employed to treat PVD. Medications employed have included intralesional interferon, corticosteroids, anesthetics, and, more recently, botulinum toxin.

Corticosteroids

While topical steroids have not been shown to be efficacious, local injection of steroids (alone or in combination with anesthetics) has been recommended in the treatment of PVD and has been reported to be successful in some patients [3]. Segal presented a case of persistent PVD that resolved following a 6-week course of submucosal injections of betamethasone and lidocaine [16]. In a case series of 22 women, Murina and colleagues found that 15 (68%) reported either marked improvement or complete relief of PVD following weekly submucosal injections of methylprednisolone and lidocaine [17]. As with other retrospective series, this study is limited by design and limited follow-up.

Anesthetics

While the use of local anesthetic injections has been endorsed for vulvar pain, evidence supporting use of such injections (again, with or without corticosteroids) is based on use in other chronic pain and myofascial pain syndromes. For example, Rapkin et al. evaluated serial multilevel nerve blocks for the treatment of PVD and found a 50% response rate in 27 women [18]. See Chapter 17 for a more thorough discussion of regional nerve blocks.

Interferon

Perhaps the most widely reported injectable therapy for PVD has been interferon, both in intralesional and systemic forms, as a single agent and in combined therapy [19–26]. In the first report of intralesional interferon use among women with vulvar pain symptoms, Horowitz noted an 88% success rate among 17 women with evidence of human papillomavirus (HPV), and lack of response among 13 women without evidence of HPV [19]. Further investigation of interferon for women believed to have HPV as the etiology for their vulvar pain symptoms did not, however, consistently support Horowitz's findings. Instead, it is possible that the mast cell inhibiting properties of interferon may be responsible for its efficacy in PVD. While a subsequent small case series found the use of intralesional interferon to improve vulvar pain and dyspareunia in 50–70% of women following treatment, systemic (subcutaneous or intramuscular) interferon provided mixed results. Treatment protocols were varied, and side effects including flu-like symptoms were common [27].

The use of interferon as an adjunct treatment has also been evaluated. Bornstein compared the use of interferon with subtotal perineoplasty to total perineoplasty and found similar improvement in both groups (7 of 10 vs. 6 of 9 with complete resolution of vulvar pain, respectively) and concluded the combination approach was as effective as total perineoplasty with fewer surgical complications [26].

Botulinum Toxin

Botulinum toxin type A (Botox™ Allergan, Irvine, CA) inhibits release of acetylcholine from the presynaptic region of the neuromuscular junction, producing chemodenervation that results in reduced muscle tone [28]. Botulinum toxin type A has been used successfully to treat movement disorders, spasticity, glandular hyperactivity, and frown lines. More recently, it has been used to treat painful conditions including trigeminal neuralgia, migraine headaches, and myofascial pain, and it has also been evaluated for the treatment of PVD and pelvic floor spasm in women. The effect of botulinum toxin type A on pain is thought to be from an inhibitory release of neuropeptides involved in pain and inflammation along with its inhibition of muscle spasticity [29].

To date, three studies have shown a potential effect from the use of botulinum toxin for the treatment of pelvic floor spasm and myalgia (vaginismus). In a small placebo-controlled study, eight women with pelvic floor spasm and hypertonicity were injected with 25 units of botulinum toxin type A directly into the bulbospongiosus muscles versus five women injected with saline [30]. Women were then surveyed at 10 months. Women in the active treatment group reported having nonpainful intromission. In another study examining 24 women with severe pelvic floor myalgia, 150–400 units of botulinum toxin type A were injected at six sites in the levator plate, including the pubococcygeus muscle [31]. After 12 months, 18/24 were cured of vaginismus and an additional 4/24 had mild pain. One woman declined follow-up examination but reported relief of pain, the remaining woman required a second injection for pain relief. In a larger randomized control trial, botulinum toxin type A was studied in 60 women with pelvic pain (including vaginismus) [32]. This group was more heterogenous, and pelvic floor myalgia was mixed amongst the other conditions causing genital pain. Injections of 80 units of botulinum toxin type A showed little improvement over placebo for dyspareunia.

The majority of studies of botulinum toxin type A in vulvar pain syndromes are targeted to pelvic floor spasm or inhibition of muscle spasticity. These studies represent some optimistic preliminary data that warrants further investigation and research in the treatment of pelvic floor myalgia and hypertonicity that often accompanies vulvovaginal pain disorders. Furthermore, it is important to note that there are three commercially available preparations of botulinum toxin that differ in potency and dose.

Thus, if considering use of botulinum toxin for the treatment of vulvar pain, one should review the available preparation and standard dosing. In addition, because of the high cost of botulinum toxin type A, some authors recommend that it should only be used to augment pelvic floor physical therapy in women with recalcitrant levator ani muscle hypertonicity [33].

Pelvic Floor Dysfunction

A final component to consider, particularly in the assessment of patients with PVD, is the concomitant role of pelvic floor myalgia. The pelvic floor changes seen in women with PVD appear to be a reactive response to pain. The pelvic floor learns a conditioned, protective guarding response, which results from repeated attempts at painful vaginal penetration [34]. While the mainstay in treatment includes pelvic floor physical therapy and biofeedback (see Chapter 13), trigger point injections have also been reported with variable success. For instance, Langford (2007) noted improvement of pain in 13 of 18 (72%) women with specific levator ani trigger points following injection of 0.25% bupivacaine (10 cc), 2% lidocaine (10 cc), and 40 mg triamcinolone (1 cc), divided into 5 cc per trigger point injection [35].

Summary

Women with vulvar pain syndromes form a heterogeneous group, and their management is often difficult for the provider and frustrating for the patient and her partner. Treatment, if possible, should be evidence-based, although for many vulvar disorders, such evidence has not yet been accrued. For a number of disorders, more than one treatment modality will often be required and treatment must be individualized.

Topical and injectable therapeutics has been investigated in the treatment of vulvar pain in part to avoid the systemic side effects of commonly employed systemic medications, with favorable clinical responses in a number of case series and small, uncontrolled trials. Injectable interferon, injectable steroids, and injectable lidocaine, topical nitroglycerin, topical lidocaine, injectable botulinum toxin, and topical capsaicin have shown some

efficacy. However, well-designed, placebo-controlled clinical trials as well as longitudinal and follow-up studies are needed.

References

1 van Ophoven A, Pokupic S, Heinecke A, et al. (2004) A prospective, randomized, placebo-controlled, double-blind study of amitriptyline for the treatment of interstitial cystitis. *Journal of Urology* **172**, 533–36.
2 McCleane G. (2000) Topical application of doxepin hydrochloride, capsaicin, and a combination of both produces analgesia in chronic human neuropathic pain: a randomized, double-blind, placebo-controlled study. *Journal of Clinical Pharmacology* **49**, 574–79.
3 Haefner HK, Collins ME, Davis GD, et al. (2005) The vulvodynia guideline. *Journal of Lower Genital Tract Disease* **9**, 40–51.
4 Updike GM, Wiesenfeld HC. (2005) Insight into the treatment of vulvar pain: a survey of clinicians. *American Journal of Obstetrics and Gynecology* **193**, 1404–09.
5 Nyirjesy P, Sobel JD, Weitz V, et al. (2001) Cromolyn cream for recalcitrant idiopathic vulvar vestibulitis: results of a placebo-controlled study. *Sexually Transmitted Infections* **77**, 53–57.
6 Zyczynski HM, Culbertson S, Gruss J, et al. (1997) Substance-P and the pathophysiology of vulvar vestibulitis. *Journal of the Society for Gynecologic Investigation* **4**, 107A.
7 Zolnoun DA, Hartmann KE, Steege JF. (2003) Overnight 5% lidocaine ointment for treatment of vulvar vestibulitis. *Obstetrics and Gynecology* **102**, 84–87.
8 Danielsson I, Torstensson T, Brodda-Jansen G, et al. (2006) EMG biofeedback versus topical lidocaine gel: a randomized study for the treatment of women with vulvar vestibulitis. *Acta Obstetricia et Gynecologica* **85**, 1360–67.
9 Bautista D, Julius D. (2008) Fire in the hole: pore dilation of the capsaicin receptor TRPV1. *Nature Neuroscience* **11**, 528–29.
10 Friedrich EG. (1988) Therapeutic studies on vulvar vestibulitis. *The Journal of Reproductive Medicine* **33**, 514–18.
11 Steinberg AC, Oyama IA, Rijba AE, et al. (2005) Capsaicin for the treatment of vulvar vestibulitis. *American Journal of Obstetrics and Gynecology* **192**, 1549–53.
12 Murina F, Radici G, Bianco V. (2004) Capsaicin and the treatment of vulvar vestibulitis syndrome: a valuable alternative? *Medscape General Medicine* **6**, 48.
13 Walsh KE, Berman JR, Berman LA, et al. (2002) Safety and efficacy of topical nitroglycerin for treatment of vulvar pain in women with vulvodynia: a pilot study. *Journal of Gender-Specific Medicine* **5**, 21–27.

14 Eva LJ, MacLean AB, Reid WM, *et al.* (2003) Estrogen receptor expression in vulvar vestibulitis syndrome. *American Journal of Obstetrics and Gynecology* **189**, 458–61.

15 Boardman LA, Cooper AS, Raker C. (2008) Topical gabapentin in the treatment of vulvodynia. *Obstetrics and Gynecology* **112**, 579–85..

16 Segal D, Tifheret H, Lazer S. (2003) Submucous infiltration of betamethasone and lidocaine in the treatment of vulvar vestibulitis. *European Journal of Obstetrics and Gynecology and Reproductive Biology* **107**, 105–6.

17 Murina F, Tassan P, Roberti P, *et al.* (2001) Treatment of vulvar vestibulitis with submucous inflitrations of methylprednisolone and lidocaine. *The Journal of Reproductive Medicine* **46**, 713–16.

18 Rapkin AJ, McDonald JS, Morgan M. (2008) Mulitlevel local anesthetic nerve blockade for the treatment of vulvar vestibulitis syndrome. *American Journal of Obstetrics and Gynecology* **198**, 41.e1–e5.

19 Horowitz BJ. (1989) Interferon therapy for condylomatous vulvitis. *Obstetrics and Gynecology* **73**, 466–68.

20 Kent HL, Wisniewski PM. (1990) Interferon for vulvar vestibulitis. *The Journal of Reproductive Medicine* **35**, 1138–40.

21 Bornstein J, Pascal B, Abramovici H. (1991) Treatment of a patient with vulvar vestibulitis by intramuscular interferon beta; a case report. *European Journal of Obstetrics and Gynecology and Reproductive Biology* **42**, 237–39.

22 Mann MS, Kaufman RH, Brown D, *et al.* (1992) Vulvar vestibulitis: significant clinical variables and treatment outcome. *Obstetrics and Gynecology* **79**, 122–25.

23 Bornstein J, Pascal B, Abramovici H. (1993) Intramuscular beta-interferon treatment for severe vulvar vestibulitis. *The Journal of Reproductive Medicine* **38**, 117–120.

24 Larsen J, Peters K, Petersen CS, *et al.* (1993) Interferon alpha-2b treatment of symptomatic chronic vulvodynia associated with koilocytosis. *Acta Dermato-Venereologica* **73**, 385–87.

25 Marinoff SC, Turner ML, Hirsch RP, *et al.* (1993) Intralesional alpha-interferon, cost-effective therapy for vulvar vestibulitis

syndrome. *The Journal of Reproductive Medicine* **38**, 19–24.

26 Bornstein J, Abramovici H. (1997) Combination of subtotal perineoplasty and interferon for the treatment of vulvar vestibulitis. *Gynecologic and Obstetric Investigation* **44**, 53–56.

27 Goldstein AT, Davies-Treene L, Hurtado S, *et al.* (2002) *Interferon Alpha Therapy for Vulvar Vestibulitis Syndrome: A Large Retrospective Trial.* Presented at the International Society for the Study of Women's Sexual Health Conference, Vancouver, BC.

28 Brown CS, Glazer HI, Vogt V, *et al.* (2006) Subjective and objective outcomes of botulinum toxin type A treatment in vestibulodynia. *The Journal of Reproductive Medicine* **51**, 635–41.

29 Dykstra DD, Presthus J. (2006) Botulinum toxin type A for the treatment of provoked vestibulodynia. *The Journal of Reproductive Medicine* **51**, 467–70.

30 Shafik A, El-Sibai O. (2000) Vaginismus: results of treatment with botulin toxin. *Journal of Obstetrics and Gynaecology* **20**, 300–2.

31 Ghazizadeh S, Nikzad M. (2004) Botulinum toxin in the treatment of refractory vaginismus. *Obstetrics and Gynecology* **104**, 922–95.

32 Abbott JA, Jarvis SK, Lyons SD, *et al.* (2006) Botulinum toxin type A for chronic pain and pelvic floor spasm in women: a randomized controlled trial. *Obstetrics and Gynecology* **108**, 915–23.

33 Burrows LJ, Goldstein AT. (2008) Vulvodynia. *The Journal of Sexual Medicine* **5**, 5–15.

34 Reissing ED, Brown C, Lord MJ, *et al.* (2005) Pelvic floor muscle functioning in women with vulvar vestibulitis syndrome. *Journal of Psychosomatic Obstetrics and Gynaecology* **26**, 107–13.

35 Langford CF, Udvari Nagy S, Ghoniem GM. (2007) Levator ani trigger point injections: an underutilized treatment for chronic pelvic pain. *Neurourology and Urodynamics* **26**, 59–62.

CHAPTER 25

Surgical Therapy: An Effective Treatment for Dyspareunia Caused by Vestibulodynia

Jacob Bornstein, Doron Zarfati

The Rappaport Faculty of Medicine, Hatechnion University, Nahariya, Israel

Pathophysiology of Vestibulodynia

The successful treatment of vestibulodynia, as with any medical condition, is dependent upon the proper identification and understanding of underlying pathophysiology. A physical, rather than psychosocial, basis for vestibulodynia is supported by abnormal histopathologic findings in the vestibule of women suffering from this condition (Figures 25.1 and 25.2). Tissue studies reveal enhanced inflammation of the vulvar vestibule [1–5], mast cell proliferation and degranulation [6, 7], hyperinnervation [6, 8–11], decreased natural killer cell activity [12], and enhanced heparanase activity [13].

The inflammation of the vestibule in vestibulodynia is related, in part, to both mast cell proliferation and hyperinnervation, acting reciprocally, and ultimately increasing local inflammation. Mast cells secrete mediators, such as nerve growth factor (NGF), histamine, and serotonin, which have been found to sensitize and induce the proliferation of C-afferent nerve fibers [6, 7, 14]. These nerve fibers release neuropeptides, including NGF, which increase the proliferation and degranulation of mast cells, cause hyperesthesia, and enhance the inflammatory response. This, in turn, increases the density of nerve fibers, leading to further activation of mast cells, and contributing to inflammation. In addition, heparanase released from mast cells degrades the basement membrane allowing increased intraepithelial hyperinnervation [13] (Figures 25.1 and 25.2). In this way, both hyperinnervation and neurogenic inflammation [15] play significant roles in the cycle resulting in chronic vulvar pain.

Surgical Technique

A number of variations have been made on Woodruff's original perineoplasty, which was first described in 1981 [16]. Due to a lack of standardization of terms, the same procedure can be referred to by different names, and the same term can refer to different procedures. The term *vestibulectomy* may be preferred over the term *perineoplasty*, which sounds like cosmetic surgery. The following are procedure names and descriptions that the authors prefer [17].

• *Vestibuloplasty*: The excision of a localized, painful area, such as the posterior vestibule. Some authors refer to this term as describing the surgical undermining of the vestibule, without tissue excision.

• *Vulvar vestibulectomy with vaginal advancement* (Figure 25.3): Vestibular excision, including both anterior and posterior aspects, with vaginal advancement.

• *Modified vestibulectomy*: Vestibular excision that is limited to the posterior of the vestibule.

Our surgical procedure is as follows: The labia majora are retracted and separated laterally revealing the entire vulvar vestibule, which is the area lying between the hymenal ring medially and Hart's line on the inner surface

Female Sexual Pain Disorders 1st edition. Edited by A. Goldstein, C. Pukall & I. Goldstein. © 2009 Blackwell Publishing, ISBN: 9781405183987.

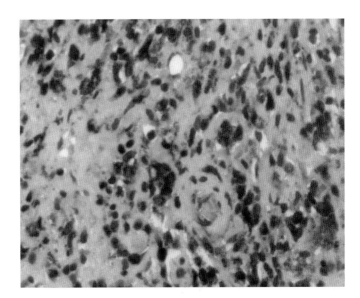

Figure 25.1 X400, Heparanase expression. Positive cytoplasmatic staining is noted in the subepithelial layer, close to the epithelial basement membrane.

of the labia minora laterally. Hart's line is the junction of the keratinized skin and mucosa and can easily be visualized on the inner aspect of the labia minora. The vulvar vestibule is then outlined using a marking pen. This is done by making parallel lines on either side of the urethra, carrying these lines superiorly to Hart's line, then inferiorly following Hart's line meeting approximately 0.7 cm on the perineum. Marcaine 0.05 % with epinephrine is used to

infiltrate the vulvar vestibular mucosa for intra-operative hemostasis and postoperative pain control.

A scalpel is used to excise the entire vulvar vestibular mucosa, approximately 3 mm deep and 5 mm past the hymenal ring, thus removing the entire hymenal ring. We advocate excision of the Bartholin's glands; however, other authors do not routinely do this as they believe that it increases intra-operative blood loss and postoperative pain.

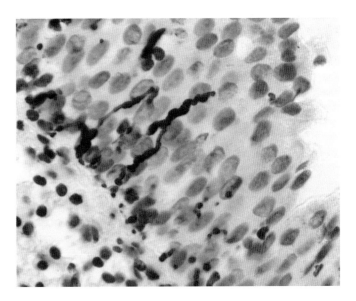

Figure 25.2 X600 staining for PGP 9.5. The nerve fibers are seen intruding into the epithelium to more than half of its depth.

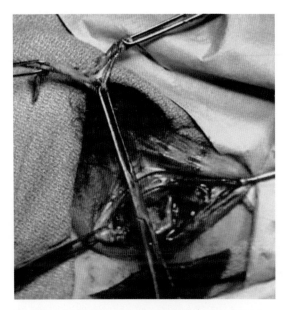

Figure 25.3 Perineoplasty: consists of excising the posterior and anterior parts of the vestibule, followed by advancement of the vagina to cover the defect.

The vaginal mucosa is grasped with two Babcock's clamps. Then approximately 1–2 cm of vaginal mucosa is gently dissected off the recto-vaginal fascia to create a vaginal advancement flap. This advancement flap will be used to cover the defect in the posterior vestibule. Caution is advised as the rectum can be injured if the surgeon is not in the correct anatomic plane.

After enough vaginal mucosa has been separated from the recto-vaginal fascia, it is anchored in an advanced position using two rows of three mattress sutures of 3-0 Vicryl. The suture passes through the vaginal mucosa and is "back-handed" through the recto-vaginal fascia and then goes back through the vaginal mucosa. It is essential that these mattress stitches go through the recto-vaginal fascia in an anterior-posterior direction so that the vaginal introital diameter will not be compromised. The mattress sutures ensure that there will not be significant tension on the suture line when the advancement flap is approximated to the perineum. In addition, these mattress sutures prevent the advancement flap from curling and prevent postoperative hematoma.

The defects in the anterior vestibule are closed with interrupted 4-0 Vicryl suture. Meticulous attention to detail is used to ensure that the urethra is not injured when clos-

ing these defects and to prevent postoperative hematoma. The advancement flap is then approximated to the labia minora and perineum using approximately 20 interrupted stitches of 4-0 Vicryl suture to complete the procedure. A digital rectal examination is performed to confirm that the mattress stitches did not go through the rectum. A vaginal packing can be inserted if the patient is to stay in the hospital overnight. The authors advocate an overnight stay in the hospital, although they recognize that the procedure can be done as an outpatient procedure.

The Extent of the Surgical Procedure

Controversy surrounds the optimal surgical approach and degree of excision during surgery. The authors conducted a controlled trial comparing vestibuloplasty, in which the vestibular tissue was undermined but not removed, to vulvar vestibulectomy with vaginal advancement. Ineffectiveness of vestibuloplasty and effectiveness of vestibulectomy led to early termination of the trial [18]. These results demonstrate that denervation in itself is not a cure for vestibulodynia.

Specialists continue to debate whether the anterior portion of the vestibule should be removed in cases in which pain is localized to the posterior aspect. Proponents of modified vestibulectomy claim that their outcomes are comparable to those of more extensive procedures, with the advantages of simplicity, minimal excision of tissue resulting in decreased operative time, and reduction in postoperative pain and complications [19, 20]. Conversely, insufficient excision has contributed to surgical failure or recurrence of symptoms [21–24]. Based on these results and our own experience, we currently recommend excision of the anterior vestibule in every surgical treatment for vulvodynia, regardless of the localization pf the pain foci. Long-term controlled studies are needed to determine the optimal extent of surgery that will achieve the best response, with minimal risk of complications and recurrence.

Postoperative Care

While the surgery can be performed as an outpatient procedure, overnight hospitalization for the administration of pain relief narcotics can be provided. The vaginal pack and the urinary catheter can be removed the morning after the operation. Pain and discomfort, generally lasting 10–14 days, are relieved by ice packs, sitz baths, and analgesics. Some surgeons advocate the use of vaginal dilators

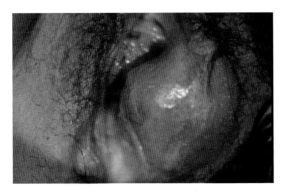

Figure 25.4 Bartholin duct cyst developed as a result of perineoplasty, with incision of the Bartholin duct and then covering it with the advanced vagina.

6–8 weeks postoperatively. In general, intercourse can be resumed after 8–12 weeks postoperatively.

Complications of Surgery

Intra-operative complications are rare. Short-term post-operative complications consist of bleeding, infection, hematoma, and partial wound separation with secondary healing. Long-term complications consist of Bartholin duct cyst formation (2–6%) (Figure 25.4), and persistent or enhanced vestibular tenderness (3–7%) [25]. The most frequent complication, reported by 25% of the women in a study of 126 women [26], was decreased lubrication during sexual intercourse.

In another study of 106 women [25], a decreased ability to achieve orgasm was reported by 8% of women postoperatively. However, in the same study, 82% had no change in their ability to achieve orgasm and 10% of women had an increased ability to have orgasm after surgery. In addition, 7% of women who had vestibulectomy thought the postoperative cosmetic changes were significant [25].

Surgical Outcomes

Outcome rates regarding surgery (vulvar vestibulectomy with vaginal advancement) vary little from study to study. The most common primary outcomes examined are the relief of pain or discomfort during sexual intercourse, the ability to engage in sexual intercourse, increased coital frequency, reduction in constant or daily vulvar discomfort, and overall satisfaction with the treatment.

Most studies have assessed success according to partial response (PR), defined as the ability to tolerate intercourse, even with pain, and complete response (CR), the ability to have intercourse without any pain. The combined sum of CR and PR from 37 studies of surgical treatment is 89% (Figure 25.5). In one study, 93% of 106 women who underwent vestibulectomy were satisfied with the surgery and would recommend surgery to another woman experiencing the same symptoms [25].

The Effect of Patient selection on Study Outcomes

Since surgery is typically performed on women who were ineffectively treated with other options, these patients may represent a more complex pain syndrome or one with a strong psychosexual component. Psychological distress in the setting of multiple failures may exacerbate their physical as well as psychological distress, making surgical cure less likely.

Data can be analysed in a way that produces skewed statistical outcomes. For example, de Jong [27] and his team conducted a follow-up on women for whom surgery failed. They did not detect long-term improvement, and subsequently concluded that surgical therapy for vulvodynia should be abandoned. Had they also examined the women for whom surgery had succeeded, they may have reached different conclusions.

While some investigators have analyzed surgical procedures on all women diagnosed with vestibulodynia according to Friedrich's criteria (erythema, point tenderness, and introital dyspareunia), others have restricted their studies to women younger than 40 [21, 26] or to those without the presence of generalized vulvodynia or pelvic floor muscle hypertonicity (pelvic floor dysfunction, vaginismus) [25]. The possibility that subject selection may play a decisive role in the success or failure of surgical treatment indicates that a variety of factors and patient characteristics may be associated with treatment outcome.

Characteristics Associated with a Successful Outcome

Though the overall success rate of vestibulectomy is very high, surgical treatment of vestibulodynia is not successful for all women. This is not surprising in light of the current understanding that this disorder has a multifactorial etiology. By identifying patient characteristics that associate with success and failure rates, we may also elucidate etiological factors for vestibulodynia.

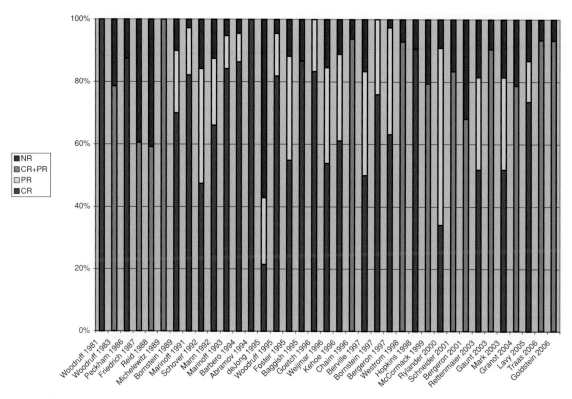

Figure 25.5 Success rates by percentage of surgeries since 1981. CR = complete response; PR = partial response. CR + PR = complete response + partial response; NR = no response. *Note*: Some researchers do no distinguish between CR and PR. See text.

A number of patient characteristics have been suggested to increase surgical success, among them: willingness to have psychological treatment, higher socio-economic status, parity [25], relatively young age [26], fewer sites of pain and absence of concomitant pain disorders, and a relatively high resting systolic blood pressure [28].

Alternatively, characteristics associated with decreased surgical success include intense premenstrual pain [29], concurrent pelvic floor dysfunction [25], a relatively low resting systolic blood pressure [28], and undiagnosed, confounding psychosexual problems. While we found the presence of human papillomavirus to be associated with surgical success [30], others have found the contrary [20].

Severity and constancy of vulvar pain are also associated with conflicting, predictive values for surgical treatment. In one study, women with more severe vestibulodynia [21] expressed greater satisfaction with surgical treatment, and were more likely to resume sexual intercourse. The authors

suggested differences in expectations and appreciation of postoperative success as an explanation. Age, the number of years of suffering, and the number of treatments undergone may also affect both women's expectations and assessment of surgical outcome. A prospective study examining the characteristics of women who chose surgery over other treatment modalities found that women who opted for surgical treatment had significantly higher pain thresholds and fewer nonvulvar pain disorders [28].

We found that women who suffer from constant vulvar pain, rather than isolated dyspareunia, experience diminished surgical response [31]. Because this group of women is generally older than those suffering from vestibulodynia, we suggested that their prolonged endurance of increasingly severe symptoms might explain the low rate of surgical success. This was later supported by another study in which delay in administration of effective treatment was shown to exacerbate symptoms [32].

Study Design

Most articles reporting outcomes for surgical treatment are actually descriptive patient reviews, some of which are wholly inclusive of clinic populations and others which utilize specific inclusion criteria. Randomized controlled studies are needed to attain a valid assessment of surgical treatment and distinguish the factors affecting treatment outcome. Only one randomized, controlled study comparing surgery with biofeedback and cognitive behavioral therapy has been published [33]. The results showed surgical treatment as having the highest success.

While randomized controlled studies afford valid assessment of associations between individual characteristics and treatment outcome, the inherent relinquishment of choice causes other difficulties. In Bergeron et al.'s randomized comparative study [33], seven (24%) of those assigned to the surgery group refused treatment after randomization. Patient preference, therefore, cannot be ignored either in study design or in treatment recommendation.

Conclusions and Future Directions

Overall, surgery for vestibulodynia is advantageous for several reasons. First, the overall success rate surpasses that of any other treatment. Second, surgery provides the only opportunity for a "true" cure (i.e., the disappearance of local sensitivity and resumption of painless sexual intercourse). Third, the rate of recurrence is minimal. For the future, randomized controlled clinical studies of well-defined candidates will help determine the optimal surgical procedure and identify characteristics that predict surgical success. Until then, an individualized treatment approach will enable women to make appropriate treatment choices.

References

1 Pyka RE, Wilkinson EJ, Friedrich EG. (1988) The histopathology of vulvar vestibulitis syndrome. *International Journal of Gynecological Pathology* 7, 249–57.
2 Chadha S, Gianotten WL, Drogendijk AC, *et al.* (1998) Histopathologic features of vulvar vestibulitis. *International Journal of Gynecological Pathology* 98, 703–6.
3 Furlonge CB, Thin RN, Evans BE, *et al.* (1991) Vulvar vestibulitis syndrome: A clinico-pathological study. *British Journal of Obstetrics and Gynecology* 98, 703–6.
4 Prayson RA, Stolar MH, Hart WR. (1995) Vulvar vestibulitis: a histopathologic study of 36 cases, including human papillomavirus in situ hybridization analysis. *American Journal of Surgical Pathology* 19, 154–60.
5 Foster DC, Piedarz KH, Murant TI, *et al.* (2007) Enhanced synthesis of proinflammatory cytokines by vulvar vestibular fibroblasts: implications for vulvar vestibulitis. *American Journal of Obstetrics and Gynecology* 196, 346.e1–e8.
6 Bornstein J, Goldschmid N, Sabo E. (2004) Hyperinnervation and mast cell activation may be used as histopathologic diagnostic criteria for vulvar vestibulitis. *Gynecological and Obstetric Investigation* 58, 171–78.
7 Metz M, Grimbaldeston MA, Nakae S, *et al.* (2007) Mast cells in the promotion and limitation of chronic inflammation. *Immunological Reviews* 217, 304–28.
8 Weström LV, Willén R. (1998) Vestibular nerve fiber proliferation in vulvar vestibulitis syndrome. *Obstetrics and Gynecology* 91, 572–76.
9 Bohm-Starke N, Hilliges M, Falconer C, *et al.* (1998) Increased intraepithelial innervation in women with vulvar vestibulitis syndrome. *Gynecological and Obstetric Investigation* 46, 256–60.
10 Tympanidis P, Terenghi G, Dowd P. (2003) Increased innervation of the vulval vestibule in patients with vulvodynia. *British Journal of Dermatology* 148, 1021–27.
11 Halperin R, Zehavi V, Ben-Ami I, *et al.* (2005) The major histopathologic characteristics in the vulvar vestibulitis syndrome. *Gynecologic and Obstetric Investigation* 59, 75–79.
12 Masterson, BJ, Galask RP, Ballas ZK. (1996) Natural killer cell function in women with vestibulitis. *The Journal of Reproductive Medicine* 41, 562–68.
13 Bornstein J, Cohen Y, Zarfati D, *et al.* (2008) Involvement of heparanase in the pathogenesis of localized vulvodynia. *International Journal of Gynecological Pathology* 27, 136–41.
14 Bohm-Starke N, Hilliges M, Brodda-Jansen G, *et al.* (2001) Psychophysical evidence of nociceptor sensitization in vulvar vestibulitis syndrome. *Pain* 94, 177–83.
15 Wesselmann U. (2001) Neurogenic inflammation and chronic pelvic pain. *World Journal of Urology* 19,180–85.
16 Woodruff JD, Genadry R, Poliakoff S. (1981) Treatment of dyspareunia and vaginal outlet distortions by perineoplasty. *Obstetrics and Gynecology* 57, 750–54.
17 Haefner HK. (2000) Critique of new gynecologic surgical procedures: surgery for vulvar vestibulitis. *Clinical Obstetrics and Gynecology* 43, 689–700.

18 Bornstein J, Zarfati D, Goldik Z, *et al.* (1995) Perineoplasty compared with vestibuloplasty for severe vulvar vestibulitis. *British Journal of Obstetrics and Gynaecology* **102**, 652–55.

19 Kehoe S, Luesley D. (1996) An evaluation of modified vestibulectomy the treatment of vulvar vestibulitis: preliminary results. *Acta Obstetricia et Gynecologica Scandinavica* **75**, 676–77.

20 Lavy Y, Lev-Sagie A, Hamani Y, *et al.* (2005) Modified vulvar vestibulectomy: simple and effective surgery for the treatment of vulvar vestibulitis. *European Journal of Obstetrics and Gynecology and Reproductive Biology* **120**, 91–95.

21 Schneider D, Yaron M, Bukovsky I, *et al.* (2001) Outcome of surgical treatment for superficial dyspareunia from vulvar vestibulitis. *The Journal of Reproductive Medicine* **46**, 227–31.

22 Rettenmaier MA, Brown JV, Micha JP. (2003) Modified vestibulectomy is inadequate treatment for secondary vulvar vestibulitis. *Journal of Gynecologic Survey* **19**, 13–17.

23 Woodruff JD, Parmley TH. (1983) Infection of the minor vestibular gland. *Obstetrics and Gynecology* **62**, 609–12.

24 Reid R, Greenberg MD, Daoud YU, *et al.* (1988) Colposcopic findings in women with vulvar pain syndromes. *The Journal of Reproductive Medicine* **33**, 523–32.

25 Goldstein AT, Klingman D, Christopher K, *et al.* (2006) Surgical treatment of vulvar vestibulitis syndrome: outcome assessment derived from a postoperative questionnaire. *The Journal of Sexual Medicine* **3**, 923–31.

26 Traas AF, Bekkers RLM, Dony JMJ, *et al.* (2006) Surgical treatment for the vulvar vestibulitis syndrome. *Obstetrics and Gynecology* **107**, 256–62.

27 de Jong JM, van Lunsen RH, Robertson EA, *et al.* (1995) Focal vulvitis: a psychosexual problem for which surgery is not the answer. *Journal of Psychosomatic Obstetrics and Gynaecology* **16**, 85–91.

28 Granot M, Friedman M, Yarnitsky D, *et al.* (2002) Enhancement of the perception of systemic pain in women with vulvar vestibulitis. *British Journal of Obstetrics and Gynaecology* **109**, 863–66.

29 Schover LR, Youngs DD, Cannata R. (1992) Psychosexual aspects of the evaluation and management of vulvar vestibulitis. *American Journal of Obstetrics and Gynecology* **167**, 630–36.

30 Bornstein J, Shapiro S, Goldshmid N, *et al.* (1997) Severe vulvar vestibulitis: relation to HPV infection. *The Journal of Reproductive Medicine* **42**, 514–18.

31 Bornstein J, Goldik Z, Stolar Z, *et al.* (1997) Predicting the outcome of surgical treatment for vulvar vestibulitis. *Obstetrics and Gynecology* **89**, 695–98.

32 Buchan A, Munday P, Ravenhill G, *et al.* (2007) A qualitative study of women with vulvodynia. I. The journey into treatment. *The Journal of Reproductive Medicine* **52**, 15–18.

33 Bergeron S, Binik YM, Khalifé S, *et al.* (2001) A randomized comparison of group cognitive-behavioral therapy, surface electromyographic biofeedback, and vestibulectomy in the treatment of dyspareunia resulting from vulvar vestibulitis. *Pain* **91**, 297–306.

CHAPTER 26

26

CHAPTER 26
Vulvar Pain: The Neurologist's View

Allan S. Gordon
University of Toronto, Toronto, Ontario, Canada

Introduction

Vulvar pain is not normally considered to be in the scope of practice of neurologists, but it should be. The pelvis, vulva, and vagina have a rich innervation with many nerves, somatic and autonomic, converging on the spinal cord and integrating with the rest of the pain system. Basic training gives neurologists an understanding of these neural systems and their function, which is important in understanding how to diagnose and treat chronic pain. In addition, neurologists are trained to conduct a relevant history and neurological examination and to perform tests to answer two questions: *where* is the lesion and *what* is the lesion? Neurologists also determine whether the pain is nociceptive or neuropathic, and what treatments are necessary. What some neurologists may lack, however, is the interest or ability to treat pain in a multidisciplinary manner.

The Wasser Pain Management Centre (WPMC) was formed in 1999. It offers a multidisciplinary, multiprofessional, and multimodal approach to pain problems with staff members in neurology, nursing, dentistry, anesthesiology, gynecology, psychiatry, sex therapy, behavioral therapy, addiction medicine, and contacts in physical therapy, urology, acupuncture, urogynecology, dermatology, and yoga. Six intertwining "programs of care" have been established: complex pharmacotherapy (e.g., antidepressants, antiepileptics, opioids, anti-inflammatories, cannabinoids); pain, addiction, and chemical dependency; pelvic and genital pain; neuro-

pathic pain; headache and facial pain; and arthritis and soft-tissue pain.

Patients referred to the WPMC fill out a detailed questionnaire including, if appropriate, a pelvic pain questionnaire. Based on the letter of referral and previous documents, the individual is triaged to see the most appropriate practitioner who does a detailed consultation and examination. Other team members may also see the patient if appropriate. Accurate diagnosis is emphasized, and multiple diagnoses may be offered. Further investigations may be ordered and then treatment plans are devised.

The female pelvic pain team can include the neurologist, gynecologist, nurse, physical therapist, anesthesiologist, and sex therapist. Evaluation includes general and neurological examination, abdominal, back and pelvic exam, vulvar examination including the cotton-swab test, and pin-prick evaluation. A drug and alcohol history is also taken.

Because of the emphasis of all aspects of chronic pain at the WPMC, the patients seen may be different, or at least evaluated differently, than in gynecology-based clinics. Examples illustrating the range of patients presenting at the WPMC include:

(1) A 55-year-old woman was referred for chronic migraine and only during the course of the evaluation did she describe a 25-year history of dyspareunia, specifically, superficial pain upon penetration.

(2) A 34-year old woman developed urgency, frequency, and dysuria. Urine cultures were negative. Investigations showed typical changes compatible with interstitial cystitis (IC). Three months later, she developed vulvar pain at rest and with intercourse. She was started on 75 mg of pregabalin twice a day, and increased to 150 mg twice a day. Her urinary symptoms improved as did her vulvar pain and dyspareunia.

Female Sexual Pain Disorders 1st edition. Edited by A. Goldstein, C. Pukall & I. Goldstein. © 2009 Blackwell Publishing, ISBN: 9781405183987.

(3) A 43-year old woman was referred with total body pain. Her vulva showed multiple cotton swab sensitivity areas, pin-prick hyperalgesia, and an exquisitely sensitive clitoris. The vulvar pain in this case was overshadowed by the widespread muscle pain to the point that she did not complain of it initially.

(4) A 45-year old woman complained of abdominal pain that started after a total abdominal hysterectomy for fibroids. Initially, the pain was restricted to the transverse lower abdominal scar on the right; over time, the pain spread down to the vulva on the right side and up to the right subcostal margin. After numerous tests, no explanation was found for this neuropathic pain other than the possible spreading effect of central sensitization from a lower abdominal segmental nerve injury. In this case, the vulvar pain was part of a larger neuropathic pain abnormality.

In addition, women presenting with provoked vestibulodynia (PVD) and/or generalized vulvodynia (GVD) and vulvar pain as part of a major genital or pelvic pain syndrome are common.

Many of our patients do not fit into the strict classification of vulvar pain offered by the International Society for the Study of Vulvovaginal Disease (ISSVD) [1]. There can be many sacral nerve functions affected and a variety of pain syndromes involved, in addition to overlap among syndromes. Therefore, treatment of vulvar pain depends on the clinical context. As such, we have developed a classification of vulvar pain based on patients presenting to the center (Table 26.1).

An Approach to Vulvar Pain Management

Our approach incorporates some broad principles of pain management. These principles are as applicable to the vulva as they are to other kinds of chronic pain syndromes. We refer to them as the five pillars of pain management (Table 26.2) [2].

Applying the Five Pillars to Vulvar Pain

Pillar One: Conduct a Risk Assessment
As a first step in treating anyone with pain or any other condition, the treating practitioner should establish treatment goals with the patient. In doing so, a risk assessment

Table 26.1 Vulvar pain classification.

I Vulvodynia
   a. vulvar vestibulitis or vestibulodynia (provoked)
   b. dysesthetic vulvodynia (unprovoked)
   c. mixed provoked and unprovoked vulvodynia
II Vulvar pain associated with other genital syndromes
   a. clitoral pain
   b. urethral pain and interstitial cystitis
   c. anal pain
III Vulvar pain associated with comorbidities
   a. fibromyalgia
   b. temporomandibular syndrome
   c. migraine
   d. irritable bowel syndrome
   e. pain and dependency issues
IV Vulvar pain as part of a larger neuropathic pain syndrome
   a. peripheral such as painful diabetic neuropathy (such as painful diabetic neuropathy)
   b. central such as multiple sclerosis (such as multiple sclerosis)
   c. part of a lumbosacral radiculopathy
V Vulvar pain stemming from a pelvic region neuropathic pain injury
VI Vulvar pain as part of pudendal neuralgia or pudendal nerve entrapment (see Chapter 17)
VII Vulvar pain as part of a pelvic pain condition
   a. endometriosis
   b. pelvic congestion syndrome
   c. fibroids
   d. adenomyosis
VII Vulvar pain as part of another entity
   a. yeast
   b. lichen sclerosus

is needed: What are the risks of treating versus not treating the patient? At the WPMC, we treat vulvar pain patients using the universal precautions approach to pain management [3] within a multidisciplinary framework. We inquire about a history of alcohol and drug abuse in the patient and family, a history of smoking or gambling addiction, a history of sexual abuse and dysfunction, prior pain and other therapies, other pain issues, anxiety and depression, and any legal and litigation issues. Between 6% and 15% of the population have an addiction [4, 5]. The more "red flags" an individual has, the more risky and difficult the treatment.

Based on this assessment, patients are divided into three groups:

Group I, low risk: little evidence to suggest addiction or psychiatric problems;

Group II, moderate risk: no active addiction but the presence of psychiatric problems; and

Table 26.2 The five pillars of pain management.

Pillar One

Risk assessment. What is the risk of treating the individual, risk to the patient, and risk to the practitioner? We apply the principles of universal precautions (Gourlay et al., 2005).

Pillar Two

Identify the underlying disease and treating it. This assumes that there are specific diseases causing pain and that there are specific treatments for those conditions and that treating the underlying condition will help the pain.

Pillar Three

Determine whether the pain is neuropathic or nociceptive (or both) and go down the evidence-based path of treatment for neuropathic and nociceptive pain. This applies more to pharmacotherapy than to nonpharmacological therapies.

Pillar Four

Treat psychosocial and comorbid conditions such as anxiety, mood and depression, addiction, sexual dysfunction, and sleep.

Pillar Five

Establish a good therapeutic alliance with the patient. Encourage and teach self-management techniques to allow the individual to take charge and share responsibility for her condition.

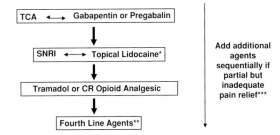

Figure 26.1 Stepwise pharamacologic management of neuropathic pain (peripheral). KEY: TCA = tricyclic antidepressant; SNRI = serotonin norepinephrine reuptake inhibitor; CR = continuous release; * 5% gel or cream, useful for focal neuropathy such as postherpetic neuralgia; ** e.g., cannabinoids, methadone, lamotrigine, topiramate, valproic acid; *** do not add SNRI to TCA. (Reproduced with permission of the Canadian Pain Society.)

Group III, high risk: serious active addiction and psychiatric issues.

Low-risk individuals can usually be easily, if not always successfully, treated by most knowledgeable practitioners. The treatment of moderate-risk patients may benefit from input from mental health and addiction specialists; at the very least, specific attention should be paid to these issues. To manage high-risk patients—the most challenging group to treat—direct input and care from experts in addiction and mental health is needed. Also, this pillar involves setting appropriate boundaries with patients: what the treatment will entail, what kind and how much medication or other treatment will be offered, and what will happen if those boundaries are broken.

Pillar Two: Identify the Underlying Disease Process and Treat It

The basis of neurological practice rests on identifying whether a neurological lesion is present. If so, its location and potential cause(s) should be determined. This process involves conducting a neurological history and physical exam, a general history and physical exam, and confirmatory tests (e.g., neurophysiology) to find the anatomical and pathological cause of the symptoms. After this has been achieved, treatment options can be considered.

Pillar Three: Diagnosing and Treating the Pain

Pain is typically classified as nociceptive or neuropathic. Nociceptive pain reflects stimulation of normal nerve endings by inflammatory substances. It may be somatic or visceral. Neuropathic pain reflects damage to the nervous system, either central or peripheral. Symptoms suggestive of neuropathic pain include burning, shooting, stabbing, or knife-like painful sensations, pain upon contact, pain produced by a usually nonpainful stimulus (allodynia), and a painful stimulus being felt more painfully than is typical (hyperalgesia). Most investigators feel that idiopathic vulvar pain is neuropathic. However, it is important to keep in mind that many different pain mechanisms may be operating in this condition.

Another way of dividing up pain reflects the axes of pain management. Pain may be acute or chronic; mild, moderate, or severe; cancer or noncancer related; and nociceptive or neuropathic. Through a complete pain assessment, we collect this pain-related information, which then guides treatment.

In the case of neuropathic pain, pharmacotherapy is based on the Canadian Neuropathic Pain Guidelines (CNPG) [6], which present a four-stage process (Figure 26.1). It is important to note that these medications have been studied extensively for neuropathic pain, but little empirical evidence exists for their effectiveness for vulvodynia.

A survey of clinicians indicated that oral medications were more likely to be used for the treatment of GVD versus PVD [7]; however, randomized, controlled treatment outcome studies are currently lacking in this area. Thus, firm conclusions cannot yet be drawn regarding the effectiveness of oral medications in the treatment of vulvodynia. This pillar also includes nerve blocks, nerve stimulation techniques, and the use of botulinum toxin; however, formal trials in vulvodynia are lacking. See Chapters 13, 17 and 24 for a discussion of these techniques.

Level 1 Medications

Tricyclic antidepressants (TCAs) are the mainstay of pharmacotherapy; these medications have the best evidence for neuropathic pain in general and have gained some support for vulvodynia. McKay [8] conducted a retrospective chart review of 20 women with GVD who were taking amitriptyline. She showed that the average dose required for symptom resolution was 60 mg and the average time required for treatment was 7 months.

Also, Munday [9] followed 32 GVD patients (11 of whom also reported PVD symptoms) on TCAs for 6 months and demonstrated that a complete response was found in 15 (47%). Only four patients (13%) obtained less than a 50% improvement in their symptoms. However, patients in this study received the TCAs as part of a comprehensive treatment program; thus, the effects cannot be solely attributable to the medication. Reed et al. [10] showed that women with vulvodynia (GVD or PVD) who were prescribed a TCA were more likely to have pain improvement compared with those women not taking these medications at follow-up. In fact, 83 women who were taking a TCA at the first follow-up improved by more than 50%.

Most practitioners begin with either amitriptyline or nortriptyline 10–25 mg at bedtime. The dose can be slowly increased either weekly or biweekly, aiming for a dose that improves the pain. It will also improve sleep, and depending upon how high the dose, possibly mood. Generally, the dose is 50–75 mg per day, although antidepressant dose levels of 150 mg are possible. It must be emphasized to patients that any improvement will come slowly and that not all patients will respond. Side effects can include weight gain, mouth dryness, sleepiness, palpitations and other cardiovascular issues, dizziness, and precipitation of glaucoma. As many women with vulvar pain have urinary symptoms, the practitioner should ask about symptoms of urinary retention.

Gabapentin and pregabalin have been found useful for neuropathic pain in general; however, their expense would likely make these two antiepileptic agents a second choice to the TCAs. The effectiveness of gabapentin has been evaluated by three groups. Bates and Timmins [11] reported improvement in two patients with GVD, and Ben-David and Bruce [12] reported that 14 of 17 patients (82%) with vulvodynia had either partial or completely relied with gabapentin therapy. Of these patients, seven had complete and seven had significant pain relief; symptom relief was typically seen between 2 and 4 weeks of treatment onset. Treatment failed in the remaining three patients. Further, a chart review indicated that 98 of 152 (64%) of women with GVD had resolution of at least 80% of their symptoms, whereas 49 (32%) did not have adequate resolution. Women with longer histories of GVD were less likely to benefit from this treatment [13].

Gabapentin is usually started at 300 mg at bedtime, increasing by 300 mg every few days, aiming at 300 mg Q8H. If there is no effect, it can be increased slowly to 600 mg Q8H and even higher. The author does not usually increase past 1800 mg per day unless some effect is noted. It may take up to several weeks to notice an effect. Side effects include weight gain, edema, dizziness, and cognitive changes. There are few, if any, drug interactions.

Pregabalin has had extensive testing in neuropathic pain (both peripheral and central). It also is of benefit for anxiety, sleep (pillar four effects; see below), central pain [14], and fibromyalgia. As such, it should be a good choice for vulvar pain patients, particularly those with significant comorbidities. Although no specific studies in vulvodynia have yet been conducted, one case report indicated that pregabalin is successful in managing the pain of GVD [15].

The recommended starting dose is 75 mg Q12H. However, in our experience, many vulvar pain patients are quite sensitive to medications, and we often start with 25 or 50 mg Q12H, increasing every week. An initial target dose would be 150–300 mg per day. Increases to 450 mg or even 600 mg per day are sometimes necessary, but note that the side effect profile will also increase. Many women complain of edema and/or weight gain, dizziness, cognitive changes, lowering of mood or libido, and muscle pain. Like gabapentin, there are few drug interactions.

Gabapentin and pregabalin both affect the alpha-2 subunit of the calcium channel, thus dampening down neurotransmitter release. However, their therapeutic effects are not identical. The highest dose for pregabalin is typically 600 mg per day, whereas gabapentin doses can reach 3600 mg, or even higher, per day. If one drug does not work, the practitioner can switch to the other. These drugs may be combined with a TCA.

Level 2 Medications

Serotonin norepinephrine reuptake inhibitors (SNRIs) have proven effective in neuropathic pain. They have not been well studied in vulvar pain [16]. Venlafaxine not only helps alleviate neuropathic pain, it also has an anxiolytic and antidepressant effect. It is available in immediate-release and extended-release formulations. The initial dosing is 37.5–75 mg OD, increasing up to 150–225 mg.

Side effects may include nausea, dizziness, insomnia, changes in blood pressure, vasodilatation, cardiac arrhythmia, GI symptoms, and sexual dysfunction. Headache is common, and there is increasing concern about the potential for suicide. The author's impression is that it is of only modest help in vulvar pain.

Duloxetine is another SNRI that is new to the market. Approved for major depression, it is also helpful in the neuropathic pain of diabetics. There are no studies of this medication in vulvar pain patients. Doses of 30–60 mg per day are used with 60 mg being the recommended dose. Drowsiness, nausea, dizziness, constipation, and dry mouth are common, and there is the possibility of serotonin syndrome if mixed with a TCA. Psychiatric symptoms and a rapid heart rate may occur.

The CNPG does not include selective serotonin reuptake inhibitors (SSRIs) (e.g., fluoxetine, citralopam), because they are not particularly effective in the treatment of neuropathic pain, including vulvar pain. However, they may be helpful for concurrent anxiety and/or depression.

Topical lidocaine, particularly in gel form, can be effective in localized neuropathic pain conditions such as postherpetic neuralgia [17]. Topical lidocaine can be helpful in PVD [18] (see Chapter 24). Of interest to us is topical capsaicin using 0.0125% applied daily over topical anesthetic. Although an initial burning sensation is common, we have achieved some good outcomes. Steinberg et al. [19] report significantly reduced discomfort and increased sexual relations using 0.025% capsaicin for PVD. The author has not been impressed with topical amitriptyline or ketamine. There has, however, been a recent positive study for topical gabapentin [20].

Level 3 Medications

Tramadol has become useful in the treatment of neuropathic pain. It is a weak tricyclic and μ-opioid agonist, and it is considered a third-line treatment approach according to the CNPG. It will be often used to treat the comorbid conditions associated with vulvar pain (e.g., fibromyalgia). There are, however, no formal studies of its effectiveness for vulvar pain. Nonetheless, practitioners should prefer its use in for vulvar pain over that of a full opioid. It may be combined with acetaminophen or be on its own in an IR or SR formulation. The maximum dose is up to 300–400 mg per day. Side effects include nausea, dizziness, headache, and sleepiness. More serious but rare side effects include seizures, and one must be cautious with its use with a TCA or SNRI as there is a risk of serotonin syndrome.

Opioids include medications such as codeine slow release, oxycodone slow release, fentanyl patch, and morphine and hydromorphone slow release. Such medications are reserved for use in complex vulvar pain patients. Short-acting agents and meperidine are discouraged. Opioids are level 3 medications for neuropathic pain. A risk assessment is necessary to decide on dosing, dispensing, and boundaries [3]. An experienced addiction specialist should be consulted if there are concerns.

Level 4 Medications

Included in this category are the "other" medications, such as carbamazepine, lamotrigine, and methadone. None of these medications have been studied for vulvar pain treatment.

Nabilone is a synthetic cannabinoid (a tetrahydrocannabinol [THC] analog). Although its use has not been studied in vulvar pain, it has been found to be effective in pain management. The pill comes in 0.5 and 1.0 mg tablets, aiming at 3–6 mg per day. Side effects of nabilone include drowsiness, dizziness, mood changes, dry mouth, unsteadiness, blurred vision, loss of appetite, and headache. In a placebo-controlled, double-blinded pilot study of 30 patients with chronic pain, there was benefit of Cesamet® [21].

Sativex® is a cannabinoid-based medication (available in Canada) approved as an adjunct for neuropathic pain and multiple sclerosis. It appears to be effective for conditions that present with allodynia [22], suggesting that it may be effective for PVD or GVD. Although it has not yet been formally tested in vulvodynia patients, we have found that several (but not all) of our patients have had some benefit (unpublished data).

Pillar Four: Treating Psychosocial and Comorbid Symptoms

Patients with chronic pain often have other issues with which to contend, including anxiety, depression, sleep disturbances, sexual dysfunction, addiction, and issues with work and finances. Attending to these problems is essential for a good quality of life and treatment outcome; pain medications generally do not work well when there are outstanding issues in these areas. The use of medications, such as the TCAs or SNRIs, can help with some of the psychosocial issues. Also, pregabalin is noted for its effect on anxiety, sleep, and mood in addition to pain [14]. However, it is important to note that many medications, such as the antiepileptics and antidepressants, interfere with sexual function. Thus, the inclusion of psychiatrists, psychologists, behavioral therapists, and sex therapists— as well as adjunct medications to offset side effects—can be helpful in pain management.

It is important to note that physical therapy could be included in pillar three, four, or even five. See Chapters 6 and 13 for information related to the assessment and treatment of vulvodynia.

Pillar Five: Establishing Good Therapeutic Alliance

Essential to a successful outcome is the inclusion of the patient as an active participant in her own management program. As such, a good therapeutic alliance is necessary for success. This process begins with establishing agreed-upon and realistic goals and continues with the assessment and management of the expectations of the patient throughout treatment. Also, it is important to emphasize that success depends on the patient, who has to learn techniques to decrease pain and improve function. Whether this is achieved through exercise, yoga, stretching, walking, or relaxation, having the patient take some control and responsibility for the outcome is essential. If the practitioner is working harder than the patient, there is something wrong.

In our vulvar pain survey [23], a significant number of women used self-management techniques (unpublished data from survey). Unfortunately, programs in cognitive behavioral therapy or mindfulness may not be easily available or may be too expensive. Still, the patient must acquire her own set of self-management skills and tools and learn what she can do for herself.

Conclusions

Vulvar pain may be caused by a number of conditions. A comprehensive overall approach is necessary if patients are to be successfully managed. The "five pillar" approach to pain management affords this kind of approach. Unfortunately, there is relatively little high-level evidence for vulvar pain treatments.

References

1 Moyal-Barracco M, Lynch PJ. (2004) 2003 ISSVD terminology and classification of vulvodynia: a historical perspective. *The Journal of Reproductive Medicine* **49**, 772–77.

2 Gordon A. (2007) Best practice guidelines for treatment of central pain after stroke. In: Henry JL, Panju A, Yashpal K (eds.) *Central Neuropathic Pain: Focus on Poststroke Pain.* IASP Press, Seattle.

3 Gourlay DL, Heit HA, Almahrezi A. (2005) Universal precautions in pain medicine: a rational approach to the treatment of chronic pain. *Pain Medicine* **6**, 107–12.

4 Passik SD, Portenoy RK, Ricketts PL. (1998) Substance abuse issues in cancer patients. Part 1: Prevalence and diagnosis. *Oncology* **12**, 517–21, 524.

5 Groerer JM, Brodsky M. (1992) The incidence of illicit drug use in the United States, 1962–1989. *British Journal of Addiction* **87**, 1345.

6 Moulin DE, Clark AJ, Gilron I, *et al.* (2007) Pharmacological management of chronic neuropathic pain: consensus statement and guidelines from the Canadian Pain Society. *Pain Research and Management* **12**, 13–21 .

7 Updike GM, Wisenfeld HC. (2005) Insight into the treatment of vulvar pain: a survey of clinicians. *American Journal of Obstetrics and Gynecology* **193**, 1404–9.

8 McKay M. (1993) Dysesthetic (essential) vulvodynia: treatment with amitriptyline. *The Journal of Reproductive Medicine* **38**, 9–13.

9 Munday PE. (2001) Response to treatment in dysaesthetic vulvodynia. *Journal of Obstetrics and Gynecology* **21**, 610–13.

10 Reed BD, Haefner HK, Cantor L. (2003) Vulvar dysesthesia (vulvodynia). A follow-up study. *The Journal of Reproductive Medicine* **48**, 409–16.

11 Bates CM, Timmins DJ. (2002) Vulvodynia: new and more effective approaches to therapy. *International Journal of STD and AIDS* **13**, 210–12.

12 Ben-David B, Friedman M. (1999) Gabapentin therapy for vulvodynia. *Anesthesia and Analgesia* **89**, 1459–60.

13 Harris G, Horowitz B, Borgida A. (2007) Evaluation of gabapentin in the treatment of generalized vulvodynia, unprovoked. *The Journal of Reproductive Medicine* **52**, 103–6.

14 Siddall PJ, Cousins MJ, Otte A, *et al.* (2006) Pregabalin in central neuropathic pain associated with spinal cord injury: a placebo-controlled trial. *Neurology* **67**, 1792–1800.

15 Jerome L. (2007) Pregabalin-induced remission in a 62-year-old woman with a 20-year history of vulvodynia. *Pain Research and Management* **12**, 212–14.

16 Haefner HK, Collins ME, Davis GD, *et al.* (2005) The vulvodynia guideline. *Journal of Lower Genital Tract Disease* **9**, 40–51.

17 Rowbotham MC, Davies PS, Field H. (1995) Topical lidocaine gel relieves postherpetic neuralgia. *Annals of Neurology* **37**, 246–53.

18 Zolnoun DA, Hartman KE, Steege JF. (2003) Overnight 5% lidocaine ointment for treatment of vulva vestibulitis. *Obstetrics and Gynecology* **102**, 84–87.

19 Steinberg AC, Oyama IA, Rejba AE, *et al.* (2005) Capsaicin for the treatment of vulvar vestibultis. *American Journal of Obstetrics and Gynecology* **192**, 1549–53.

20 Boardman LA, Cooper AS, Blais LR, *et al.* (2008) Topical gabapentin in the treatment of localized and generalized vulvodynia. *Obstetrics and Gynecology* **112**, 579–85.

21 Pinsger M, Schimetta W, Volc D, *et al.* (2006). Benefits of an add-on treatment with the synthetic cannabinomimetic nabilone on patients with chronic pain: randomized controlled trial. *Wiener Klinische Wochenschrift* **118**, 327–35.

22 Nurmikko TJ, Serpell M, Hoggart B, *et al.* (2007) Sativex® successfully treats neuropathic pain characterized by allodynia: a randomized double blind, placebo controlled trial. *Pain* **133**, 210–20.

23 Gordon AS, Panahian-Jand M, McComb F, *et al.* (2003) Characterists of women with vulvar pain disorders: responses to a web-based survey. *Journal of Sex and Marital Therapy.* **29**, 45–58.

CHAPTER 27

Mast Cells and Their Role in Sexual Pain Disorders

Alessandra Graziottin

Center of Gynecology and Medical Sexology, H. San Raffaele Resnati, Milan, Italy

Introduction

Mast cells play a key role in many sexual pain disorders including interstitial cystitis (IC), provoked vestibulodynia (PVD), and endometriosis. Mast cells are ubiquitous, present in virtually all organs and vascularized tissue where they work to modulate the immune response. In addition, mast cells are present in, and recruited to, sites of inflammation, where they orchestrate key steps in the inflammatory response. Granules released by mast cells contain angiogenic, pro-inflammatory, and neurotrophic factors. These granules are heterogenous and different substances are released depending on the type, location, and timing of the damaging event or agent. When persistently up-regulated, mast cells maintain chronic inflammation, leading to a shift between nociceptive and neuropathic pain. This chapter reviews the biochemical complexity of mast cells to illustrate their role in sexual pain disorders.

The Importance of Mast Cells

Although mast cells were discovered over 100 years ago, they still represent a "biological enigma" [1]. Mast cells possess a series of biochemical and functional properties that place them at the center of both the inflammatory and immune responses. Mast cells are activated by stimuli of "agonists" and released by means of degranulation, a

wide array of biologically active mediators. These mediators can be synthesized at the time of the stimulus, or can be immediately released from storage vesicles called cytoplasmic granules [2, 3]. Mast cells are able to respond to a wide range of agonist stimuli, and to differentially release biochemical mediators [4]. It is this heterogeneity that enables mast cells to have a functional role in a wide range of problems including sexual pain disorders, ranging from inflammatory conditions (e.g., IC), to neuropathic pain syndromes (e.g., PVD), to fibrotic involutions (endometriosis) [5–8].

Mast cells contain, and selectively release, biochemicals that mediate the typical signs and symptoms of local inflammation including erythema, edema, increased local temperature, pain, and functional impairment as first described by ancient Roman physicians in "rubor, tumor, calor, dolor, functio laesa." These changes can be seen during a cystoscopic examination of a woman with IC or vulvoscopic (see Chapter 7) examination of a woman with PVD. Mast cells also contain "neurotrophins" that activate the nerve endings of pain fibers, inducing proliferation and growth toward the epidermis of the nerve terminals in the inflamed mucosa. These changes are the morphological correlates, respectively, of hyperalgesia and allodynia. These alterations in pain perceptions are typical of sexual pain disorders including PVD, generalized vulvodynia (GVD), and IC.

The Morphology of Mast Cells

Selye was the first to describe the human mast cell as rounded elements with an oval nucleus and cytoplasm

Female Sexual Pain Disorders 1st edition. Edited by A. Goldstein, C. Pukall & I. Goldstein. © 2009 Blackwell Publishing, ISBN: 9781405183987.

filled with spherical metachromatic granules, located in the dermis, adjacent to blood vessels, nerve endings, glandular ducts, and hair follicles. Historically, Toluidine blue and Giemsa stains were used to visualize mast cells microscopically [9, 10]. Unfortunately, these stain techniques inadequately demonstrated the presence of mast cells in inflamed tissue, but with newer immunostaining techniques (immunotryptase), mast cells are more easily seen. This increased visualization has yielded evidence of mast cell proliferation in the initial stages of several sexual pain disorders including PVD, IC, irritable bowel syndrome (IBS), and endometriosis. In later stages of these diseases, when the chronic inflammation has led to fibrosis, mast cells may almost disappear from the functionally deserted tissue.

Mast cells are currently divided into three groups based on their immunocytochemical characteristics [11, 12]. Specifically, there are mucosal mast cells containing only tryptase (mast cell$_T$); connective tissue mast cells containing tryptase, chymase, carboxypeptidase, and cathepsin G (mast cell$_{TC}$); and mast cells that can be found in several different tissues containing chymase and carboxypeptidase (mast cells$_C$). Although dermal mast cells have traditionally been thought of as indigenous only to the dermis, mast cells have a migratory capacity and demonstrate extraordinary functional adaptation in response to disturbances of tissue homeostasis [2].

The density of mast cells in inflamed tissue changes over time. In tissue where there is an acute inflammatory response, the concentration of mast cells is high. As the inflammation becomes more chronic, the number of mast cells decreases and may even disappear late in the fibrotic process. However, as the density of mast cells decreases, there is an increase in neuronal proliferation. At this late stage of the inflammatory process, neuropathic symptoms, such as spontaneous hyperalgesia, become prominent.

Functional Role of Mast Cells

Dermal mast cells, which are strategically located between vessels and nerves, are directly stimulated by immunological signals from cytokines, immunoglobulin E, complement fractions, and neuropeptides [2, 13–15]. These activated dermal mast cells play several crucial roles in mediating the inflammatory responses discussed below:

(a) **Neurogenic inflammation:** Neuropeptide nerve growth factor (NGF), calcitonin gene-related peptide (CGRP), and somatostatin are released by stimulated or damaged dermo-epidermal nerve endings. These neuropeptides activate local mast cells, causing degranulation [14]. In addition, physical, chemical, or mechanical stimuli also act to trigger mast cell degranulation [16, 17]. Once released from the mast cells, cytokines, growth factors, vasoactive amines, and proteolytic enzymes influence the surrounding cellular elements, thereby coordinating the biological response to tissue injury with both defensive and reparative effects.

(b) **The mast cell–mediated vascular response:** Mast cells that adhere to the walls of blood vessels are part of a vascular control system responsible for constantly monitoring microcirculatory homeostasis [18]. Through the release of vasoactive mediators such as histamine, protease, tumor necrosis factor (TNF), and metabolites of arachidonic acid, mast cells induce vasodilation and increase vascular permeability, leading to tissue edema and erythema [19, 20].

(c) **The mast cell–directed inflammatory response:** As the inflammatory process develops, mast cells play a crucial role in the recruitment of circulating leukocytes, neutrophils, basophils, and eosinophils to the area of injury [21]. Specifically, mast cells release TNF, leukotrienes, proteases, and cytokines (especially interleuken-8) that mediate leukocyte marginalization and migration [22]. These leukocytes, along with resident macrophages, perform specific defence functions including phagocytosis and debridement.

(d) **The mast cell–mediated neurogenic response:** Local innervation is influenced by the functional state of the mast cell [23]. Specifically, NGF released by mast cells causes a reduction in the nociceptive threshold. This is the key mechanism responsible for the hyperalgesia in sexual pain disorders [24–26].

(e) **Mast cell–mediated neovascularization and re-epithelialization:** Mast cells coordinate neovascularization in injured tissue by influencing the regrowth potential of endothelial cells. Specifically, histamine, heparin, TNF, interleuken-6, interleuken-8, platelet–derived growth factor, vascular endothelial–derived growth factor, transforming growth factor-beta, and fibroblast growth factor represent the "angiogenic pool" rapidly released by activated mast cells by means of degranulation. This angiogenic pool modulates the various stages of new vessel formation [27–30]. In addition, mast cells also act to influence the re-epithelialization process by mediating keratinocyte migration and proliferation around the wound edges, leading to the formation of new epithelium [31, 32].

(f) **Mast cells role in scarring:** Mast cells play an essential role in initiating scar tissue formation by mediating the activity of fibroblasts. The mast cells release substances with specific fibroproliferative activity including histamine, interleuken-1, interleuken-4, NGF, tryptase, fibroblast growth factor, and transforming growth factor-beta [33–38]. Therefore, mast cells possess the biological signals needed to stimulate chemotaxis, migration, phenotype differentiation, and biosynthetic activity of fibroblasts. In addition, there are gap junctions between fibroblasts and mast cells that enhance the functional synergy between these two cell types [27].

Clinical Significance of Mast Cells

As shown above, mast cells show extraordinary complexity and heterogeneity in the content of their granules. More importantly, they are able to selectively release different granules depending on the stage of the inflammatory process, the site of tissue damage, and the response of the other cells participating to the inflammatory process. Disinhibition of the inflammatory process and/or persistence of inflammatory stimuli may alter the healing process, maintaining an upregulation of the mast cell's response. This intensifies neurogenic inflammation and tissue damage, with two major consequences. First, there is progressive functional and anatomic damage associated with prominent tissue scarring, exemplified by the natural history of endometriosis. Second, there is upregulation of nerve pain, with morphological and functional changes. This may contribute to the shift from the typical inflammatory response as seen in "early" PVD where mast cells are significantly increased in the vestibular mucosa, to "late" PVD where there is increased density of C-afferent nociceptors in the vestibular mucosa. In these later stages, pain shifts from nociceptive pain toward neuropathic pain.

Conclusions

Understanding the role of mast cells in the pathophysiology of local inflammation is critical if physicians hope to move from symptomatic, late interventions in conditions such as PVD, to etiologically based multimodal treatments. Mast cells play a significant role as the sophisticated directors of the immune and inflammatory response; they can influence a positive or negative outcome, according to genetic, local, and contextual factors. Physicians can change the natural history of many inflammatory conditions that lead to chronic and aggressive pain disorders if they consider the critical role of mast cells and intervene in two ways: by reducing *agonist* stimuli that cause mast cell upregulation and damaging degranulation, and by testing/using drugs that may act as *antagonist* modulators of mast cells, thereby reducing the release of inflammatory and neurotrophic substances [39].

References

1 Ehrlich P. (1879) Beitrage zur Kenntnis der granulierten Bindegewebszellen und der eosinophilen leukocyten. *Archiv für Anatomie und Physiologie* **3**, 166–69.
2 Galli SJ. (1993) New concepts about the mast cell. *The New England Journal of Medicine* **328**, 257–65.
3 Bradding P. (1996) Human mast cell cytokines. *Clinical and Experimental Allergy* **26**, 13–19.
4 Theoharides C, Kempuraj D, Tagen M, *et al.* (2007) Differential release of mast cell mediators and the pathogenesis of inflammation. *Immunological Reviews* **217**, 65–78.
5 Letourneau R, Sant GR, el-Mansoury M, *et al.* (1992) Activation of bladder mast cells in interstitial cystitis. *International Journal of Tissue Reactions* **14**, 307–12.
6 Bornstein J, Goldschmid N, Sabo E. (2004) Hyperinnervation and mast cell activation may be used as histopathologic diagnostic criteria for vulvar vestibulitis. *Gynecologic and Obstetric Investigation* **58**, 171–78.
7 Bornstein J, Cohen Y, Zarfati D, *et al.* (2008) Involvement of heparanase in the pathogenesis of localized vulvodynia. *International Journal of Gynecological Pathology* **27**, 136–41.
8 Sugamata M, Ihara T, Uchiide I. (2005) Increase of activated mast cells in human endometriosis. *American Journal of Reproductive Immunology* **53**, 120–25.
9 Enerback L. (1996) Mast cells in rat gastrointestinal mucosa. I. Effects of fixation. *Acta Pathologica Microbiologica Scandinavica* **66**, 289–302.
10 Enerback L. (1996) Mast cells in rat gastrointestinal mucosa. II. Dye-binding and metachromatic properties. *Acta Pathologica Microbiologica Scandinavica* **66**, 303–12.
11 Benyon RC, Lowman MA, Church MK. (1987) Human skin mast cells: their dispersion, purification, and secretory characterization. *Journal of Immunology* **138**, 861–68.

12 Bienenstock J, Befus AD, Demburg JA. (1986) Mast cell heterogeneity. In: Befus AD, Bienenstock J, Demburg JA. (eds.) *Mast Cell Differentiation and Heterogeneity.* Raven Press, New York, pp. 391–402.

13 Bienenstock J, MacQueen G, Sestini P, *et al.* (1991) Mast cell/nerve interactions in vitro and in vivo. *American Review of Respiratory Diseases* **143**, S55–S58.

14 Williams RM, Bienenstock J, Stead RH. (1995) Mast cells: the neuroimmune connection. *Chemical Immunology* **61**, 208–35.

15 Beaven MA, Baumgartner RA. (1996) Downstream signals initiated in mast cells by FceRI and other receptors. *Current Opinion in Immunology* **8**, 766–72.

16 El Sayed SO, Dyson M. (1993) Responses of dermal mast cells to injury. *Journal of Anatomy* **182**, 369–76.

17 Malaviya R, Morrison AR, Pentland AP. (1996) Histamine in human epidermal cells is induced by ultraviolet light injury. *Journal of Investigative Dermatology* **106**, 785–89.

18 Waltner-Romen M, Falkensammer G, Rabl W, *et al.* (1998) A previously unrecognized site of local accumulation of mononuclear cells: the vascular-associated lymphoid tissue. *The Journal of Histochemistry and Cytochemistry* **46**, 1347–50.

19 Valent P, Sillaber C, Baghestanian M, *et al.* (1998) What have mast cells to do with edema formation, the consecutive repair and fibrinolysis? *International Archives on Allergy and Applied Immunology* **115**, 2–8.

20 Huang C, Sali A, Stevens RL. (1998) Regulation and function of mast cell proteases in inflammation. *Journal of Clinical Immunology* **18**, 169–83.

21 Kanwar S, Kubes P. (1994) Ischemia/reperfusion-induced granulocyte influx is a multistep process mediated by mast cells. *Microcirculation* **1**, 175–82.

22 Ribeiro RA, Souza-Filho M, Souza M, *et al.* (1997) Role of resident mast cells and macrophages in the neutrophil migration induced by LTB[4], fMLP, and C5a. *International Archives on Allergy and Applied Immunology* **112**, 27–35.

23 Schaffer M, Beiter T, Dieter Becker H, *et al.* (1998) Neuropeptides: mediators of inflammation and tissue repair? *Archives of Surgery* **133**, 1107–16.

24 Leon A, Buriani A, Dal Toso R, *et al.* (1994) Mast cells synthesize, store, and release nerve growth factor. *Proceedings of the National Academy of Sciences* **91**, 3739–43.

25 Lewin GR, Rueff A, Mendell LM. (1994) Peripheral and central mechanisms of NGF-induced hyperalgesia. *European Journal of Neuroscience* **6**, 1903–12.

26 Tal M, Liberman R. (1997) Local injection of nerve growth factor (NGF) triggers degranulation of mast cells in rat paw. *Neuroscience Letters* **221**, 129–32.

27 Metcalfe DD, Baram D, Mekori YA. (1997) Mast cells. *Physiological Reviews* **77**, 1033–79.

28 Levi-Schaffer F, Kupietzky A. (1990) Mast cells enhance migration and proliferation of fibroblasts into an in vitro wound. *Experimental Cell Research* **188**, 42–49.

29 Katayama I, Yokozeki H, Nishioka K. (1992) Mast cell–derived mediators induce epidermal cell proliferation: clue for lichenified skin lesion formation in atopic dermatitis. *International Archives on Allergy and Applied Immunology* **98**, 410–14.

30 Nicosia RF, Bonnano E, Smith M. (1993) Fibronectin promotes the elongation of microvessels during angiogenesis in vitro. *Journal of Cellular Physiology* **154**, 654–61.

31 Clark RAF. (1993) Biology of dermal wound repair. *Dermatologic Clinics* **11**, 647–66.

32 Woodley DT, Chen JD, Kim JP, *et al.* Re-epithelialization: human keratinocyte locomotion. *Dermatologic Clinics* **11**, 641–46.

33 Russell JD, Russell SB, Trupin KM. (1977) The effect of histamine on the growth of cultured fibroblasts isolated from normal and keloid tissue *Journal of Cellular Physiology* **93**, 389–94.

34 Kupietzky A, Levi-Schaffer F. (1996) The role of mast cell–derived histamine in the closure of an in vitro wound. *Inflammation Research* **45**, 176–80.

35 Kovacs EJ. (1991) Fibrogenic cytokines: the role of immune mediators in the development of scar tissue. *Immunology Today* **12**, 17–23.

36 Gruber BL, Kew RR, Jelaska A, *et al.* (1997) Human mast cells activate fibroblasts. Tryptase is a fibrogenic factor stimulating collagen messenger ribonucleic acid synthesis and fibroblast chemotaxis. *The Journal of Immunology* **158**, 2310–17.

37 Bressler RB, Lesko J, Jones ML, *et al.* (1997) Production of IL-5 and granulocyte–macrophage colony-stimulating factor by naive human mast cells activated by high-affinity IgE receptor ligation. *Journal of Allergy and Clinical Immunology* **99**, 508–14.

38 Qu Z, Kayton RJ, Ahmadi P, *et al.* (1998) Ultrastructural immunolocalization of basic fibroblast growth factor in mast cell secretory granules: morphological evidence for bFGF release through degranulation. *The Journal of Histochemistry and Cytochemistry* **46**, 1119–28.

39 D'Cruz OJ, Uckun FM. (2007) Targeting mast cells in endometriosis with janus kinase 3 inhibitor, JANEX-1. *American Journal of Reproductive Immunology* **58**, 75–97.

CHAPTER 28

Hormonal Factors in Women's Sexual Pain Disorders

Irwin Goldstein

Alvarado Hospital, San Diego, CA, USA

Introduction

There are multiple proposed pathophysiological processes, both psychological and biological, involved in female sexual pain disorders [1–16]. These disorders involve central and peripheral genital/reproductive tissues, including specific central nervous system nuclei such as the medial preoptic area, nucleus paragigantocellularis, paraventricular nucleus, and specific peripheral structures such as the mons pubis, labia majora, labia minora, clitoris, prepuce, frenulum, labia minora, hymen, vulvar vestibule, minor vestibular glands, Skene's glands, urethral meatus, and vagina (Figures 28.1–28.3).

Central [17–23] and peripheral genital tissues [24–31] utilize sex steroid hormones (androgens, estrogens, and progestins) for structure and function. Thus, it is possible that sexual pain disorders can occur in women with abnormalities in sex steroid hormones. This chapter reviews the measurement of sex steroid hormones, the physiology and pathophysiology of sex steroids, and the treatment of women with sexual dysfunction. When relevant, hormones and sexual pain disorders—provoked vestibulodynia (PVD) and atrophic vaginitis [32–41]—are examined.

Clinical Measurement of Sex Steroids

Currently, there is no consensus regarding sex steroid hormone blood tests for women's sexual health concerns.

Female Sexual Pain Disorders 1st edition. Edited by A. Goldstein, C. Pukall & I. Goldstein. © 2009 Blackwell Publishing, ISBN: 9781405183987.

Because there are several types of androgens, estrogens, and progesterone, multiple sex steroid hormones should be measured in women with all types of sexual dysfunction, including dyspareunia. In addition, other endocrine assessments should be pursued; pituitary function can be assessed by determination of prolactin, follicle-stimulating hormone (FSH), and lutenizing hormone (LH) levels, and thyroid function can be assessed by measuring thyroid-stimulating hormone levels [42, 43].

The following androgen values may be measured if considered appropriate in women with sexual dysfunctions: dehydroepiandrosterone sulphate (DHEA-S), androstenedione, total testosterone, and dihydrotestosterone. Assessment of DHEA-S and androstenedione values may provide insight as to the function of the adrenal gland zona reticularis. DHEA is usually measured in the sulfated form, DHEA-S, because the half-life is much longer, resulting in more stable levels. Both DHEA-S and androstenedione levels remain stable over the various phases of the menstrual cycle [44]. The glycoprotein, sex hormone binding globulin (SHBG) should be measured if the woman with dyspareunia has taken exogenous estrogen steroids, such as ethinyl estradiol (in oral contraceptive pills) [45–48] or estradiol (in menopausal hormone therapy) [49, 50], or has a history of hyperthyroidism [51], liver disease [52], anorexia nervosa [53], or other nonestradiol drug use (e.g., phentoin) [54].

These conditions are recognized causes of increased SHBG values. It is clinically important to record SHBG values in women with dyspareunia as this globulin binds to testosterone. Androgens circulate in the bloodstream, bound mostly to SHBG and to serum albumin. Only 1–2% of androgens are unbound, and thus biologically

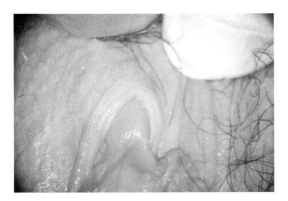

Figure 28.1 Normal anatomy of the clitoris.

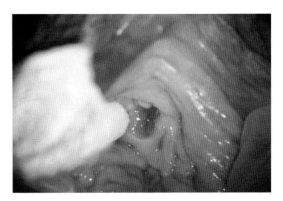

Figure 28.3 Normal anatomy of the urethral meatus.

active to enter cells in structures such as the clitoris, vagina, and minor vestibular glands and activate the cytoplasmic androgen receptor. This hormone–receptor complex becomes a transcriptional agent that enters the nucleus and induces protein synthesis [27]. Critical proteins such as vascular endothelial growth factor, nerve growth factor, and nitric oxide synthase are androgen-dependent. Of note, SHBG also binds estradiol, while progesterone is bound by transcortin.

When recording androgen levels in women with sexual pain, several caveats should be mentioned. There are universal accuracy limitations to the measurement of total testosterone in both genders [55]. In women—who physiologically have approximately 10% of the testosterone values as compared to men—it is recognized that more accurate and reliable testosterone assays are needed. The U.S. Food and Drug Administration, however, has permitted equilibrium dialysis free testosterone and bioavailable testosterone assays in clinical trials of testosterone treatment trials in women [56].

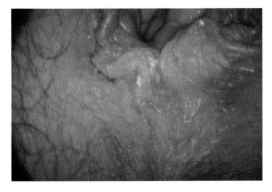

Figure 28.2 Normal anatomy of the perineal region.

Several laboratories offer mass spectroscopy after column chromatography separation of the steroids. Mass spectroscopy is utilized to obtain a higher level of accuracy with total testosterone measurements [57]. This is relevant especially because equilibrium dialysis free testosterone and the bioavailable testosterone measurements depend on the accuracy of the total testosterone determination. In women with sexual pain, a calculated free testosterone value may also be determined [58–60], which takes into account total testosterone, SHBG, and albumin. A calculator for this value is available online at http://www.issam.ch/freetesto.htm. This method has high reliability and sensitivity to equilibrium dialysis-free testosterone values [58–60].

Unbound free testosterone values may also be estimated using the free androgen index, which is defined as the total testosterone concentration (in nmol/L; multiply testosterone units in ng/dL × 3.47 = nmol/L) divided by the concentration of SHBG (in nmol/L). Finally, the timing of the measurement may be of importance, especially in premenopausal women. Testosterone levels reach a peak during the early follicular phase, with small but less significant variation across the rest of the cycle [44]. Thus, blood may be drawn after day 8 of the cycle, and preferably before day 20.

Sex steroid hormones undergo metabolism by critical intracellular cytosolic enzymes (5-α-reductase) and undergo binding to critical cytosolic hormone receptors (androgen receptors) for physiologic genomic action. These cytoplasmic and nuclear physiologic processes are variable in individuals and determine individual tissue exposure, tissue sensitivity, and tissue responsiveness. For example, within individuals, there are variations in the activity of critical cytosolic enzymes such as 5-α-reductase. There are also variations in androgen receptor sequencing within individuals. For example, the number of repeat sequences of cytosine, adenine, and guanine nucleotides (CAG repeats) in the deoxyribonucleic acid molecule coding for the sex steroid hormone receptor may vary widely in individuals [61]. Thus, independent of the values of plasma testosterone values, the unique variations in critical enzymes and sex steroid hormone receptors result in individual differences in how testosterone is utilized and metabolized. So, the health care provider needs to be aware that measurement of plasma testosterone values are only the tests "currently clinically available." In the future, there will be better, and more accurate, sensitive, and clinically meaningful measurements of androgen metabolism in women [62].

The blood test for dihydrotestosterone may be of interest if women with dyspareunia report side effects of acne [63] or alopecia [64] following treatment with testosterone for the management of androgen insufficiency syndrome associated with oral contraceptive pill use. If dihydrotestosterone is elevated, a 5α-reductase inhibitor may be considered to lower the level and reduce the symptoms.

Estrogen values such as estradiol and estrone may be assessed with the understanding that estradiol is the most biologically active form of estrogen. It should be noted that the blood levels of estradiol may not reflect exogenous estrogen administration in women on exogenous conjugated equine estrogens or exogenous ethinyl estradiol, since the latter estrogens are not bio-identical and therefore cannot be accurately assessed in serum. If a woman with sexual pain is perimenopausal, three determinations of estradiol, progesterone, LH, and FSH every 10 days during a month, will assess ovarian and ovulatory integrity.

The "normal range" for sex steroid blood test values in women with sexual pain has not been defined. Normative androgen data for women without sexual health problems have been published in a large study of over 1,400 women (aged 18–75) separated into age-related cohorts [65]. Normative androgen data have also been reported in a subset of premenopausal healthy women without sexual health concerns [66]. Both normative data sets correlate well with each other.

Concerning the relation of androgens to aging, a prospective longitudinal study of serum testosterone, DHEA-S, and SHBG levels through the menopause transition [67], as well as a study of androgen levels in women of all ages using mass spectrometry [68] both demonstrated a marked decline in serum concentrations of adrenal C19 sex steroid precursors and conjugated androgen metabolites with increasing age.

DHEA-S and total and unbound testosterone values also decrease with age in women [67, 69, 70]. Zumoff et al. [70] reported that the testosterone concentration of women aged 20–29 years was twice the value of women aged 40–49 years. Guay et al. [66] examined androgen values in women "without sexual dysfunction." Androgen concentrations were highest in the women aged 20–29 years. The calculated free testosterone in these women was 0.6–0.8 ng/dL for women aged 20–29 years and 0.4–0.6 ng/dL for women between the ages of 30 and 49 years.

Androgens: Physiology and Pathophysiology

DHEA is an adrenal precursor sex steroid hormone that is converted to other androgens, such as δ androstenediol, $δ^4$-androstenedione, and testosterone via the enzymes 3β- and 17β-hydroxysteroid dehydrogenase, and ultimately to estradiol via aromatase or to dihydrotestosterone via 5α-reductase. Any positive effects of DHEA on sexual function must take into account all the actions of DHEA: DHEA alone, and as a precursor of androgens and estrogens. DHEA receptors have been found on endothelial cells, implying that DHEA is involved in the process of vascular smooth muscle relaxation [71]. The physiologic process of vascular smooth muscle relaxation is intimately involved with peripheral sexual arousal [27].

$δ^5$-androstenediol acts on its own receptors on the vaginal mucosa and is involved in the mucin content of vaginal lubrication [72, 73]. It may be possible that low values of $δ^5$-androstenediol are associated with sexual arousal and sexual pain disorders.

Testosterone has been linked to the central regulation of female sexual behavior. Animal studies reveal that neurons containing androgen receptors are widely distributed in the hypothalamus and telencephalon, which are thought to play a key role mediating the hormonal control of sexual behavior. These regions provide strong input to the medial preoptic and ventromedial nuclei, areas also associated with sexual behavior [74–77].

Androgens are critical in maintaining peripheral genital tissue structure and function [27]. Androstenedione and testosterone levels have been shown to be linked to vaginal physiologic function [72, 73]. Androgen receptors have been reported in the vagina and vulvar vestibule [78, 79]; these may play a critical role in vaginal and vulvar health. Multiple preclinical studies in ovariectomized animals (rabbits and rats) have been performed [27]. These investigations have shown that androgen treatment enhances vaginal tissue nitric oxide synthase expression and activity, facilitates vaginal smooth muscle relaxation, increases vaginal blood flow [72], enhances vaginal mucification [73], and maintains the health and integrity of the vaginal muscularis layer [27]. Androgens contribute to other sexual and nonsexual physiologic functions, such as bone and skeletal muscle metabolism, cognition, energy, and feelings of well-being [80].

In premenopausal women with regular menstrual cycles, there is a rise in testosterone and androstenedione in the late follicular phase of the menstrual cycle and in the luteal phase. In women, approximately 50% of testosterone synthesis occurs directly in the ovaries and in the adrenal glands, and the remaining 50% occurs from testosterone precursors such as androstenedione and DHEA in the peripheral tissues.

There is a slow and progressive decline in serum testosterone levels as women age [66–70], which is in sharp contrast to estrogen and progesterone levels that fall abruptly with menopause. In the late reproductive years, the midcycle rise in free testosterone, a hallmark of the menstrual cycle in young ovulating women, begins to diminish. The level of adrenal precursors that serve as a prehormone for approximately half of ovarian testosterone production as serum DHEA-S and DHEA, also falls with increasing age [68]. Thus, after menopause, androgen insufficiency occurs, in part due to contributions from reduced synthetic function in both the adrenal and the ovaries. Furthermore, SHBG increases in postmenopausal women, especially in women who are treated with oral estrogen therapy [46, 47]. The net effect of a diminished androgen synthesis and an increase in SHBG is a reduced amount of free unbound testosterone. Low androgens are associated with decreased sexual interest, impaired sexual functioning including decreased lubrication, muscle wasting, osteoporosis, loss of energy, changes in mood, and depression [81–83].

A series of investigations [84–87] have found correlations with diminished levels of androgens and female sexual dysfunctions, including sexual pain [87]. Correlations

between total testosterone, free testosterone, and DHEA-S were found in one study using the Female Sexual Function Index [88]. A significant correlation between androgens, sexual desire, and sexual arousal was demonstrated in a study of perimenopausal women [84]. Braunstein and colleagues found a significant correlation between sexual desire and total testosterone, as well as with free testosterone, bioavailable testosterone, and dihydrotestosterone [85]. Finally, in a small group of healthy premenopausal women with and without symptoms of sexual dysfunction, those who had sexual disorders had a significant decrease in the concentrations of δ^5-androgenic steroids, predominantly in the adrenal gland [86]. However, Davis and colleagues were unable to demonstrate a correlation between total testosterone plasma levels and symptoms of sexual function [89].

There are several relevant clinical presentations associated with low testosterone levels. The one most relevant to premenopausal women with dyspareunia is the use of oral contraceptives [36–40, 47, 48]. In women on oral contraceptives, there is suppression of ovarian testosterone production and increased SHBG synthesis. This combination of effects leads to low calculated free testosterone values. Hyperprolactinemia, which may occur either secondary to a prolactinoma or to psychotropic medications, may result in hypogonadotrophic hypogonadism which causes reduced testosterone and sexual dysfunction. Adrenal insufficiency may result in diminished DHEA sulphate and total testosterone values. Cushing's disease, or endogenous or exogenous glucocorticosteroid excess, may lead to adrenal suppression and androgen insufficiency. Hyperthyroidism can raise SHBG, thus reducing unbound, free testosterone values [90, 91].

A multinational expert panel assessed the role of androgen insufficiency in women with sexual health concerns, including sexual pain [83]. Androgen insufficiency was defined as a pattern of characteristic clinical symptoms in the presence of decreased bioavailable or free testosterone. These symptoms include a diminished sense of well-being or dysphoric mood, persistent unexplained fatigue, changes in sexual function (including decreased libido, sexual receptivity, and pleasure), vasomotor instability, and decreased vaginal lubrication (even with adequate estrogen treatment). The inclusion of inadequate lubrication in the constellation of androgen insufficiency symptoms makes this especially important to women with sexual pain [83].

Androgens: Clinical Data

Administration of DHEA to women has been shown to increase testosterone levels. One placebo-controlled randomized clinical trial involved a 4-month crossover design of 24 women with adrenal insufficiency [92]. Compared to those subjects who received 50 mg/day of DHEA versus placebo, the active drug increased serum testosterone from below normal to the normal range and significantly increased physical satisfaction. While this trial did not specifically measure sexual pain, this author's clinical experience is that women with sexual pain improve on DHEA therapy [93]. A retrospective open-label study of DHEA treatment (50 mg/day) in 113 healthy women with sexual dysfunction noted significant increases in lubrication and satisfaction compared to baseline function [93]. Baulieu et al. reported that DHEA treatment doubled total testosterone values and also significantly increased sexual activity and sexual satisfaction after 12 months [94].

Several clinical studies have examined the relationship between serum testosterone levels and sexual activity. In two studies of premenopausal women [95, 96], transdermal testosterone therapy significantly improved many aspects of sexual function and behavior including sexual motivation, fantasy, frequency of sexual activity, pleasure, orgasm, and satisfaction. In postmenopausal women [56, 85, 97–99], transdermal testosterone patches significantly increased free testosterone, bioavailable testosterone, and dihydrotestosterone from the lower limit of the normal range to higher values within the normal range.

The frequency of sexual activity and pleasure was significantly greater than placebo in one study, and in another, significant increases were noted in total satisfying sexual activity, arousal, orgasm, pleasure, and body image following testosterone transdermal patch versus placebo in postmenopausal women. Women assigned to testosterone also reported a significant decrease in distress related to sexual function. The symptom improvements in sexual function were considered clinically relevant [98]. Improvement in sexual pain was not specifically noted as the presence of clinically significant sexual pain was an exclusion criterion in these studies. Goldstein and Burrows have reported that administration of testosterone to women with androgen insufficiency syndrome and sexual pain is associated with symptom improvement [100].

Any woman with sexual pain treated with androgen therapy needs to be thoroughly counseled regarding risks and benefits and the need for routine follow-up and blood test surveillance testing [101]. Safety issues for DHEA and androgen administration include acne and hirsutism [56, 85, 92–94, 97–99, 101]. Side effects such as balding, voice deepening, cliteromegaly, and polycythemia were not noted in clinical trials. There was no evidence that exogenous testosterone increases the risk of endometrial cancer or endometriosis. No significant adverse effects were noted from baseline on measures of blood lipids, including total cholesterol, high-density lipoprotein cholesterol, low-density lipoprotein cholesterol, or triglycerides [56, 85, 92–94, 97–99, 101].

Estrogens/Progestins: Physiology and Pathophysiology

Throughout the reproductive years, the primary source of estradiol is cyclical synthesis by the ovaries, which are under the control of the pituitary via FSH and inhibin. There is a rise in estradiol in the late follicular phase of the menstrual cycle and in the luteal phase. The luteal phase is characterized by a rise in progesterone, whose primary source of synthesis is the corpus luteum of the ovary. As long as the premenopausal woman continues to regularly ovulate, estrogen and progesterone levels are maintained until the time of menopause. When ovulation ceases at the time of menopause, estradiol and progesterone levels fall abruptly. Outside of the ovary, estrogen synthesis occurs via adrenal and ovarian androgen precursors. In addition, estrogen continues to be synthesized in the periphery (e.g., skin, adipose tissue, bone, muscle) in postmenopausal women through conversion of androstenedione to estrone and testosterone to estradiol, but the amount of estradiol synthesized depends, in part, on the enzymatic activity of aromatase.

Premenopausal women with sexual dysfunction, including dyspareunia, who do not have regular, normal menstrual cycles and are otherwise amenorrheic, dysmenorrheic, or menorrhagic, should have the underlying pathophysiology managed. Other medical issues during the premenopausal years that interfere with cyclical estrogen and progesterone production include rapid weight loss and anorexia nervosa [102]. It has been well documented that estrogen and progesterone levels fall in these conditions and women may exhibit sexual dysfunction including dyspareunia.

Estrogens and other sex steroids act via cytosolic receptors in a genomic process that utilizes transcription to induce protein synthesis directed to specific central nervous system or peripheral genital tissue structure and function. Estradiol acts in a nongenomic fashion with direct interactions with numerous central neurotransmitter systems including catecholaminergic, serotonergic, cholinergic and Γ-aminobutyric acidergic systems [103]. The high concentrations of estradiol in the hypothalamus and the preoptic area suggest that it is involved in sexual behaviors [104, 105].

Less is known about the relationship of progesterone with sexual function [105–110]. Progesterone has genomic activity via progesterone receptors that modulates gene expression and thus regulates neuronal networks that control sexual behavior. Of note, estradiol increases the expression of progesterone receptors that in turn function as a critical coordinator of sexual response [105–110].

Estrogens/Progestins: Clinical Data

Should there be the need for exogenous estrogen and progesterone, there are many treatment options. Bioidentical and synthetic forms of estradiol and progesterone are available via multiple delivery systems including oral, transdermal, transvaginal, or parenteral. The choice of estrogen and progesterone utilized (synthetic or nonsynthetic) may have important implications on the woman's sex steroid hormonal milieu, especially SHBG and androgen values. Thus, the choice of estrogen and/or progesterone may adversely influence sexual function. This is especially pertinent for synthetic progestin agents [111].

For example, for reversible pharmacologic birth control, premenopausal women who are otherwise healthy, have no sexual health issues, and have normal menstrual cycles may elect to use exogenous potent synthetic estrogen (ethinyl estradiol) in combination with various synthetic progestogens. These oral contraceptives diminish FSH and LH levels and reduce metabolic activity of the ovary, including suppression of ovulation. Circulating levels of androgens are decreased by oral contraceptives by two separate mechanisms: (i) direct inhibition of androgen production in the ovaries and (ii) marked increase in the hepatic synthesis of SHBG. The combination of these two mechanisms may lead to very low circulating levels of free and bioavailable testosterone. Several studies have already reported negative effects of oral contraceptives on sexual function, including sexual pain and vestibulodynia [36–40].

Sexual Pain Disorders

Provoked Vestibulodynia (PVD)

One highly prevalent form of dyspareunia is PVD (previously called vulvar vestibulitis syndrome) (see Chapter 12). It is characterized by severe burning at the vaginal entrance in response to contact during both sexual and nonsexual situations [100, 112, 113]. There are multiple pathophysiologic theories concerning the sensitivity of the vulvar vestibule to contact [100, 112, 113]. Women with PVD may experience anxiety and hypervigilance to painful stimuli [114], resulting in increased pelvic floor muscle tension [115]. Some histological examinations reveal inflammatory infiltrates in vestibular tissue, which may be related to a history of repeated yeast infections [116] and/or altered vestibular tissue properties [117]. These changes in vestibular tissue include increased density of intraepithelial nerve fibers, increased nociceptor sensitization, increased expression of receptors, and increased presence of calcitonin gene-related peptide in pain fibers. In some women with PVD, a genetic predisposition exists for the persistence of the chronic vestibular inflammation. Women with PVD have more frequent expression of alleles associated with severe and prolonged inflammatory immune responses [118–120].

This author has observed women who present with PVD and androgen insufficiency syndrome (low total testosterone, low calculated free testosterone, and elevated SHBG). In these women, a noted reduction in pain symptoms following androgen therapy with systemic testosterone was observed (Figures 28.4 and 28.5) [100].

A review of the literature revealed that, in addition to the pathophysiologic factors listed above, hormonal factors related to estrogen and testosterone may also play a role in PVD [36–41]. Women who used oral contraceptives had an increased risk of developing PVD later in life (Figures 28.6). Early menarche is also associated with increased risk. Women with PVD have significantly decreased estrogen receptor-α expression [113, 121]. The sex steroids are critical for genital tissue structure and function, including vestibular tissue. While Eva et al. described the presence of estrogen receptors in vestibular tissue, there is a paucity of information related to the presence of androgen receptors in vestibular tissue [113, 121].

In contrast to the established estrogen hormonal dependence of female genital tissues, such as the uterus, fallopian tubes, vagina, clitoris, or labia, there are limited

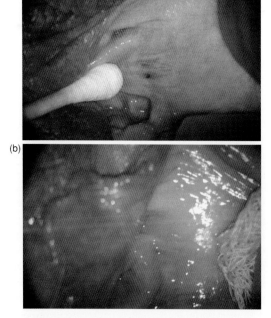

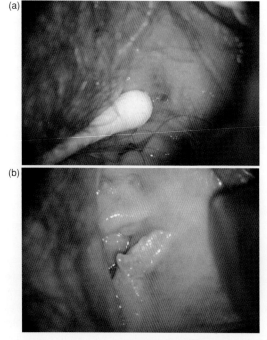

Figure 28.4 A woman with PVD before (a) and after (b) hormone treatment.

Figure 28.5 A woman with PVD before (a) and after (b) hormone treatment.

data on the presence or absence of the various sex steroid hormonal receptors in human vestibular tissue. Vestibular tissue is embryologically derived from the urogenital sinus. In particular, the minor vestibular glands that line the labial–hymenal junction share embryologic origin with the glands of Littre within the anterior urethra of the male, a well-established androgen-dependent glandular tissue involved in mucin secretion during sexual foreplay.

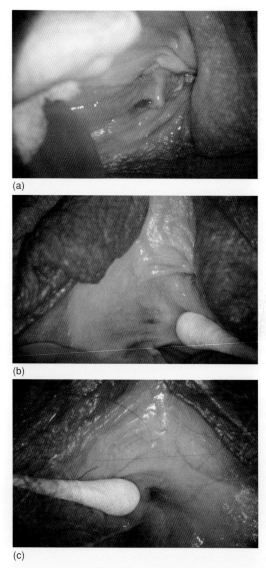

Figure 28.6 The vulva of women with PVD on oral contraceptive pills.

Sutherland et al. [122] performed preliminary histologic and immunohistochemical analysis of human vestibular tissue for androgen receptors in women with PVD and dyspareunia. Immunohistochemical data for androgen receptors in vestibular tissue from women with PVD and sexual dysfunction were compared to vestibular tissue from women who underwent radical vestibulectomy for vulvar cancer. Androgen receptors were significantly lower in tissue from women with PVD. It is hypothesized that women on oral contraceptives with abnormally low values of free testosterone fail to synthesize androgen receptors in cells of the minor vestibular glands. Minor vestibular glands with low androgen receptor content would therefore not release mucin during sexual arousal. Organisms not cleared by mucous release could elicit an inflammatory response that, in some women, could theoretically lead to PVD. This hypothesis relating a potential hormonal mechanism for oral contraceptive–associated dyspareunia needs further investigation.

Treatment of women on oral contraceptives who complain of sexual pain or symptoms consistent with androgen insufficiency syndrome should consider alternate contraception methods [123], such as the intrauterine device with local progesterone (Mirena). If the calculated free testosterone values remain low despite discontinuation of the oral contraceptive, one should consider administering systemic bioidentical testosterone at a dose that re-establishes calculated free testosterone in the normal range [95, 96]. Transdermal drug delivery, which avoids first-pass metabolism through the liver, is being studied for safety and efficacy in reducing sexual symptoms in premenopausal women with testosterone insufficiency syndrome [95, 96].

Bioidentical testosterone for women is currently approved by the European Regulatory Authority (Europe Medicines Agency) for the treatment of hypoactive sexual desire disorder in surgically menopausal women (bilaterally oophorectomized and hysterectomized) on concomitant estrogen. Until this medication is available elsewhere, a common treatment option is to use bioidentical testosterone in 1% concentration in a gel form (a government-approved delivery system for men). One strategy is to place 0.5 mL daily to the back of the calf. Children should not come into contact with this topical testosterone, and the patient should not swim or shower for several hours after application.

The levels of calculated free testosterone in the blood should be monitored, with blood tests of total testosterone and SHBG at 3-month intervals. There are various safety concerns regarding the use of systemic bioidentical testosterone, primarily related to minor androgenic effects [95, 96]. Current data for women with sexual dysfunction show that there are no increased risks of impaired liver function, sleep apnea, aggression, endometrial stimulation, or cardiovascular concerns, but long-term data are needed [95, 96]. Systemic testosterone appears to have a protective effect against the development of breast cancer, but more data are needed [101]. There are no double-blind placebo-controlled safety and efficacy data with the use of bioidentical testosterone in women with PVD.

Atrophic Vaginitis (with or without Urethral Prolapse)

Estrogens are required for genital structure and function [124–127]. Estrogens act on estrogen receptors that are prominent in the genital tissues, including epithelial/endothelial cells and the smooth muscle cells of the vagina, vestibule, labia, and urethra. Estrogen provides vaginal health and protection from sexual pain. Diminished estrogen production in the transition/menopause renders these genital tissues highly susceptible to atrophy.

Following exposure of peripheral genital tissue to low estradiol, atrophic changes can be identified, many of which can lead to dyspareunia [128]. Genital tissue structural changes and cellular dysfunctions that occur in the genital tissues as a result of estrogen deficiency are as follows. Specifically in the vagina, estrogen deficiency leads to vaginal atrophy and an alteration of the normally acidic vaginal pH (Figure 28.7) [129] that usually discourages

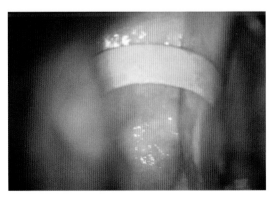

Figure 28.7 Normal vaginal pH.

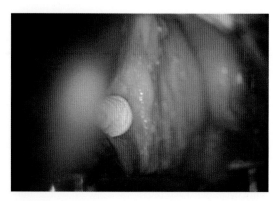

Figure 28.8 Absent rugae.

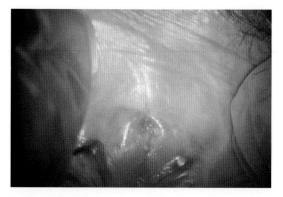

Figure 28.9 Clitoral phimosis.

growth of pathogenic bacteria. In an estrogen-rich environment, glycogen from sloughed epithelial cells is hydrolyzed into glucose and then metabolized to lactic acid by normal vaginal flora.

In postmenopausal women, epithelial thinning reduces the available glycogen. The change to an alkaline pH value leads to a shift in the vaginal flora resulting in the likelihood of vaginal yeast infections, discharge, odor, and dyspareunia. In addition, the epithelium and vascular, muscular, and connective tissues of the vagina atrophy. This leads to the vaginal vault becoming pale or colorless in appearance with loss of multiple folds or rugae (Figure 28.8) [130] normally present in the estrogenized vagina. The atrophy of the lamina propria blood vessels leads to diminished blood flow to the tissues, decreased lubrication, vaginal dryness, and dyspareunia. The thinning of the vaginal epithelial layer leads to increased friability and lowered elasticity of vaginal tissues. When coital activity is attempted in the presence of estrogen deficiency, the marked shortening and narrowing of the vaginal vault may make sexual activity unpleasant, unsatisfactory, and/or painful.

Estrogen deficiency also adversely affects other genital tissues. The clitoral hood may become phimotic (Figure 28.9) [131] and the glans clitoris may atrophy and become fibrosed with persistent estrogen deficiency and diminished genital blood flow and sexual pain. The labia majora atrophy (Figure 28.10) as there is decreased subcutaneous fat and skin elasticity. It is common for women to experience itching and pain as tissues atrophy. The endocervical glandular tissue produces less mucin, further contributing to vaginal dryness and dyspareunia.

Estrogen deficiency also adversely affects the bladder and urethral meatus [132, 133]. Women frequently note dysuria, urinary frequency, urgency, incontinence, postcoital urinary tract infections, and dyspareunia. In particular, prolapse of the urethral mucosa out the urethral lumen is associated with estrogen deficiency states [134]. It is not uncommon for women with urethral prolapse to note spotting of blood on the toilet paper after wiping following voiding. The abnormal voiding history is often accompanied by a unique sexual history: women with urethral prolapse often have the ability to have full sexual pleasure and satisfaction during self-stimulation of the clitoris; however, during sexual activity with the partner or with a mechanical device, she experiences pain and/or urgency to urinate and/or inability to have orgasm secondary to pain. Physical examination of a urethral prolapse reveals a beefy red, erythematous, protruding, inflamed, and edematous mucosa prolapsing from the meatus in different degrees. Conservative treatment options include topical or systemic estrogens. If necessary, surgical excision may be required.

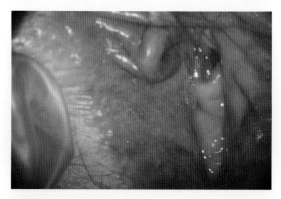

Figure 28.10 Labial atrophy.

Local estrogen therapy can, within weeks to months, effectively restore vaginal epithelium and relieve atrophy [135, 136]. There are a variety of local vaginal estrogen therapies such as creams consisting of conjugated equine estrogen, estradiol, and estriol. Other forms of local estrogen delivery systems include rings and tablets [137–139]. A 2-mg estradiol ring, placed in the vagina for 3 months, slowly releases the estradiol locally. A 17β-estradiol tablet in a 25 μg or a low-dose 10-μg single vaginal dose applicator is administered several times per week.

Several studies have shown restoration of vaginal cytology and improvement of vaginal atrophy and dryness. A randomized clinical trial found that among postmenopausal women with vaginal atrophy, a continuous low-dose estradiol-releasing vaginal ring provided relief and was more acceptable compared to conjugated equine estrogen vaginal cream. Another comparative study of menopausal women found that local 25 hydroxy, 17-β estradiol vaginal tablets, and conjugated equine estrogen vaginal cream were equally efficacious in relieving vaginal atrophy, but the vaginal tablets produced less endometrial proliferation and were more favorable than the cream. Higher estrogen dosages of vaginal creams can result in increased systemic estrogen concentrations due to the bolus absorption of the product [137–139].

Conservative treatment involves the use of local topical vestibular and/or intravaginal estrogen. There are multiple products on the market including intravaginal rings, pills, and creams. In the first 10–14 days, until the vaginal epithelium thickens, plasma estradiol levels may increase to values similar to systemic estrogen administration; thus, early monitoring is required as indicated by the physician [140–142]. Also, some patients are allergic to the additives in the topical estradiol product. For example, some women react negatively to propylene glycol. There are also multiple estrogen alternatives, such as soy, black cohosh, wild yam, chaste berry, angelica, damiana, nettle, red clover, and saw palmetto, although there are limited double-blind placebo controlled safety and efficacy trials with these products.

Conclusion

Sexual pain is common and has multifactorial pathophysiologies. It is hypothesized that hormonal factors are associated with the pathophysiology of several sexual

pain disorders including atrophic vaginitis (with or without urethral prolapse) and PVD. Additional research is needed in this important aspect of women's sexual health.

References

1 Weijmar Schultz W, Basson R, Binik Y, *et al.* (2005) Women's sexual pain and its management. *The Journal of Sexual Medicine* **2**, 301–16.

2 Graziottin A, Leiblum SR. (2005) Biological and psychosocial pathophysiology of female sexual dysfunction during the menopausal transition. *The Journal of Sexual Medicine* **2**, 133–45.

3 Pukall C, Kandyba K, Amsel R, *et al.* (2007) Effectiveness of hypnosis for the treatment of vulvar vestibulitis syndrome: a preliminary investigation. *The Journal of Sexual Medicine* **4**, 417–25.

4 Mascherpa F, Bogliatto F, Lynch PJ, *et al.* (2007) Vulvodynia as a possible somatization disorder: more than just an opinion. *The Journal of Reproductive Medicine* **52**, 107–10.

5 Bergeron S, Khalifé S, Glazer HI, *et al.* (2008) Surgical and behavioral treatments for vestibulodynia: two-and-one-half year follow-up and predictors of outcome. *Obstetrics and Gynecology* **111**, 159–66.

6 Desrosiers M, Bergeron S, Meana M, *et al.* (2008) Psychosexual characteristics of vestibulodynia couples: partner solicitousness and hostility are associated with pain. *The Journal of Sexual Medicine* **5**, 418–27.

7 Payne KA, Binik YM, Amsel R, *et al.* (2005) When sex hurts, anxiety and fear orient attention towards pain. *European Journal of Pain* **9**, 427–36.

8 Reissing ED, Binik YM, Khalifé S, *et al.* (2004) Vaginal spasm, pain, and behavior: an empirical investigation of the diagnosis of vaginismus. *Archives of Sexual Behavior* **33**, 5–17.

9 Kandyba K, Binik YM. (2003) Hypnotherapy as a treatment for vulvar vestibulitis syndrome: a case report. *Journal of Sex and Marital Therapy* **29**, 237–42.

10 Reissing ED, Binik YM, Khalifé S, *et al.* (2003) Etiological correlates of vaginismus: sexual and physical abuse, sexual knowledge, sexual self-schema, and relationship adjustment. *Journal of Sex and Marital Therapy* **29**, 47–59.

11 Binik YM, Reissing E, Pukall CF, *et al.* (2002) The female sexual pain disorders: genital pain or sexual dysfunction? *Archives of Sexual Behavior* **31**, 425–29.

12 Bergeron S, Brown C, Lord MJ, *et al.* (2002) Physical therapy for vulvar vestibulitis syndrome: a retrospective study. *Journal of Sex and Marital Therapy* **28**, 183–92.

13 Pukall CF, Binik YM, Khalifé S, *et al* (2002) Vestibular tactile and pain thresholds in women with vulvar vestibulitis syndrome. *Pain* **96**, 163–75.

14 Bergeron S, Binik YM, Khalifé S, *et al.* (2001) A randomized comparison of group cognitive-behavioral therapy, surface electromyographic biofeedback, and vestibulectomy in the treatment of dyspareunia resulting from vulvar vestibulitis. *Pain* **91**, 297–306.

15 Binik YM, Pukall CF, Reissing ED, *et al.* (2001) The sexual pain disorders: a desexualized approach. *Journal of Sex and Marital Therapy* **27**, 113–16.

16 Binik YM, Meana M, Berkley K, *et al.* (1999) The sexual pain disorders: is the pain sexual or is the sex painful? *Annual Review of Sexual Research* **10**, 210–35.

17 Blaustein JD. (2008) Progesterone and progestin receptors in the brain: the neglected ones. *Endocrinology* **149**, 2737–38.

18 Blaustein JD. (2008) Neuroendocrine regulation of feminine sexual behavior: lessons from rodent models and thoughts about humans. *Annual Review of Psychology* **59**, 93–118.

19 Jyotika J, McCutcheon J, Laroche J, *et al.* (2007) Deletion of the Bax gene disrupts sexual behavior and modestly impairs motor function in mice. *Developmental Neurobiology* **67**, 1511–19.

20 Molenda-Figueira HA, Williams CA, Griffin AL, *et al.* (2006) Nuclear receptor coactivators function in estrogen receptor– and progestin receptor–dependent aspects of sexual behavior in female rats. *Hormones and Behavior* **50**, 383–92.

21 Turcotte JC, Hunt PJ, Blaustein JD. (2005) Estrogenic effects of zearalenone on the expression of progestin receptors and sexual behavior in female rats. *Hormones and Behavior* **47**, 178–84.

22 Becker JB, Arnold AP, Berkley KJ, *et al.* (2005) Strategies and methods for research on sex differences in brain and behavior. *Endocrinology* **146**, 1650–73.

23 Lonstein JS, Blaustein JD. (2004) Immunocytochemical investigation of nuclear progestin receptor expression within dopaminergic neurones of the female rat brain. *Journal of Neuroendocrinology* **16**, 534–43.

24 Huang A, Yaffe K, Vittinghoff E, *et al.* (2008) The effect of ultralow-dose transdermal estradiol on sexual function in postmenopausal women. *American Journal of Obstetrics and Gynecology* **198**, 265.

25 van der Stege JG, Groen H, van Zadelhoff SJ, *et al.* (2008) Decreased androgen concentrations and diminished general and sexual well-being in women with premature ovarian failure. *Menopause* **15**, 23–31.

26 Cayan F, Dilek U, Pata O, *et al.* (2008) Comparison of the effects of hormone therapy regimens, oral and vaginal estradiol, estradiol + drospirenone and tibolone, on sexual function in healthy postmenopausal women. *The Journal of Sexual Medicine* **5**, 132–38.

27 Giraldi A, Marson L, Nappi R, *et al.* (2004) Physiology of female sexual function: animal models. *The Journal of Sexual Medicine* **1**, 237–53.

28 Traish AM, Kim N, Min K, *et al.* (2002) Role of androgens in female genital sexual arousal: receptor expression, structure, and function. *Fertility and Sterility* **77**, S11–18.

29 Pessina MA, Hoyt RF Jr., Goldstein I, *et al.* (2006) Differential effects of estradiol, progesterone, and testosterone on vaginal structural integrity. *Endocrinology* **147**, 61–69.

30 Traish AM, Kim SW, Stankovic M, *et al.* (2007) Testosterone increases blood flow and expression of androgen and estrogen receptors in the rat vagina. *The Journal of Sexual Medicine* **4**, 609–19.

31 Pessina MA, Hoyt RF Jr, Goldstein I, *et al.* (2006) Differential regulation of the expression of estrogen, progesterone, and androgen receptors by sex steroid hormones in the vagina: immunohistochemical studies. *The Journal of Sexual Medicine* **3**, 804–14.

32 Bachmann G, Lobo RA, Gut R, *et al.* (2008) Efficacy of low-dose estradiol vaginal tablets in the treatment of atrophic vaginitis: a randomized controlled trial. *Obstetrics and Gynecology* **111**, 67–76.

33 Suckling J, Lethaby A, Kennedy R. (2006) Local oestrogen for vaginal atrophy in postmenopausal women. *Cochrane Database of Systematic Reviews.* **18**, CD001500.

34 Castelo-Branco C, Cancelo MJ, Villero J, *et al.* (2005) Management of postmenopausal vaginal atrophy and atrophic vaginitis. *Maturitas* **15**, S46–52.

35 Caruso S, Agnello C, Intelisano G, *et al.* (2005) Prospective study on sexual behavior of women using 30 mg ethinylestradiol and 3 mg drospirenone oral contraceptive. *Contraception* **72**, 19–23.

36 Berglund AL, Nigaard L, Rylander E. (2002) Vulvar pain, sexual behavior, and genital infections in a young population: a pilot study. *Acta Obstetricia et Gynecologica Scandinavica* **81**, 738–42.

37 Harlow BL, Vitonis AF, Stewart EG. (2008) Influence of oral contraceptive use on the risk of adult-onset vulvodynia. *The Journal of Reproductive Medicine* **53**, 102–10.

38 Bouchard C, Brisson J, Fortier M, *et al.* (2002) Use of oral contraceptive pills and vulvar vestibulitis: a case-control study. *American Journal of Epidemiology* **156**, 254–61.

39 Sjöberg I, Nylander Lundqvist EN. Vulvar vestibulitis in the north of Sweden: an epidemiologic case-control study. *The Journal of Reproductive Medicine* **42**, 166–68.

40 Greenstein A, Ben-Aroya Z, Fass O, *et al.* (2007) Vulvar vestibulitis syndrome and estrogen dose of oral contraceptive pills. *The Journal of Sexual Medicine* **4**, 1679–83.

41 Panzer C, Wise S, Fantini G, *et al.* (2006) Impact of oral contraceptives on sex hormone–binding globulin and androgen levels: a retrospective study in women with sexual dysfunction. *The Journal of Sexual Medicine* **3**, 104–13.

42 Goldstein I. (2007) Current management strategies of the postmenopausal patient with sexual health problems. *The Journal of Sexual Medicine* **4**, 235–53.

43 Goldstein I, Alexander JL. (2005) Practical aspects in the management of vaginal atrophy and sexual dysfunction in perimenopausal and postmenopausal women. *The Journal of Sexual Medicine* **2**, 154–65.

44 Salonia A, Pontillo M, Nappi RE, *et al.* (2008) Menstrual cycle–related changes in circulating androgens in healthy women with self-reported normal sexual function. *The Journal of Sexual Medicine* **5**, 854–63.

45 O'Connell K, Westhoff C. (2008) Pharmacology of hormonal contraceptives and acne. *Cutis* **81**, 8–12.

46 Sitruk-Ware RL, Menard J, Rad M, *et al.* (2007) Comparison of the impact of vaginal and oral administration of combined hormonal contraceptives on hepatic proteins sensitive to estrogen. *Contraception* **75**, 430–37.

47 White T, Ozel B, Jain JK, *et al.* (2006) Effects of transdermal and oral contraceptives on estrogen-sensitive hepatic proteins. *Contraception* **74**, 293–96.

48 Warnock JK, Clayton A, Croft H, *et al.* (2006) Comparison of androgens in women with hypoactive sexual desire disorder: those on combined oral contraceptives (COCs) vs. those not on COCs. *The Journal of Sexual Medicine* **3**, 878–82.

49 Lee JS, Lacroix AZ, Wu L, *et al.* (2008) Associations of serum sex hormone–binding globulin and sex hormone concentrations with hip fracture risk in postmenopausal women. *Journal of Clinical Endocrinology and Metabolism* **93**, 1796–1803.

50 Shifren JL, Rifai N, Desindes S, *et al.* (2008) A comparison of the short-term effects of oral conjugated equine estrogens versus transdermal estradiol on C-reactive protein, other serum markers of inflammation, and other hepatic proteins in naturally menopausal women. *Journal of Clinical Endocrinology and Metabolism* **93**, 1702–10.

51 Zähringer S, Tomova A, von Werder K, *et al.* (2000) The influence of hyperthyroidism on the hypothalamic–pituitary–gonadal axis. *Experimental and Clinical Endocrinology and Diabetes* **108**, 282–89.

52 Luppa PB, Thaler M, Schulte-Frohlinde E, *et al.* (2006) Unchanged androgen-binding properties of sex hormone–binding globulin in male patients with liver cirrhosis. *Clinical Chemistry and Laboratory Medicine* **44**, 967–73.

53 Pascal N, Amouzou EK, Sanni A, *et al.* (2002) Serum concentrations of sex hormone binding globulin are elevated in kwashiorkor and anorexia nervosa but not in marasmus. *American Journal of Clinical Nutrition* **76**, 239–44.

54 Isojärvi JI, Taubøll E, Herzog AG. (2005) Effect of antiepileptic drugs on reproductive endocrine function in individuals with epilepsy. *CNS Drugs* **19**, 207–23.

55 Rosner W, Auchus RJ, Azziz R, *et al.* (2007) Position statement: utility, limitations, and pitfalls in measuring testosterone: an Endocrine Society position statement. *Journal of Clinical Endocrinology and Metabolism* **92**, 405–13.

56 Shifren JL, Braunstein GD, Simon JA, *et al.* (2000; 2005) Transdermal testosterone treatment in women with impaired sexual function after oophorectomy. *New England Journal of Medicine* **343**, 682–88; **165**, 1582–89.

57 Turpeinen U, Linko S, Itkonen O, *et al.* (2008) Determination of testosterone in serum by liquid chromatography-tandem mass spectrometry. *Scandinavian Journal of Clinical and Laboratory* **68**, 50–57.

58 Vermeulen A, Verdonck L, Kaufman JM. (1999) A critical evaluation of simple methods for the estimation of free testosterone in serum. *Journal of Clinical Endocrinology and Metabolism* **84**, 3666–72.

59 DeVan ML, Bankson DD, Abadie JM. (2008) To what extent are free testosterone (FT) values reproducible between the two Washingtons, and can calculated FT be used in lieu of expensive direct measurements? *American Journal of Clinical Pathology* **129**, 459–63.

60 Rinaldi S, Geay A, Déchaud H, *et al.* (2002) Validity of free testosterone and free estradiol determinations in serum samples from postmenopausal women by theoretical calculations. *Cancer Epidemiology Biomarkers and Prevention* **11**, 1065–71.

61 Xita N, Georgiou I, Lazaros L, *et al.* (2008) The role of sex hormone–binding globulin and androgen receptor gene variants in the development of polycystic ovary syndrome. *Human Reproduction* **23**, 693–98.

62 Labrie F, Bélanger A, Bélanger P, *et al.* (2006) Androgen glucuronides, instead of testosterone, as the new markers of androgenic activity in women. *Journal of Steroid Biochemistry and Molecular Biology* **99**, 182–88.

63 Cappel M, Mauger D, Thiboutot D. (2005) Correlation between serum levels of insulin-like growth factor 1, dehydroepiandrosterone sulfate, and dihydrotestosterone and acne lesion counts in adult women. *Archives of Dermatology* **141**, 333–38.

64 Tosti A, Piraccini BM, Iorizzo M, *et al.* (2005) The natural history of androgenetic alopecia. *Journal of Cosmetic Dermatology* **4**, 41–43.

65 Davison SL, Bell R, Donath S, *et al.* (2005) Androgen levels in adult females: changes with age, menopause, and oophorectomy. *Journal of Clinical Endocrinology and Metabolism* **90**, 3847–53.

66 Guay A, Munarriz R, Jacobson J, *et al.* (2004) Serum androgen levels in healthy premenopausal women with and without sexual dysfunction: Part A. Serum androgen levels in women aged 20–49 years with no complaints of sexual dysfunction. *International Journal of Impotence Research* **16**, 112–20.

67 Burger HG, Dudley EC, Cui J, *et al.* (2000) A prospective longitudinal study of serum testosterone, dehydroepiandrosterone sulfate, and sex hormone–binding globulin levels

through the menopause transition. *Journal of Clinical Endocrinology and Metabolism* **85**, 2832–38.

68 Labrie F, Bélanger A, Cusan L, *et al.* (1997) Marked decline in serum concentrations of adrenal C19 sex steroid precursors and conjugated androgen metabolites during aging. *Journal of Clinical Endocrinology and Metabolism* **82**, 2396–2402.

69 McTiernan A, Wu L, Barnabei VM, *et al.*; WHI Investigators. (2008) Relation of demographic factors, menstrual history, reproduction and medication use to sex hormone levels in postmenopausal women. *Breast Cancer Research and Treatment* **108**, 217–31.

70 Zumoff B, Strain GW, Miller LK, *et al.* (1995) Twenty-four-hour mean plasma testosterone concentration declines with age in normal premenopausal women. *Journal of Clinical Endocrinology and Metabolism* **80**, 1429–30.

71 Liu D, Si H, Reynolds KA, *et al.* (2007) Dehydroepiandrosterone protects vascular endothelial cells against apoptosis through a G α i protein-dependent activation of phosphatidylinositol 3-kinase/Akt and regulation of antiapoptotic Bcl-2 expression. *Endocrinology* **148**, 3068–76.

72 Traish AM, Kim NN, Huang YH, *et al.* (2003) Sex steroid hormones differentially regulate nitric oxide synthase and arginase activities in the proximal and distal rabbit vagina. *International Journal of Impotence Research* **15**, 397–404.

73 Traish AM, Huang YH, Min K, *et al.* (2004) Binding characteristics of [3H]delta(5)-androstene-3β,17β-diol to a nuclear protein in the rabbit vagina. *Steroids* **69**, 71–78.

74 Bodo C, Rissman EF. (2008) The androgen receptor is selectively involved in organization of sexually dimorphic social behaviors in mice. *Endocrinology*.

75 Dakin CL, Wilson CA, Kalló I, *et al.* (2008) Neonatal stimulation of 5-HT(2) receptors reduces androgen receptor expression in the rat anteroventral periventricular nucleus and sexually dimorphic preoptic area. *European Journal of Neuroscience* **27**, 2473–80.

76 Yague JG, Wang AC, Janssen WG, *et al.* (2008) Aromatase distribution in the monkey temporal neocortex and hippocampus. *Brain Research* **1209**, 115–27.

77 Graziottin A, Leiblum SR. (2005) Biological and psychosocial pathophysiology of female sexual dysfunction during the menopausal transition. *The Journal of Sexual Medicine* **3**, 133–45.

78 Taylor AH, Guzail M, Al-Azzawi F. (2008) Differential expression of oestrogen receptor isoforms and androgen receptor in the normal vulva and vagina compared with vulval lichen sclerosus and chronic vaginitis. *British Journal of Dermatology* **158**, 319–28.

79 Hodgins MB, Spike RC, Mackie RM, *et al.* (1998) An immunohistochemical study of androgen, oestrogen and progesterone receptors in the vulva and vagina. *British Journal of Obstetrics and Gynaecology* **105**, 216–22.

80 Davis SR. (1999) The therapeutic use of androgens in women. *Journal of Steroid Biochemistry and Molecular Biology* **69**, 177–84.

81 Braunstein GD. (2006) Androgen insufficiency in women. *Growth Hormone and IGF Research* **16**, S109–117.

82 Rivera-Woll LM, Papalia M, Davis SR, *et al.* (2004) Androgen insufficiency in women: diagnostic and therapeutic implications. *Human Reproduction Update* **10**, 421–32.

83 Bachmann G, Bancroft J, Braunstein G, *et al.* (2002) Female androgen insufficiency: the Princeton consensus statement on definition, classification, and assessment. *Fertility and Sterility* **77**, 660–65.

84 Santoro N, Torrens J, Crawford S, *et al.* (2005) Correlates of circulating androgens in midlife women: the study of women's health across the nation. *Journal of Clinical Endocrinology and Metabolism* **90**, 4836–45.

85 Braunstein GD, Sundwall DA, Katz M, *et al.* (2005) Safety and efficacy of a testosterone patch for the treatment of hypoactive sexual desire disorder in surgically menopausal women: a randomized, placebo controlled trial. *Archives of Internal Medicine* **165**, 1582–89.

86 Guay A, Jacobson J, Munarriz R, *et al.* (2004) Serum androgen levels in healthy premenopausal women with and without sexual dysfunction: Part B: Reduced serum androgen levels in healthy premenopausal women with complaints of sexual dysfunction. *International Journal of Impotence Research* **16**, 121–29.

87 Song YS, Yang HJ, Song ES, *et al.* (2008) Sexual function and quality of life in Korean women with chronic renal failure on hemodialysis: case-control study. *Urology* **71**, 243–46.

88 Turna B, Apaydin E, Semerci B, *et al.* (2005) Women with low libido: correlation of decreased androgen levels with female sexual function index. *International Journal of Impotence Research* **17**, 48–53.

89 Davis SR, Davison SL, Donath S, *et al.* (2005) Circulating androgen levels and self-reported sexual function in women. *Journal of the American Medical Association* **294**, 91–96.

90 Krassas GE, Tziomalos K, Papadopoulou F, *et al.* (2008) Erectile dysfunction in patients with hyper- and hypothyroidism: how common and should we treat? *Journal of Clinical Endocrinology and Metabolism* **93**, 1815–19.

91 Carani C, Isidori AM, Granata A, *et al.* (2005) Multicenter study on the prevalence of sexual symptoms in male hypo- and hyperthyroid patients. *Journal of Clinical Endocrinology and Metabolism* **90**, 6472–79.

92 Arlt W, Callies F, van Vlijmen JC, *et al.* (1999) Dehydroepiandrosterone replacement in women with adrenal insufficiency. *New England Journal of Medicine* **341**, 1013–20.

93 Munarriz R, Talakoub L, Flaherty E, *et al.* (2002) Androgen replacement therapy with dehydroepiandrosterone for androgen insufficiency and female sexual dysfunction:

androgen and questionnaire results. *Journal of Sex and Marital Therapy* **28**, 165–73.

94 Baulieu EE, Thomas G, Legrain S, *et al.* (2000) Dehydroepiandrosterone (DHEA), DHEA sulfate, and aging: contribution of the DHEAge Study to a sociobiomedical issue. *Obstetrical and Gynecological Survey* **55**, 695.

95 Davis S, Papalia MA, Norman RJ, *et al.* (2008) Safety and efficacy of a testosterone metered-dose transdermal spray for treating decreased sexual satisfaction in premenopausal women: a randomized trial. *Annals of Internal Medicine* **148**, 569–77.

96 Goldstat R, Briganti E, Tran J, *et al.* (2003) Transdermal testosterone therapy improves well-being, mood, and sexual function in premenopausal women. *Menopause* **10**, 390–98.

97 El-Hage G, Eden JA, Manga RZ. (2007) A double-blind, randomized, placebo-controlled trial of the effect of testosterone cream on the sexual motivation of menopausal hysterectomized women with hypoactive sexual desire disorder. *Climacteric* **10**, 335–43.

98 Kingsberg S, Shifren J, Wekselman K, *et al.* (2007) Evaluation of the clinical relevance of benefits associated with transdermal testosterone treatment in postmenopausal women with hypoactive sexual desire disorder. *The Journal of Sexual Medicine* **4**, 1001–8.

99 Kingsberg S. (2007) Testosterone treatment for hypoactive sexual desire disorder in postmenopausal women. *The Journal of Sexual Medicine* **4**, 2.

100 Goldstein AT, Burrows L. (2008) Vulvodynia. *The Journal of Sexual Medicine* **5**, 5–14.

101 Braunstein GD. (2007) Management of female sexual dysfunction in postmenopausal women by testosterone administration: safety issues and controversies. *The Journal of Sexual Medicine* **4**, 859–66.

102 Fenichel RM, Warren MP. (2007) Anorexia, bulimia, and the athletic triad: evaluation and management. *Current Osteoporosis Reports* **5**, 160–64.

103 Wessler S, Otto C, Wilck N, *et al.* (2006) Identification of estrogen receptor ligands leading to activation of non-genomic signaling pathways while exhibiting only weak transcriptional activity. *Journal of Steroid Biochemistry and Molecular Biology* **98**, 25–35.

104 Bakker J, Baum MJ. (2008) Role for estradiol in female-typical brain and behavioral sexual differentiation. *Frontiers in Neuroendocrinology* **29**, 1–16.

105 Blaustein JD. (2008) Neuroendocrine regulation of feminine sexual behavior: lessons from rodent models and thoughts about humans. *Annual Review of Psychology* **59**, 93–118.

106 White MM, Sheffer I, Teeter J, *et al.* (2007) Hypothalamic progesterone receptor-A mediates gonadotropin surges, self-priming, and receptivity in estrogen-primed female mice. *Journal of Molecular Endocrinology* **38**, 35–50.

107 Petralia SM, Frye CA. (2006) In the ventral tegmental area, cyclic AMP mediates the actions of progesterone at dopamine type 1 receptors for lordosis of rats and hamsters. *Journal of Neuroendocrinology* **18**, 902–14.

108 Frye CA, Walf AA, Petralia SM. (2006) Progestins' effects on sexual behaviour of female rats and hamsters involving D1 and GABA(A) receptors in the ventral tegmental area may be G-protein-dependent. *Behavioral Brain Research* **172**, 286–93.

109 Molenda-Figueira HA, Williams CA, Griffin AL, *et al.* (2006) Nuclear receptor coactivators function in estrogen receptor– and progestin receptor–dependent aspects of sexual behavior in female rats. *Hormones and Behavior* **50**, 383–92.

110 Frye CA, Walf AA, Petralia SM. (2006) In the ventral tegmental area, progestins have actions at D1 receptors for lordosis of hamsters and rats that involve GABA A receptors. *Hormones and Behavior* **50**, 332–37.

111 Pazol K, Northcutt KV, Wilson ME, *et al.* (2006) Medroxyprogesterone acetate acutely facilitates and sequentially inhibits sexual behavior in female rats. *Hormones and Behavior* **49**, 105–13.

112 Landry T, Bergeron S, Dupuis MJ, *et al.* (2008) The treatment of provoked vestibulodynia: a critical review. *Clinical Journal of Pain* **24**, 155–71.

113 Johannesson U, Sahlin L, Masironi B, *et al.* (2008) Steroid receptor expression and morphology in provoked vestibulodynia. *American Journal of Obstetrics and Gynecology* **198**, 311.

114 Green J, Hetherton J. (2005) Psychological aspects of vulvar vestibulitis syndrome. *Journal of Psychosomatic Obstetrics and Gynecology* **26**, 101–6.

115 Reissing ED, Brown C, Lord MJ, *et al.* (2005) Pelvic floor muscle functioning in women with vulvar vestibulitis syndrome. *Journal of Psychosomatic Obstetrics and Gynecology* **26**, 107.

116 Nyirjesy P. (2001) Chronic vulvovaginal candidiasis. *American Family Physician* **63**, 697–702.

117 Bohm-Starke N, Hilliges M, Brodda-Jansen G, *et al.* (2001) Psychophysical evidence of nociceptor sensitization in vulvar vestibulitis syndrome. *Pain* **94**, 177–83.

118 Babula O, Linhares IM, Bongiovanni AM, *et al.* (2008) Association between primary vulvar vestibulitis syndrome, defective induction of tumor necrosis factor-α, and carriage of the mannose-binding lectin codon 54 gene polymorphism. *American Journal of Obstetrics and Gynecology* **198**, 101.

119 Babula O, Danielsson I, Sjoberg I, *et al.* (2004) Altered distribution of mannose-binding lectin alleles at exon I codon 54 in women with vulvar vestibulitis syndrome. *American Journal of Obstetrics and Gynecology* **191**, 762–66.

120 Foster DC, Sazenski TM, Stodgell CJ. (2004) Impact of genetic variation in interleukin-1 receptor antagonist and

melanocortin-1 receptor genes on vulvar vestibulitis syndrome. *The Journal of Reproductive Medicine* **49**, 503–9.

121 Eva LJ, MacLean AB, Reid WM, *et al.* (2003) Estrogen receptor expression in vulvar vestibulitis syndrome. *American Journal of Obstetrics and Gynecology* **189**, 458–61.

122 Sutherland S, Stankovic M, Cerda S, *et al.* (2004) Female sexual dysfunction secondary to sexual pain: androgen influence on the pathophysiology of vulvar vestibulitis syndrome. Podium #26. Presented to the Annual ISSWSH Meeting Oct 28–31, Atlanta.

123 ESHRE Capri Workshop Group. (2008) Intrauterine devices and intrauterine systems. *Human Reproduction Update* **14**, 197–208.

124 Suckling J, Lethaby A, Kennedy R. (2006) Local oestrogen for vaginal atrophy in postmenopausal women. *Cochrane Database of Systematic Reviews* **18**, CD001500.

125 Castelo-Branco C, Cancelo MJ, Villero J, *et al.* (2005) Management of postmenopausal vaginal atrophy and atrophic vaginitis. *Maturitas* **52**, S46–52.

126 Mainini G, Scaffa C, Rotondi M, *et al.* (2005) Local estrogen replacement therapy in postmenopausal atrophic vaginitis: efficacy and safety of low-dose 17β-estradiol vaginal tablets. *Clinical and Experimental Obstetrics and Gynecology* **32**, 111–13.

127 Ballagh SA. (2005) Vaginal hormone therapy for urogenital and menopausal symptoms. *Seminars in Reproductive Medicine* **23**, 126–40.

128 Greendale GA, Zibecchi L, Petersen L, *et al.* (1999) Development and validation of a physical examination scale to assess vaginal atrophy and inflammation. *Climacteric* **2**, 197–204.

129 Kulp JL, Chaudhry S, Wiita B, *et al.* (2008) The accuracy of women performing vaginal pH self-testing. *Journal of Womens Health* **17**, 523–26.

130 Whiteside JL, Barber MD, Paraiso MF, *et al.* (2005) Vaginal rugae: measurement and significance. *Climacteric* **8**, 71–75.

131 Munarriz R, Talakoub L, Kuohung W, *et al.* (2002) The prevalence of phimosis of the clitoris in women presenting to the sexual dysfunction clinic: lack of correlation to disorders of desire, arousal and orgasm. *Journal of Sex and Marital Therapy* **28**, 18.

132 Ballagh SA. (2005) Vaginal hormone therapy for urogenital and menopausal symptoms. *Seminars in Reproductive Medicine* **23**, 126–40.

133 Ouslander JG, Greendale GA, Uman G, *et al.* (2001) Effects of oral estrogen and progestin on the lower urinary tract among female nursing home residents. *Journal of the American Geriatrics Society* **49**, 803–07.

134 Abouzeid H, Shergill IS, Al-Samarrai M. (2007) Successful medical treatment of advanced urethral prolapse. *Journal of Obstetrics and Gynaecology* **27**, 634–35.

135 Society of Obstetricians and Gynaecologists of Canada. (2004) SOGC clinical practice guidelines. The detection and management of vaginal atrophy. *International Journal of Gynaecology and Obstetrics* **88**, 222–28.

136 Crandall C. (2002) Vaginal estrogen preparations: a review of safety and efficacy for vaginal atrophy. *Journal of Women's Health* **11**, 857–877

137 Santen RJ, Pinkerton JV, Conaway M, *et al.* (2002) Treatment of urogenital atrophy with low-dose estradiol: preliminary results. *Menopause* **9**, 179–87.

138 Manonai J, Theppisai U, Suthutvoravut S, *et al.* (2001) The effect of estradiol vaginal tablet and conjugated estrogen cream on urogenital symptoms in postmenopausal women: a comparative study. *Journal of Obstetrics and Gynaecology Research* **27**, 255–60.

139 Manonai J, Theppisai U, Chittacharoen A. (2001) Effect and safety of 17β-estradiol vaginal tablet in postmenopausal women with urogenital symptoms. *Journal of the Medical Association of Thailand* **84**, 1015–20.

140 Taechakraichana N, Intraragsakul A, Panyakhamlerd K, *et al.* (1997) Estradiol and follicle-stimulating hormone levels in oophorectomized women using vaginal estrogen. *Journal of the Medical Association of Thailand* **80**, 626–30.

141 Dew JE, Wren BG, Eden JA. (2003) A cohort study of topical vaginal estrogen therapy in women previously treated for breast cancer. *Climacteric* **6**, 45–52.

142 Kendall A, Dowsett M, Folkerd E, *et al.* (2006) Caution: Vaginal estradiol appears to be contraindicated in postmenopausal women on adjuvant aromatase inhibitors. *Annals of Oncology* **17**, 584–87.

CHAPTER 29

Lieomyomas and Adnexal Masses: Are They a Significant Cause of Dyspareunia?

Denniz Zolnoun, Caitlin Shaw
University of North Carolina, Chapel Hill, NC, USA

Introduction

Upper genital pathologies, such as fibroids and ad-nexal masses, are common diagnoses in reproductive-aged women, affecting up to 25% of this population [1]. Though in practice these pathologies are believed to cause dyspareunia, this association may in fact be coincidental [2]. Certainly, such pathologies can present with dyspareunia, specifically deep pain. However, more often than not, dyspareunia attributed to these pathologies may be due to other comorbid conditions such as endometriosis (see Chapter 19), adenomyosis, and pelvic inflammatory disease (see Chapter 20). This chapter reviews the research examining the association between two of the most common gynecological conditions—ovarian mass and uterine lieomyoma—and dyspareunia.

Ovarian Mass

Ovarian masses are common findings in women of all ages, affecting about 8% of reproductive-aged women [3]. Ovarian mass can be categorized into two broad categories: functional (e.g., follicular or luteal cyst) or neoplastic. Approximately 70% of the identified masses in reproductive women are functional [3]. They occur due to ovulatory disruptions. In the process of normal ovulation,

a follicle develops to maturity and then ruptures to release an ovum; this is followed by formation and subsequent involution of the corpus luteum. Follicular cysts arise when rupture does not occur and the follicle continues to grow; corpus luteum cysts occur when the corpus luteum fails to involute and continues to enlarge after ovulation. These cysts are therefore called physiologic or functional [1], and they affect approximately 7% of reproductive-aged women [3].

Ovarian neoplasms arise from the surface epithelium, germ cells, and sex-cord-stromal tissue, and may be benign or malignant. An overwhelming majority are benign; the risk of malignancy of an adnexal mass is only 6–11% in premenopausal women and 29–35% in postmenopausal women [1, 4]. In women aged 20–39, the three most frequent types of benign ovarian masses are: (i) serous and mucinous cystadenoma (arising from surface epithelium), (ii) endometrioma (a.k.a. "chocolate cysts" arising from ectopic endometrial tissue) [1], and (iii) mature cystic teratoma (a.k.a. dermoid cyst arising from the germ cell layers) [5].

Recent advances in ultrasonographic technology have played a pivotal role in questioning the validity of our age-old assumptions with regards to the clinical significance of an ovarian mass. Cystic ovarian masses in premenarchial females, once viewed as pathologic and associated with premature puberty, are now known to be common [6]. In general, ultrasonographic evaluations and imaging of the upper genital tract should not be used routinely as a screening tool, especially with respect to the evaluation of dyspareunia.

Ovarian Mass and Dyspareunia

Because an ovarian mass is a common finding in women of reproductive age, its mere presence should not be thought as causative in painful intercourse. In fact, although commonly blamed as the cause of sexual pain in clinical practice, ovarian cysts are rarely associated with persistent dyspareunia [2]. Nevertheless, functional ovarian cysts can be associated with acute and/or cyclical pain and, less commonly, dyspareunia [3], and in cases in which symptoms of intermittent dyspareunia exist simultaneously with ovarian mass, deep dyspareunia is the most likely subtype to be found.

A common cause of deep dyspareunia is due to Mittleshmertz (a.k.a. ovulatory pain), which may last anywhere from 2 hr to 2 days. It may occur spontaneously or can be precipitated with intercourse in midcycle. Women with ovulatory pain may report cyclical pain that may be positional and exacerbated with deep thrusting. When examined, pain and discomfort with cervical movement and abdominal pressure is often noted during the painful episode. Upon ultrasound evaluation, an ovulatory cyst with a small amount of free peritoneal fluid is commonly found. Mittleshmertz is a self-limiting condition and spontaneously resolves with supportive therapy (e.g., heat application) and use of nonsteroidal anti-inflammatory drugs (NSAIDS). Hormonal suppression with oral contraceptive therapy is empirically [7, 8] used for the treatment of recurrent symptoms.

Other causes of deep dyspareunia may include tubo-ovarian abscess, adnexal torsion, and benign ovarian neoplasm [9]. These causes, in addition to other infection- and pregnancy-related causes, should always be ruled out before attributing the diagnosis to an adnexal mass. The first two conditions present with systemic signs of inflammation, such as fever and an elevated white blood cell count, as well as severe pain. Benign ovarian neoplasms, on the other hand, can enlarge without the presence of pain. In contrast, malignant neoplasms are indolent and more likely to present with vague abdominal pain and ascites.

Overall, radiological imaging (most commonly ultrasound examination) of the upper genital tract should be reserved for cases presenting with deep dyspareunia and/or findings of tenderness in the uterus, adnexa, and/or with cervical movement (commonly known as cervical motion tenderness). Ectopic pregnancy and infectious etiologies of deep dyspareunia should always be ruled out first. In our experience, even when an ovarian cyst is present, it is likely that other conditions such as endometriosis [10] are responsible for the dyspareunia.

Uterine Leiomyomata

With a lifetime prevalence of greater than 50%, uterine leiomyomata (a.k.a. uterine fibroids) are the most common gynecological reason for surgery, accounting for one-third of hysterectomies each year in the United States [11]. Uterine leiomyomatas (i.e., fibroids) are benign monoclonal tumors arising from the smooth muscle cells of the myometrium. They contain a large amount of extracellular matrix and are surrounded by a thin pseudocapsule of areolar tissue and compressed muscle fibers.

The myomatous uterus is irregularly shaped and can cause specific symptoms due to pressure from fibroids in particular locations. Common symptoms of fibroids can be placed into three main categories: increased uterine bleeding (menorrhagia), reproductive dysfunction such as infertility, and bulk-related symptoms. Bulk-related symptoms include pelvic pressure and pain resulting from fibroids in particular locations, such as constipation from fibroids pushing on the rectum and dyspareunia from cervical fibroids proximate to the vagina [12]. Despite conventional wisdom and a number of case reports suggesting a relationship between fibroids and dyspareunia, this notion is not substantiated in large-scale population level studies.

Fibroids and Dyspareunia

The correlation between uterine fibroids and other associated gynecological disorders such as menorrhagia, dysmenorrhea, dyspareunia, and pelvic pain is primarily based on indirect evidence and a handful of case reports. For example, associations as high as 59% have been reported between uterine fibroids and pelvic pain [2, 11, 13]. However, as is often the case with such "clinical relics," their validity is often challenged with the advent of large-scale, population-based studies. In the case of leiomyomatas and gynecological pain, this did not happen until 2003 when Lippman's findings challenged the validity of our age-old "clinical wisdom" [2, 11].

Lippman [11] and Ferrero [2] were the first investigators to examine the relationship between gynecological pain and uterine fibroids in population-based studies in 2003 and 2006, respectively. Unlike Ferrero who found no significant associations between deep dyspareunia and uterine fibroids, Lippman reported an association. Her group noted that women with dyspareunia were more likely to have an associated fibroid [11]. However, it is important to note that 80% of those with dyspareunia were fibroid-free. In a combined cohort of over 1000 women, there were no significant associations between the number, location, and size of fibroids and gynecological pain, specifically deep dyspareunia and chronic pelvic pain. Thus, in the absence of reproducible pain upon examination, uterine fibroids are unlikely to be etiologic when identified. When present on examination, reproducible pain is more likely to be associated with other coincidental pathologies, such as endometriosis and adenomyosis, than with isolated uterine fibroids [11].

Nevertheless, a small association between uterine fibroids and dyspareunia may exist and needs to be explored on a case-by-case basis. Okolo et al. found that a familial prevalence of uterine fibroids is associated with distinct clinical and molecular features that differ from those found when fibroids occur sporadically. When compared with families with sporadic fibroids, familial prevalence of fibroids was associated with a higher incidence of dyspareunia [14]. This study highlights the importance of a comprehensive assessment of symptom complexes in order to provide a biological context for assessing the degree to which a given gynecological finding may be etiologic or incidental.

Treatment of Fibroids

Treatment for uterine fibroids should be guided by a number of clinical factors such as the nature and severity of presenting symptoms, patient characteristics (e.g., age, desire for future fertility), and preference. In general, treatment options fall into the two broad categories of interventional and noninterventional therapies.

Interventional treatments for fibroids can be categorized as noninvasive, minimally invasive, and invasive. Advances in interventional radiology have significantly shifted the state of art in treatment of fibroids away from invasive surgical options to noninvasive interventions, such as uterine artery embolization and magnetic resonance-guided focused ultrasound surgery (e.g., Ex-Ablate 2000). Myomectomy, in lieu of hysterectomy, continues to be the mainstay of treatment for women of child-

bearing age (specifically those with infertility) [12]. There has been a steady, though slow, shift away from the invasive abdominal myomectomy to that of minimally invasive robotic- and laparoscopic-assisted procedures.

With increasing popularity and refinements in techniques, a significant decrease in the morbidity associated with myomectomy is likely to be seen in the future. However, for women who are not concerned with fertility, endometrial ablation and myolysis—alone or in combination—remain the preferred minimally invasive therapy for the treatment of fibroids and associated bleeding [12].

The most common noninterventional therapies for the treatment of fibroids are hormonal therapy (oral and injectable) and intrauterine implants. The three most common forms of hormonal therapies are oral contraceptives, androgenic steroids (e.g., danazol), and antiprogestins (e.g., mefiprogestrone), with gonadotropin-releaiting hormone (GnRH) agonists such as Depo-Lupron® being the most common injectable therapy. In general, hormonal therapies exert their therapeutic benefit via direct and indirect "thinning" of the endometrial lining, which subsequently results in decreased menstrual flow. Other benefits, such as the reduction in the number and size of myomas, have also been reported.

Androgenic steroids such as danazol are not frequently recommended due to their frequent side effects such as weight gain, muscle cramps, acne, hirsutism, oily skin, mood changes, and depression [12]. In recent years, novel hormonal therapies such as antiprogesterone agents [e.g., mifepristone (RU-486)] have been gaining increasing popularity for the treatment of fibroids. These agents are reported to reduce uterine volume by 26–74% in women, and lower doses can treat heavy bleeding while maintaining cyclicity and avoiding the side effects of high doses [15]. Even though there is accumulating evidence that mifepristone provides symptomatic relief and improved quality of life, fibroid regrowth occurs slowly following cessation of the drug [16].

Lastly, levonorgestrel-releasing intrauterine contraception (Mirena IUD®) has received considerable attention in large part due to its long-term (5-year) localized effect with documented reduction in both bulk-related and menorrhagia symptoms. The device is widely used and is endorsed for these indications by many experts but is not recommended for women with intracavitary leiomyomas amenable to hysteroscopic resection [12].

Conclusion

Although significant strides in understanding the role of the biological and psychological aspects of dyspareunia have been made, the underlying pathophysiology is sometimes difficult to ascertain. In the absence of a conceptual framework built by empirical evidence, clinicians often resort to costly and ineffective evaluation and treatment (e.g., laparoscopy) modalities. These treatments are often instigated by "incidental" ultrasonographic findings. In our experience, imaging studies such as ultrasound, computed tomography (CT), or magnetic resonance imaging (MRI) have rarely led to a well-defined etiology of pain. Pursuing a host of imaging modalities to find a cause, in our experience, only leads to incidental findings of common gynecological disorders that may not be associated with pain. Therefore, symptom-based, case-by-case assessments of patients are warranted, bearing in mind that uterine leiomyomata and ovarian masses are frequently only incidental findings.

References

1 Hoffman MS. (2008) Differential diagnosis of the adnexal mass. In: Rose BD (ed.) UpToDate. Waltham, MA.

2 Ferrero S, Abbamonte LH, Giordano M, *et al.* (2006) Uterine myomas, dyspareunia, and sexual function. *Fertility and Sterility* **86**, 1504–10.

3 Borgfeldt C, Andolf E. (1999) Transvaginal sonographic ovarian findings in a random sample of women 25–40 years old. *Ultrasound in Obstetrics and Gynecology* **13**, 345–50.

4 Kinkel K, Lu Y, Mehdizade A, *et al.* (2005) Indeterminate ovarian mass at US: incremental value of second imaging test for characterization: meta-analysis and Bayesian analysis. *Radiology* **236**, 85–94.

5 Killackey M, Neuwirth, RS. (1988) Evaluation and management of the pelvic mass: a review of 540 cases. *Obstetrics and Gynecology* **71**, 319.

6 Norris HJ, Jensen RD. (1972) Relative frequency of ovarian neoplasms in children and adolescents. *Cancer* **30**, 713–19.

7 Spanos WJ. (1973) Preoperative hormonal therapy of cystic adnexal masses. *American Journal of Obstetrics and Gynecology* **116**, 551–56.

8 Holt VL, Daling JR, McKnight B, *et al.* (1992) Functional ovarian cysts in relation to the use of monophasic and triphasic oral contraceptives. *Obstetrics and Gynecology* **79**, 529–33.

9 ACOG PB. (2004) *Chronic Pelvic Pain.* American College of Obstetrics and Gynecology, Washington, DC, p. 17.

10 Sinaii N, Plumb K, Cotton L, *et al.* (2008) Differences in characteristics among 1000 women with endometriosis based on extent of disease. *Fertility and Sterility* **89**, 538–45.

11 Lippman SA, Warner M, Samuels S, *et al.* (2003) Uterine fibroids and gynecologic pain symptoms in a population-based study. *Fertility and Sterility* **80**, 1488–94.

12 Stewart EA. (2008) Epidemiology, clinical manifestations, diagnosis, and natural history of uterine leiomyomas. In: Rose BD (ed.) UpToDate, Waltham, MA.

13 Hickey M, Farquhar CM. (2003) Update on treatment of menstrual disorders. *Medical Journal of Australia* **178**, 625–29.

14 Okolo SO, Gentry CC, Perrett CW, *et al.* (2005) Familial prevalence of uterine fibroids is associated with distinct clinical and molecular features. *Human Reproduction* **20**, 2321–24.

15 Fiscella K, Eisinger SH, Meldrum S, *et al.* (2006) Effect of mifepristone for symptomatic leiomyomata on quality of life and uterine size: a randomized controlled trial. *Obstetrics and Gynecology* **108**, 1381–1387.

16 Eisinger SH, Bonfiglio T, Fiscella K, *et al.* (2005) Twelve-month safety and efficacy of low-dose mifepristone for uterine myomas. *Journal of Minimally Invasive Gynecology* **12**, 227–33.

CHAPTER 30
Animal Models of Dyspareunia

Melissa A. Farmer, Yitzchak M. Binik, Jeffrey S. Mogil
McGill University Health Centre, Montréal, Québec, Canada

Introduction

In recent years, the development and application of new animal models of disease processes has been a popular scientific trend [1]. However, few of these models have focused on sexuality, and fewer still have modeled pain conditions that impact sexuality. Urogenital and abdominal pain conditions associated with dyspareunia impact a staggering percentage of women, yet very few of these conditions are well understood. Although imaging studies have greatly advanced human research in this area [2], experimental options using human subjects are still limited. Animal models allow experimental manipulations to evaluate the causal relationships between pathological causes and physiological effects. These models are convenient and cost-effective, and they permit the testing of hypotheses that are otherwise ethically implausible in humans. The development of viable animal models for conditions that are associated with painful intercourse, such as endometriosis, interstitial cystitis (IC), irritable bowel syndrome (IBS), and provoked vestibulodynia (PVD) might have profound implications for our understanding of the etiology, maintenance, and treatment of these debilitating conditions.

Evaluation of Animal Models of Pain

Pain in animals is defined as "an aversive sensory experience caused by actual or potential injury that elicits progressive motor and vegetative reactions, results in

learned avoidance behavior, and may modify species-specific behavior, including social behavior" [3]. Animals cannot verbally rate their pain intensity, quality, or location, nor can they communicate the impact of emotion on pain. Instead, researchers infer the presence of pain from abnormal behaviors that are (hopefully) unique to the experimentally induced nociceptive state. The difficulty in measuring an animal's emotional or cognitive responses to pain suggests that we are largely using *nociceptive models*, rather than true pain models [4]. However, just because we can't measure something doesn't mean it isn't there. Nevertheless, the word *pain* will be used throughout this chapter.

Pain can be typified as spontaneous or provoked, depending on whether or not it is elicited by exogenous stimulation. Many existing animal models of pain are limited in their duration; chronic, spontaneous pain—the most clinically relevant form—has proved particularly difficult to model in animals [5]. Pain conditions can also be visceral or somatic in nature. Visceral pain originates from the internal organs contained within the chest and abdomen, and it is characterized by increased autonomic reactivity, emotional salience, and diffuse pain that may be referred to other visceral or somatic tissue that shares common innervation at the level of the spinal cord [6]. Referred pain is perceived in areas distal from the site of injury that receives common spinal input as the region where pain originates [7, 8]. The majority of animal models of pain conditions associated with dyspareunia are visceral in nature, including uterine inflammation, vaginal and uterine distension, endometriosis, and abdominal pain (including cystitis and colitis).

In animal models, behavioral responses may reflect the location of the pain in the case of somatic tissue (e.g., withdrawal of a heated hind paw), whereas visceral pain

Female Sexual Pain Disorders 1st edition. Edited by A. Goldstein, C. Pukall & I. Goldstein. © 2009 Blackwell Publishing, ISBN: 9781405183987.

may be manifested as referred somatic pain [7]. Patterns of pain behavior can increase in frequency or magnitude with higher levels of noxious stimulation. Abnormal behaviors that show temporal correspondence with tissue injury or inflammation are thought to reflect injury-specific pain, although the correlation may not be strong. For visceral pain in particular, the *absence* of behavior may be indicative of pain, as evidenced by reduced mobility or motivation to engage in normal activity [9]. In addition, estrous cyclicity may significantly impact some behaviors [10], but many indices of behavioral pain show equal variability when male versus female animals are used [11]. Empirical validation that a behavior is specific to pain is often achieved via the administration of known analgesics, such as nonsteroidal anti-inflammatory drugs, lidocaine, or morphine.

Ultimately, many behaviors have been associated with pain in rodents. Table 30.1 lists behaviors that have been linked to animal models of dyspareunia. Notably, the criteria for dyspareunia vary between models. Whereas some models directly measure vaginal sensitivity to noxious stimuli, other models induce pain conditions associated with dyspareunia. Ideally, pain behaviors are unique to an experimental manipulation, easily quantifiable with minimal need for interpretation, frequent enough to allow for statistical comparisons between groups, and reliably observed in afflicted animals (and rare in healthy animals). Such behavior should coincide with the duration and severity of injury and be mitigated by analgesics in a dose-dependent manner. Most importantly, the validity of an animal model of pain relies on whether the researchers have accurately identified a pain behavior that closely parallels the clinical characteristics of the condition it is intended to model. This chapter will be limited to reviewing rodent models of female urogenital and abdominal pain that include the measurement of pain *behavior*, not electrophysiological or electromyographic proxies, as a primary outcome measure [4].

Animal Models of Dyspareunia

Ureteral Calculosis
Women with dysmenorrhea, or painful menstruation, often report dyspareunia and are more likely to experience urinary calculosis (kidney stones). Based on this comorbidity, animal models of ureteral calculosis (UC) may in-

directly induce dyspareunia, although this link has never been formally tested.

The first detailed behavioral characterization of UC-induced visceral pain was conducted by Giamberardino's laboratory [12]. Within a day of implantation of an artificial stone into the left ureter, rats displayed a variety of spontaneous pain behaviors including stretching, hunched back, abdominal/flank licking, flank muscle contractions accompanied by ipsilateral inward hindlimb motions, lower abdominal squashing (against the floor), and the adoption of a supine position with the left hindlimb retracted into the abdomen. These behaviors slowly decreased in frequency and duration over four days postimplantation. Rats with frequent visceral pain behaviors were more likely to vocalize to electrical stimulation of the ipsilateral oblique muscles, indicative of referred pain. These behaviors are similar to the protracted abdominal stretching observed in early visceral pain models [13, 14]. Pain behaviors were reduced with intraperitoneal 5 mg/kg/day morphine. Giamberardino's model established a typology for abnormal pain behaviors associated with visceral pain that would be replicated or modified by the majority of subsequent abdominal visceral pain models.

Based on preliminary human evidence linking dysmenorrhea, endometriosis, and UC [15], Giamberardino and colleagues [16] developed a dual rat model of endometriosis with UC to investigate whether abdominal pain behaviors found in either condition are enhanced by the comorbidity. Animals with endometrial autografts plus stone implantations showed significantly longer bouts of pain behavior compared to stone implantation only or sham groups. Although all animals developed some referred hyperalgesia caused by the presence of a ureteral stone, the endometriosis + UC group displayed the greatest magnitude of referred pain as indicated by reduced vocalization threshold in response to electrical stimulation of the left oblique muscles.

Uterine Inflammation
Wesselmann and colleagues [17] characterized pain behavior associated with uterine inflammation in the rat. The pain behaviors they examined were based on the Giamberardino model of UC [12]. To induce inflammation, 10% mustard oil and a mineral oil vehicle were injected into the uterine lumen, and pain behaviors were videotaped for seven days postsurgery. Of animals receiving

Table 30.1 Common pain behaviors used in animal models of dyspareunia.

Pain Behaviors	Type of Pain	Condition Modeled	References
Pushing abdomen against floor ("stretch-flat" position)	Spontaneous, visceral	Ureteral calculosis, endometriosis, uterine inflammation, colitis, parturition	12, 16, 17, 41, 49
Lifting abdomen off floor	Spontaneous, visceral	Colitis	42–43
Sharp back hunch ("lambda" position)	Spontaneous, visceral	Ureteral calculosis, endometriosis, uterine inflammation	12, 16–17
Abdomen pressed against floor with nose facing toward tail of afflicted side ("alpha" position)	Spontaneous, visceral	Ureteral calculosis, endometriosis, uterine inflammation	12, 16–17
Lower abdomen pressed against floor while standing/sitting ("squash-pelvic" position)	Spontaneous, visceral	Ureteral calculosis, endometriosis, uterine inflammation, parturition	12, 16–17, 49
Stretching (back arched)	Spontaneous, visceral, mechanical distension	Ureteral calculosis, uterine inflammation, uterine distension, cystitis, colitis	12, 17–18, 32, 41-43
Experimenter observed abdominal contractions	Spontaneous, visceral	Cystitis, colitis	32–33, 41–44
Hunched posture	Spontaneous, visceral, mechanical distension	Ureteral calculosis, uterine inflammation, uterine distension, cystitis, parturition	12, 17–18, 31, 33, 35–36, 49
Inward turning of hindlimb	Spontaneous, visceral	Ureteral calculosis, uterine inflammation, parturition	12, 17, 49
Jumping or retreating from palpation/pressure	Provoked, mechanical or thermal or electrical, referred	Ureteral calculosis, referred hypersensitivity from: uterine inflammation, cystitis, colitis, ovariectomy, YIST model	12, 17, 34–35, 37, 41, 43–44, 46–47
Operant response	Provoked mechanical distension, spontaneous, referred	Vaginal and uterine distension, endometriosis, ovariectomy	18, 20–21, 24–25, 29
Licking afflicted area	Spontaneous or provoked	Ureteral calculosis, uterine inflammation, cystitis, colitis, parturition	12, 17, 31–34, 41, 49
Writhing	Spontaneous, visceral, tonic		13–14
Reduced physical activity	Spontaneous	Cystitis, uterine inflammation, colitis	7, 17, 32, 41–42
Vocalization	Spontaneous or provoked	Ureteral calculosis + endometriosis, uterine inflammation, uterine distension	12, 16–18
Piloerection	Spontaneous	Cystitis (rat model only)	31–35
Abnormal defecation/urination	Spontaneous or provoked	Colitis	43
Facial expression (eye squint, blink)	Spontaneous	Cystitis	36

uterine inflammation, 79% displayed prolonged periods of spontaneous pain behavior, with behavior frequency peaking two days after surgery. Dramatic individual differences were found in the frequency and duration of pain behaviors, and animals with uterine inflammation showed reductions in overall mobility. Of animals displaying spontaneous pain behavior, 66% also showed referred muscle hypersensitivity in the lower back and flanks that actually outlasted the occurrence of spontaneous pain behaviors.

Wesselmann's study was especially significant in that it established that pain from distinct viscera—the ureter and the uterus—resulted in very similar behaviors, including behavioral evidence of referred pain. Although this behavioral similarity may support the validity of these behaviors as being specific to pain, it also indicates that the behaviors are not specific enough to distinguish between visceral pains of different origins. The poor localization of visceral pain, however, makes it very unlikely that different visceral pains would be manifested in unique behavioral patterns.

Vaginal and Uterine Distension

Berkley and colleagues [18] established one of the earliest rat models of reproductive tract pain using vaginal and uterine distension. The elegance of this model relies on the novel operant task devised by the authors, which required rats to learn that a discrete behavioral response (extending the nose to interrupt a photocell circuit) would terminate an aversive stimulus (vaginal or uterine mechanical distension with a latex balloon). The authors argued that the rats' motivation to perform the escape behavior in response to high levels of distension indicated that intense mechanical distension constituted an aversive stimulus to the rats. The intense level of stimulation employed by this model is in contrast to innocuous levels of vaginal stimulation, which have positively reinforcing and analgesic properties in rodents [19].

Berkley et al. [18] validated this behavioral pain model in adult virgin female rats with low levels of ovarian hormones (i.e., Metestrus), to control for the potentially confounding effects of estrous cycle hormone fluctuations. Rats reliably escaped distension with increasing speed and frequency as the vaginal distension volume increased, and this response pattern held throughout the estrous cycle [20]. The rats' ability to detect and escape from uterine distension, however, was less predictable—many rats produced operant responses during control trials when distension volumes were minimal, and a large minority of animals did not show behavioral discomfort with maximum levels of uterine distension. The authors noted that rats often responded to uterine distension with stretching behavior.

Interestingly, escape behaviors increased in response to higher vaginal and uterine pressures when estrogen levels were low during Metestrus and Diestrus [20]. Similarly, ovariectomy (OVX) also induced moderate to high levels of vaginal hyperalgesia that were promptly reversed with 17β-estradiol replacement [21]. This pattern of estrogen-dependent vaginal sensitivity has adaptive reproductive significance. The increased tolerance to vaginal pressure, such as that induced by penile penetration, would be functionally important during the height of sexual activity in late proestrus, after estrogen and progesterone levels have peaked.

The development of this model exemplifies the successes and hazards of validating reliable behavioral correlates of pain. The authors succeeded in identifying a reliable pattern of behaviors for vaginal distension, yet uterine distension pain proved more difficult to characterize. Escape responding during uterine distension correlated with a prominent visceral pain behavior, which lends support to the aversive quality of the distension stimulus. One strength of this model is that it relies on an organized motor response that requires cerebral processing, which is thought to more accurately reflect the sensory perception of pain compared to simple reflex responses [4].

Endometriosis

Endometriosis is a painful condition defined by dysmenorrhea, dyspareunia, infertility, and chronic abdominal and low back pain [22]. To induce endometriosis, a segment of uterine horn is removed (i.e., hysterectomy), and pieces of endometrial tissue from the uterine horn (or fat for sham-operated controls) are autotransplanted onto blood vessels in the left ovary, the internal lower abdominal wall, or the cascade mesenteric arteries. Cysts rapidly develop at uterine transplant sites. The endometriosis rat model shares important similarities with endometriosis in women, including pelvic pain, infertility, in vitro and in vivo tissue and cell properties, and treatment responses [23].

Berkley and colleagues [24] combined the distension-induced pain model with the endometriosis rat model.

Animals subjected to the endometriosis surgery showed a significant increase in escape behavior in response to vaginal distension compared to baseline, whereas sham-operated animals without cysts showed no change in behavior. The findings of increased hypersensitivity to vaginal distension in rats with endometriosis have immense clinical relevance given the comorbidity of endometriosis and dyspareunia [22].

In a follow-up study, Cason and colleagues [25] found time- and estrous cycle–dependent changes in distension-induced vaginal hypersensitivity following endometriosis surgery. When postsurgical data from all stages of the estrous cycle were pooled together, the rate of escape responding to vaginal distension steadily increased for eight weeks in proportion to the growth of endometrial cysts. When specific stages of the estrous cycle were examined, rats with endometriosis increased escape responding from vaginal distension during Metestrus, Diestrus, and Proestrus (but not Estrus).

This finding is interesting for two reasons: First, the robust impact of endometriosis on vaginal sensitivity is fully reversed for about a day during the estrous cycle; second, this effect appears to be independent of normal patterns of vaginal hypersensitivity wherein moderate and high levels of estrogen during estrus and proestrus enhance tolerance to vaginal pressure [20]. The difference may be that nonpathological fluctuations in vaginal sensitivity are due to the direct effects of estrogen on vaginal tissue [26–27], whereas the pathological mechanisms underlying endometriosis-induced vaginal hyperalgesia may become centrally mediated [28]. Even a profound drop in ovarian hormones due to OVX does not change endometriosis-induced vaginal hyperalgesia [29], suggesting that either a reduction in estrogen levels does not alter the mechanisms underlying the hyperalgesia or that the capacity for both endometriosis plus OVX to produce hyperalgesia is not additive. Estrogen replacement following endometriosis plus OVX reverses the vaginal hypersensitivity, and this reversal may in part be due to central effects of estrogen [29].

Interstitial Cystitis

Interstitial cystitis (IC) is highly comorbid with dyspareunia and may be accompanied by a burning or aching vaginal pain [30]. Animal models of cystitis use a variety of irritants to induce bladder inflammation, including cyclophosphamide (an antitumor agent), turpentine, and even bacteria.

The cystitis-induced visceral pain model was first developed in the rat [31] and then in the mouse [9, 32]. Following cystitis induction, spontaneous pain behaviors progressively increased in frequency and were correlated with increasing severity of bladder inflammation [31–33]. Cystitis pain behaviors may be more pronounced in the rat compared to the mouse, with the former exhibiting spontaneous abnormal behaviors (i.e., hunched posture, abdominal licking and contractions, reduced locomotion) and the latter exhibiting a general reduction in physical activity [9, 31, 32], although one study found comparable hunching behaviors in the mouse [34]. Rat and mouse models show that cystitis produces referred pain to other areas receiving common innervation, such as the tail, hindpaw, and abdomen [9, 34–36]. In both species, cystitis-induced referred mechanical and thermal hypersensitivity were dose-dependently reduced with morphine [9, 34, 35]. The development of cystitis-induced behaviors does not vary across estrous stages, but interestingly, the onset of pain behaviors progresses more rapidly in female compared to male rats [33].

A model of bacteria-induced cystitis demonstrated that mice showed reduced hindpaw-withdrawal latencies to noxious radiant heat for 14 days following *Escherichia coli* administration, whereas otherwise genetically similar mice but with deficient Toll-like receptor 4 (TLR-4) function failed to show this thermal hypersensitivity [37]. Toll-like receptors are part of the innate immune defence against foreign pathogens, and TLR-4 recognizes bacterial wall components, contributing to nuclear factor-kappa B (NF-κB) activation and subsequent increases in proinflammatory cytokine expression [38]. Central TLR-4 has also been implicated in behavioral hypersensitivity to neuropathic pain [39, 40]. These findings indicate that a bacterium is a sufficient inflammatory irritant to induce experimental, TLR-4-dependent cystitis.

Colitis

In order to model functional abdominal pain like IBS, an animal model of visceral pain from colitis was developed by the Cervero laboratory which measured behavioral responses to colonic irritation from capsaicin and mustard oil [41]. Colonic irritation rapidly and dose-dependently produced abdominal pain behaviors (i.e., abdominal licking and hunching postures), as well as increased mechanical sensitivity on abdominal, tail, and hindpaw tissues indicative of referred pain. Abdominal pain behaviors were dose-dependently reduced by morphine. Similar models that correlated colonic irritation with increased acute and chronic abdominal pain behaviors showed no apparent structural damage to colonic mucosa [42, 43]. Furthermore, a minority of animals (about one-quarter) may develop chronic mechanical and thermal hypersensitivity lasting up to 16 weeks after severe colitis, indicating the presence of referred pain long after colitis-associated inflammation has resolved [44]. Due to the production of abdominal pain without detectable colonic pathology, these animal models are thought to mimic the clinically important characteristics of IBS, including visceral hypersensitivity and referred somatic pain [45].

Estrogen levels may play an important role in visceral pain. Sanoja and Cervero [46, 47] demonstrated that OVX mice developed robust mechanical, thermal, and visceral allodynia and hyperalgesia in abdominal, hindpaw, and proximal tail skin within a month of OVX surgery. Compared to control groups, the OVX group showed significantly greater numbers of referred visceral pain behaviors following intracolonic capsaicin (including abdominal licking, stretching, squashing, and retractions). This shift in pain sensitivity was reversed with 17β-estradiol replacement. A potential mechanism for this model involves serotonin, which is implicated in the descending inhibitory modulation of pain [48].

Parturition

One of the most commonly encountered forms of visceral pain occurs during labor, when the lower uterus and cervix are stretched and sometimes even torn to permit passage of the offspring. A rat model of parturition pain found that pain behaviors observed in the 1.5 hr preceding birth are similar to behaviors outlined in other animal models of visceral pain [49]. Rats in labor displayed frequent abdominal straining and squashing and an inward turning of the hindpaw, and the rate of these behaviors increased proportionately with labor duration. Systemic oxytocin (10 μg/kg) reduced the labor duration and increased the rate of pain behaviors, which were reduced with epidural morphine (30 ug/10 μL).

Yeast-Induced Sensitization to Touch (YIST) Model

Provoked vulvar pain—involving somatic tissue—is the most common cause of dyspareunia, and yet the majority of existing animal models of pain conditions that cause dyspareunia in women are visceral. We have developed a method of testing vulvar mechanical sensitivity in order to evaluate a mouse model of PVD. The testing method is an adaptation of the classic von Frey [50] psychophysical test and involves stimulation of mouse posterior vulvar tissue, located ventrally from the anogenital ridge, with calibrated nylon monofilaments (0.009–2.0 g). Mice display varying intensities of behavior in response to vulvar stimulation, including sniffing or licking of the vulva, body repositioning, or jumps. Because a rapid, full jump (all four paws off the ground) was the behavior most reliably elicited (albeit at high levels of applied force), we adopted this behavior as the criterion for an aversive response to mechanical stimulation.

Based on multiple reports that women with PVD are significantly more likely to have experienced recurrent vulvovaginal candidiasis (RVVC) [51–53], we developed a mouse model of provoked vulvar pain following three successive vulvovaginal infections with Candida albicans. For each infection, mice were vaginally inoculated with yeast, and four days following inoculation the infections were verified and eliminated with seven days of oral fluconazole. Following three weeks of consistently negative cultures from vaginal lavage fluid, mechanical sensitivity measurements were taken and compared to baseline measurements. After three yeast infections, significant differences in vulvar mechanical sensitivity were found between RVVC mice exposed to vulvovaginal yeast compared to fluconazole and saline controls. No changes in hindpaw mechanical sensitivity were found, indicating that increases in sensitivity were specific to the vulvar tissue exposed to yeast. We are hopeful that our model may allow an improved understanding of the mechanisms underlying provoked vulvar pain, as well as the development of novel treatments for clinical use.

Validity of Animal Models of Dyspareunia

As outlined in Table 30.2, the animal models we have reviewed do not meet the proposed criteria for

Table 30.2 Evaluation of the validity of behavioral outcome measures presented by model.

Pain Conditions	Behavior Specific to Condition?	Reliable	Frequently Observed?	Behavior Time Course	Related to Pathology?	Reversible with Analgesics?	Human Condition Modeled?
Ureteral calculosis	No	Yes	Varies between individuals	Onset in 1st day, reduces within 4 days	Unknown	Yes	Urinary calculosis (kidney stones)
Uterine inflammation	No	Yes	Varies between individuals	Onset in 2–4 days of mustard oil	No	N/A	Various uterine pathologies
Vaginal distension	Yes	Yes	Yes	Within sec of noxious distension	Yes, in case of endometriosis	N/A	Vaginal dyspareunia
Uterine distension	Sometimes	No	Varies	Within sec of noxious distension	Unknown	N/A	Unknown
Endometriosis	No	Yes	Yes	Abnormal sensitivity by 1–2 mo	Yes, behavior correlates with cyst growth	Yes	Endometriosis
Cystitis	No	Yes	Yes	Gradually increases in 1–4 hrs	Yes, behavior correlates with bladder inflammation	Yes	Cyclophosphamide-induced cystitis
Colitis	No	Yes	Yes	Onset within 1 hr, several days referred pain	No	Yes	Irritable bowel syndrome
Parturition	No	Yes	Yes	Onset 1.5 hr before birth	N/A	Yes	Labor pain
YIST model	Yes	Yes	Yes	Following three infections	Unknown	N/A	Yeast infection–induced provoked vulvar pain

accurately modeling clinical symptoms of dyspareunia and its associated disorders, as the visceral pain behaviors used in most models are not specific to any particular pain stimulus. Only vaginal distension and vulvar mechanical sensitivity behaviors are unique to a stimulus. Most models produce reliable and frequent pain behaviors, although much individual variation may exist [12, 17, 18].

Pain models vary from acute onset [18] to tonic inflammatory [17, 32] and chronic referred pain [44]. A correlation between behavior and physical pathology is largely absent, with the exception of endometriosis and cystitis models [24, 25, 31–33], and most models are reversible with known analgesics. Each of these models requires substantial development, including a refinement of

pain behavior patterns, improved understanding of corresponding physiological pathology, and identification of clinically relevant symptoms specific to dyspareunia.

References

1 Crawley JN. (2008) Behavioral phenotyping strategies for mutant mice. *Neuron* **57**, 809–18.

2 Pukall CF, Strigo IA, Binik YM, *et al.* (2005) Neural correlates of painful genital touch in women with vulvar vestibulitis syndrome. *Pain* **115**, 118–27.

3 Zimmermann M. (1986) Behavioral investigations of pain in animals. In: Duncan IJH, Molony Y (eds.) *Assessing Pain in Farm Animals.* Office for Official Publications of the European Communities, Bruxelles, pp. 16–29.

4 Le Bars D, Gozariu M, Cadden SW. (2001) Animal models of nociception. *Pharmacological Reviews* **53**, 597–652.

5 Mogil JS, Crager S. (2004) What should we be measuring in behavioral studies of chronic pain in animals? *Pain* **112**, 12–15.

6 Ness TJ, Gebhart GF. (1990) Visceral pain: a review of experimental studies. *Pain* **41**, 167–234.

7 Head H. (1893) On disturbances of sensation with special reference to the pain of visceral disease. *Brain* **16**, 1–133.

8 Gebhart GF. (2000) Pathobiology of visceral pain: molecular mechanisms and therapeutic implications, IV. Visceral afferent contributions the pathobiology of visceral pain. *American Journal of Physiology: Gastrointestinal and Liver Physiology* **278**, G834–38.

9 Bon K, Lichtensteiger CA, Wilson SG, *et al.* (2003) Characterization of cyclophosphamide cystitis, a model of visceral and referred pain, in the mouse: species and strain differences. *Journal of Urology* **170**, 1008–12.

10 Fillingim RB, Ness TJ. (2000) Sex-related hormonal influences on pain and analgesic responses. *Neuroscience and Biobehavioral Reviews* **24**, 485–501.

11 Mogil JS, Chanda ML. (2005) The case for the inclusion of female subjects in basic science studies of pain. *Pain* **117**, 1–5.

12 Giamberardino MA, Valente R, de Bigontina P, *et al.* (1995) Artificial ureteral calculosis in rats: behavioral characterization of visceral pain episodes and their relationship with referred lumbar muscle hyperalgesia. *Pain* **61**, 459–69.

13 Siegmund E, Cadmus R, Lu G. (1957) A method for evaluating both non-narcotic and narcotic analgesics. *Proceedings of the Society for Experimental Biology* **95**, 729–31.

14 Van der Wende C, Margolin S. (1956) Analgesic tests based upon experimentally induced acute abdominal pain in rats. *Federation Proceedings* **15**, 494.

15 Giamberardino MA, De Laurentis S, Affaitati G, *et al.* (2001) Modulation of pain and hyperalgesia from the urinary tract by algogenic conditions of the reproductive organs in women. *Neuroscience Letters* **304**, 61–64.

16 Giamberardino MA, Berkley KJ, Affaitati G, *et al.* (2002) Influence of endometriosis on pain behaviors and muscle hyperalgesia induced by a ureteral calculosis in female rats. *Pain* **95**, 247–57.

17 Wesselmann U, Czakanski PP, Affaitati G, *et al.* (1998) Uterine inflammation as a noxious visceral stimulus: behavioral characterization in the rat. *Neuroscience Letters* **246**, 73–76.

18 Berkley KJ, Wood E, Scofield SL, *et al.* (1995) Behavioral responses to uterine or vaginal distension in the rat. *Pain* **61**, 121–31.

19 Komisaruk BR, Whipple B. (2000) How does vaginal stimulation produce pleasure, pain and analgesia? In: Fillingim ERB (ed.) *Sex, Gender, and Pain. Progress in Pain Research and Management.* IASP Press, Seattle, pp. 109–34.

20 Bradshaw HB, Temple JL, Wood E, *et al.* (1999) Estrous variations in behavioral responses to vaginal and uterine distention in the rat. *Pain* **82**, 187–97.

21 Bradshaw HB, Berkley, KJ. (2002) Estrogen replacement reverses ovariectomy-induced vaginal hyperalgesia in the rat. *Maturitas* **41**, 157–65.

22 Evans S, Moalem-Taylor G, Tracey DJ. (2007) Pain and endometriosis. *Pain* **132**, S22–S25.

23 Sharpe-Timms KL. (2002) Using rats as a research model for the study of endometriosis. *Annals of the New York Academy of Sciences* **955**, 318–27.

24 Berkley KJ, Cason A, Jacobs H, *et al.* (2001) Vaginal hyperalgesia in a rat model of endometriosis. *Neuroscience Letters* **306**, 185–88.

25 Cason AM, Samuelson CL, Berkley KJ. (2003) Estrous changes in vaginal nociception in a rat model of endometriosis. *Hormones and Behavior* **44**, 123–31.

26 Pessina MA, Hoyt RF, Goldstein I, *et al.* (2006) Differential effects of estradiol, progesterone, and testosterone on vaginal structural integrity. *Endocrinology* **147**, 61–69.

27 Ting AY, Blacklock AD, Smith PG. (2004) Estrogen regulates vaginal sensory and autonomic nerve density in the rat. *Biology of Reproduction* **71**, 1397–1404.

28 Nagabukuro H, Berkley KJ. (2007) Influence of endometriosis on visceromotor and cardiovascular responses induced by vaginal distension in the rat. *Pain* **132**, S96–S103.

29 Berkley KJ, McAllister SL, Accius BE, *et al.* (2007) Endometriosis-induced vaginal hyperalgesia in the rat: effect of estropause, ovariectomy, and estradiol replacement. *Pain* **132**, S150–S159.

30 Bogart LM, Berry SH, Clemens JQ. (2007) Symptoms of interstitial cystitis, painful bladder syndrome, and similar diseases in women: a systematic review. *Journal of Urology* **177**, 450–56.

31 Lantéri-Minet M, Bon K, de Pommery J, *et al.* (1995) Cyclophosphamide cystitis as a model of visceral pain in rats: model elaboration and spinal structures involved as revealed by the expression of c-Fos and Krox-24 proteins. *Experimental Brain Research* **105**, 220–32.

32 Olivar T, Laird JMA. (1999) Cyclophosphamide cystitis in mice: behavioral characterization and correlation with bladder inflammation. *European Journal of Pain* **3**, 141–49.

33 Bon K, Lantéri-Minet M, Menétrey D, *et al.* (1997). Sex, time-of-day, and estrous variations in behavioral and bladder histological consequences of cyclophosphamide-induced cystitis in rats. *Pain* **73**, 423–29.

34 Wantuch C, Piesla M, Leventhal L. (2007) Pharmacological validation of a model of cystitis pain in the mouse. *Neuroscience Letters* **421**, 250–52.

35 Jaggar SI, Scott HCF, Rice ASC. (1999). Inflammation of the rat urinary bladder is associated with a referred thermal

hyperalgesia which is nerve growth factor dependent. *British Journal of Anaesthesia* **83**, 442–48.

36 Meen M, Coudore-Civiale MA, Eschalier A, *et al.* (2001) Involvement of hypogastric and pelvic nerves for conveying cystitis induced nociception in conscious rats. *Journal of Urology* **166**, 318–22.

37 Bjorling DE, Wang Z, Boldon K, *et al.* (2008) Bacterial cystitis is accompanied by increased peripheral thermal sensitivity in mice. *Journal of Urology* **179**, 759–63.

38 Tsan MF, Gao B. (2004) Endogenous ligands of Toll-like receptors. *American Journal of Physiology* **286**, C739–C744.

39 Wadachi R, Hargreaves KM. (2006) Trigeminal nociceptors express TLR-4 and CD14: a mechanism for pain due to infection. *Journal of Dental Research* **85**, 49–53.

40 Tanga FY, Nutile-McMenemy N, DeLeo JA. (2005). The CNS role of Toll-like receptor 4 in innate neuroimmunity and painful neuropathy. *PNAS* **102**, 5856–61.

41 Laird JMA, Martinez-Caro L, Garcia-Nicas E, *et al.* (2001) A new model of visceral pain and referred hyperalgesia in the mouse. *Pain* **92**, 335–42.

42 Al-Chaer ED, Kawasaki M, Pasricha PJ. (2000) A new model of chronic visceral hypersensitivity in adult rats induced by colon irritation during postnatal development. *Gastroenterology* **119**, 1276–85.

43 Bourdu S, Dapoigny M, Chapuy E, *et al.* (2005) Rectal instillation of butyrate provides a novel clinically relevant model of noninflammatory colonic hypersensitivity in rats. *Gastroenterology* **128**, 1996–2008.

44 Zhou Q, Price DD, Caudle RM, *et al.* (2008) Visceral and somatic hypersensitivity in a subset of rats following TNBS-induced colitis. *Pain* **134**, 9–15.

45 Verne GN, Robinson ME, Price DD. Hypersensitivity to visceral and cutaneous pain in the irritable bowel syndrome. *Pain* **93**, 7–14.

46 Sanoja R, Cervero F. (2005) Estrogen-dependent abdominal hyperalgesia induced by ovariectomy in adult mice: a model of functional abdominal pain. *Pain* **118**, 243–53.

47 Sanoja R, Cervero F. (2008) Estrogen modulation of ovariectomy-induced hyperalgesia in adult mice. *European Journal of Pain* **12**, 573–81.

48 Ito A, Takeda M, Furue H, *et al.* (2004) Administration of estrogen shortly after ovariectomy mimics the antinociceptive action and change in 5-HT_{1A}-like receptor expression induced by calcitonin in ovariectomized rats. *Bone* **35**, 697–703.

49 Catheline G, Touquet B, Besson JM, *et al.* (2006). Parturition in the rat: a physiological pain model. *Anesthesiology* **104**, 1257–65.

50 von Frey M. (1922) Zur physiologie der juckemfindung. *Archives Néerlandaises de Physiologie de l'Homme et des Animaux* **7**, 142–45.

51 Mann MS, Kaufman RH, Brown D, Adam E. (1992) Vulvar vestibulitis: significant variables and treatment outcome. *Obstetrics and Gynecology* **79**, 122–25.

52 Marinoff SC, Turner MLC. (1991) Vulvar vestibulitis syndrome: an overview. *American Journal of Obstetrics and Gynecology* **165**, 1228–33.

53 Pukall CF, Binik YM, Khalifé S, *et al.* (2002) Vestibular tactile and pain thresholds in women with vulvar vestibulitis syndrome. *Pain* **96**, 163–75.

CHAPTER 31

Psychological and Relational Aspects of Dyspareunia

Kelly B. Smith, Caroline F. Pukall, Stéphanie C. Boyer

Queen's University, Kingston, Ontario, Canada

Introduction

Paraphrased.

Dyspareunia, by definition, is pain that occurs during sexual intercourse, and, by its very nature, occurs in an intimate context. Women with dyspareunia often experience psychological distress and sexual difficulties, and partners may also be negatively impacted by the pain. This chapter examines sexual, relationship, and psychological factors associated with dyspareunia resulting from a variety of conditions, including provoked vestibulodynia (PVD), vulvodynia, vaginismus, interstitial cystitis (IC), endometriosis, and chronic pelvic pain (CPP). Although still preliminary, research in this area has increased substantially over the past decade and has provided some understanding of the links between dyspareunia and psychosocial functioning.

Sexual Aspects

One of the most investigated psychosocial aspects of dyspareunia is that of sexual functioning. Sexual intercourse is explicitly linked to the experience of pain among women with dyspareunia, and other sexual difficulties may develop as intercourse becomes associated with negative, rather than pleasurable, outcomes. In addition, women may anticipate the pain in intimate contexts, thereby reducing their ability to become aroused or experience enjoyment. Accordingly, several studies have

Female Sexual Pain Disorders 1st edition. Edited by A. Goldstein, C. Pukall & I. Goldstein. © 2009 Blackwell Publishing, ISBN: 9781405183987.

indicated that all components of the sexual response cycle are negatively affected by the pain. Women with dyspareunia experience lower levels of sexual desire, arousal, and satisfaction, less vaginal lubrication, and lower frequencies of sexual intercourse, orgasm, and masturbation in comparison to nonaffected women [1–4]. Also, recent surveys report that 80% of vulvodynia sufferers and 49% of women with IC indicate that the pain significantly and negatively affects their sexual functioning [5, 6].

Although prospective studies are lacking, the onset of pain during intercourse appears to be highly associated with altered sexual functioning. For example, 78% of women with PVD reported negative changes in sexual activity and satisfaction after pain onset, with most stating that they felt less able to participate in sexual activity [7]. In addition, compared to premorbid functioning, women with IC reported significant declines in level of sexual desire and frequency of orgasm [8]. The experience of pain may even lead some women to avoid or discontinue sexual activity [5, 9, 10]: in one sample, 90% of women with vulvodynia reported having to stop sexual activity at least once because of the pain, and 56% ceased penetrative activities altogether [5]. However, some women with dyspareunia continue to engage in intercourse for reasons that include feeling obligated to please their partners or experiencing emotional and physical pleasure from intimacy that outweighs the pain [11].

Women with dyspareunia also experience higher levels of erotophobia (feelings of guilt and fear related to sex) and more negative feelings toward sex as compared to women without such pain [1, 3, 7, 12]. Heightened fear of pain during sexual intercourse has also been documented in dyspareunia sufferers [8, 13]. Consistent with these findings, studies have found that women with dyspareunia are less likely to make sexual advances, more likely to refuse their partner's advances, and more likely to participate in sexual activity without wanting to do so [3, 7, 14, 15]. Affected women also are more likely to report feeling guilty or inadequate as a result of not being able to perform sexually and are less likely to feel relaxed or fulfilled after sexual activity [3, 7, 9, 14]. Not surprisingly, women with dyspareunia report less sexual satisfaction [15, 16] and perceive their partners to be more sexually dissatisfied in comparison to nonaffected women [15].

Relationship Aspects

Clinical reports make reference to the devastating impact that dyspareunia has on intimate relationships [17–20]. Despite having theoretical and intuitive draw, surprisingly little research has systematically examined the sexual relationships of women with dyspareunia. Of the existing research, evidence regarding decreased relationship adjustment is mixed: several studies have found no differences in relationship functioning between women with dyspareunia and control women [1, 12, 21–24], whereas others report less relationship satisfaction among affected women [15, 25].

Most women with PVD report that their intimate relationships have been impacted by the pain [26, 27]. Specifically, 40% reported severe and negative changes in their intimate relationships [7], and 77% reported fears that the pain would ruin their relationship [11]. These findings may be related to feelings, on the part of the women with dyspareunia, that their partners are less sexually satisfied [15, 28] and that they themselves are less sexually desirable to their partners [7]. In addition, pain severity and relationship adjustment appear to be differentially associated: Meana et al. [29] found that affected women who reported better relationship adjustment also reported less pain. The link between dyspareunia and relationship functioning is likely complex and moderated by several factors, many of which have yet to be investigated empirically.

Very little is known about the sexual and psychological characteristics of partners of women with dyspareunia. A recent study found no deficits with regards to self-reported erectile function or relationship satisfaction in male partners of women with vaginismus; this same study indicated that male partners also reported more

sexual and overall satisfaction in comparison to normative data [30]. Other research, however, has reported increased depression among partners of women with PVD, and feelings of helplessness, anger, and low mood among partners of women with endometriosis [26, 31]. To date, it is not known how partner-specific factors influence dyspareunia-affected couples, nor is it well understood how partner responses to the pain contribute to women's experiences with dyspareunia, or vice versa. However, recent evidence suggests that women who perceive their male partners to be more solicitous (i.e., more supportive or attentive) in response to the dyspareunia experience more intense pain during intercourse [32]; although seemingly paradoxical, this is consistent with findings from the general chronic pain literature.

While much of the reviewed research has focused on the negative relational impact of dyspareunia, one study found that the most frequently reported source of emotional support was an understanding partner [11]. Furthermore, a recent qualitative study of endometriosis-affected couples suggested a variety of ways that couples may adapt to the experience of chronic pain, some of which may serve to strengthen the relationship [33]. For example, couples may explore different ways to fulfill each partner's sexual needs or may develop a sense of humor in relation to challenges that arise.

Psychological Aspects

The effects of pain and dsypareunia can pervade many aspects of women's lives; dyspareunia has been linked to reduced quality of life and decreased emotional well-being [5, 7, 34–37]. Symptoms of psychological distress, in particular depression and anxiety, have also been found to be significantly higher in women with dyspareunia as compared with pain-free women [1, 7, 16, 26, 38–44]. Rates of clinical depression, however, are not necessarily heightened in women who experience painful intercourse [5, 38]. When certain dyspareunic conditions are compared, women with CPP report worse mental and physical well-being in comparison to those with vulvodynia [23, 45]. However, comparisons of multiple types of dyspareunia with regard to sexual and psychosocial functioning are needed.

Pain-related cognitions and behaviors may explain why some individuals experience increased distress when faced with pain [46], and, in turn, more severe or frequent pain may influence psychological functioning among women with dyspareunia. Meana et al. [47] found that women who attributed the cause of their dyspareunic pain to psychosocial (i.e., anxiety) versus physical factors experienced increased pain. Furthermore, women with PVD exhibit significantly higher pain catastrophizing and hypervigilance [48, 49] and demonstrate more defensive behaviors in painful situations than control women [50].

Chronic pain may also affect psychological functioning through its daily interference; this issue may be especially true of conditions such as endometriosis that involve persistent deep abdominal pain in addition to dyspareunia. Research has shown that endometriosis interferes significantly more with daily functioning as compared to chronic migraine pain [34] and as compared to other dyspareunia subtypes [37]. Indeed, feeling a lack of control over the pain due to its relentlessness may also contribute to worsened quality of life among women with dyspareunia; to this end, one study found that many affected women felt out of control of their bodies and lives [5]. Psychological functioning may also be reduced due to the negative impact of the pain on self-esteem, as research has found an association between vulvar pain and decreased self-concept and body image [3, 7, 11, 41].

Future Directions

Despite the fact that dyspareunia is often elicited by a partner in an intimate situation, little is known about relationship quality and partner functioning in affected couples. Controlled studies including qualitative, quantitative, and observational data would greatly contribute to the existing literature. In addition, an investigation of genital pain complaints in same-sex female couples may also reveal novel findings related to dyspareunia. For example, it may be that lesbians experience less dyspareunia-related sexual difficulties due to decreased focus on penetrative activities within their relationships. Finally, the systematic comparison of various dyspareunic conditions may indicate whether these conditions differ in terms of their specific psychosocial outcomes. Such research may help identify important areas for the assessment and management of dyspareunia, and, using rigorous and multifaceted methodologies, would improve our understanding of the psychosocial issues associated with the pain.

References

1 Meana M, Binik YM, Khalifé S, et al. (1997) Biopsychosocial profile of women with dyspareunia. Obstetrics and Gynecology 90, 583–89.
2 Ottem DP, Carr LK, Perks AE, et al. (2007) Interstitial cystitis and female sexual function. Urology 69, 608–10.
3 Reed BD, Advincula AP, Fonde KR, et al. (2003) Sexual activities and attitudes of women with vulvar dysesthesia. Obstetrics and Gynecology 102, 325–31.
4 Verit FF, Verit A, Yeni E. (2006) The prevalence of sexual dysfunction and associated risk factors in women with chronic pelvic pain: a cross-sectional study. Archives of Gynecology and Obstetrics 274, 297–302.
5 Arnold LD, Bachmann GA, Rosen RA, et al. (2006) Vulvodynia: characteristics and associations with comorbidities and quality of life. Obstetrics and Gynecology 107, 617–24.
6 Tincello DG, Walker ACH. (2005) Interstitial cystitis in the UK: results of a questionnaire survey of members of the Interstitial Cystitis Support Group. European Journal of Obstetrics and Gynecology 118, 91–95.
7 Sackett S, Gates E, Heckman-Stone C, et al. (2001) Psychosexual aspects of vulvar vestibulitis. The Journal of Reproductive Medicine 46, 593–98.
8 Peters KM, Killinger KA, Carrico DJ, et al. (2007) Sexual function and sexual distress in women with interstitial cystitis: a case-control study. Urology 70, 543–47.
9 Ferrero S, Esposito F, Abbamonte LH, et al. (2005) Quality of sex life in women with endometriosis and deep dyspareunia. Fertility and Sterility 83, 573–79.
10 Webster D. (1997) Recontextualizing sexuality in chronic illness: women and interstitial cystitis. Health Care for Women International 18, 575–70.
11 Gordon A, Panahian-Jand M, McComb F, et al. (2003) Characteristics of women with vulvar pain disorders: responses to a web-based survey. Journal of Sex and Marital Therapy 29, 45–58.
12 Reissing ED, Binik YM, Khalifé S, et al. (2003). Etiological correlates of vaginismus: sexual and physical abuse, sexual knowledge, sexual self-schema, and relationship adjustment. Journal of Sex and Marital Therapy 29, 47–59.
13 Smith KB, Pukall CF, Chamberlain S, et al. (Submitted) Pain-related anxiety and catastrophizing among women with provoked vestibulodynia.
14 Gates EA, Galask RP. (2001) Psychological and sexual functioning in women with vulvar vestibulitis. Journal of Psychosomatic Obstetrics and Gynecology 22, 221–28.
15 White G, Jantos M. (1998) Sexual behavior changes with vulvar vestibulitis syndrome. The Journal of Reproductive Medicine 43, 783–89.

16 Kaya B, Unal S, Ozenli Y, *et al.* (2006) Anxiety, depression and sexual dysfunction in women with chronic pelvic pain. *Sexual and Relationship Therapy* **21**, 187–96.

17 Graziottin A, Brotto LA. (2004) Vulvar vestibulitis syndrome: a clinical approach. *Journal of Sex and Marital Therapy* **30**, 125–39.

18 McCormick, NB. (1999) When pleasure causes pain: living with interstitial cystitis. *Sexuality and Disability* **17**, 7–17.

19 Baggish MS, Miklos JR. (1995) Vulvar pain syndrome: a review. *Obstetrical and Gynecological Survey* **50**, 618–27.

20 Davis HJ, Reissing ED. (2007) Relationship adjustment and dyadic interaction in couples with sexual pain disorders: a critical review of the literature. *Sexual and Relationship Therapy* **22**, 245–54.

21 Bornstein J, Zarfati D, Goldik Z, *et al.* (1999) Vulvar vestibulitis: physical or psychosexual problem? *Obstetrics and Gynecology* **93**, 876–80.

22 van Lankveld JJDM, Weijenborg PTM, ter Kuile MM. (1996) Psychologic profiles of and sexual function in women with vulvar vestibulitis and their partners. *Obstetrics and Gynecology* **88**, 65–70.

23 Reed BD, Haefner HK, Punch MR, *et al.* (2000) Psychosocial and sexual functioning in women with vulvodynia and chronic pelvic pain: a comparative evaluation. *The Journal of Reproductive Medicine* **45**, 624–632.

24 Schover LR, Youngs DD, Cannata R. (1992) Psychosexual aspects of the evaluation and management of vulvar vestibulitis. *American Journal of Obstetrics and Gynecology* **167**, 630–36.

25 Masheb RM, Brondolo E, Kerns RD. (2002) A multidimensional, case-control study of women with self-identified chronic vulvar pain. *Pain Medicine* **3**, 253–59.

26 Nylanderlundqvist E, Bergdahl J. (2003) Vulvar vestibulitis: evidence of depression and state anxiety in patients and partners. *Acta Dermato-Venereologica* **83**, 369–73.

27 Bergeron S, Binik YM, Khalifé S, *et al.* (2001) A randomized comparison of group cognitive-behavioral therapy, surface electromyographic biofeedback, and vestibulectomy in the treatment of dyspareunia resulting from vulvar vestibulitis. *Pain* **91**, 297–306.

28 Danielsson I, Sjoberg I, Wikman, M. (2000) Vulvar vestibulitis: medical, psychosexual, and psychosocial aspects, a case-control study. *Acta Obstetricia et Gynecologica Scandinavica* **79**, 872–78.

29 Meana M, Binik YM, Khalifé S, *et al.* (1998) Affect and marital adjustment in women's rating of dyspareunic pain. *Canadian Journal of Psychiatry* **43**, 381–85.

30 van Lankveld JJ, ter Kuile MM, de Groot HE, *et al.* (2006) Cognitive-behavioral therapy for women with lifelong vaginismus: a randomized waiting list–controlled trial of efficacy. *Journal of Consulting and Clinical Psychology* **74**, 168–78.

31 Fernandez I, Reid C, Dziurawiec S. (2006) Living with endometriosis: the perspective of male partners. *Journal of Psychosomatic Research* **61**, 433–38.

32 Desrosiers M, Bergeron S, Meana M, *et al.* (2008) Psychosexual characteristics of vestibulodynia couples: partner solicitousness and hostility are associated with pain. *The Journal of Sexual Medicine* **5**, 418–27.

33 Butt FS, Chesla C. (2007) Relational patterns of couples living with chronic pelvic pain from endometriosis. *Qualitative Health Research* **17**, 571–85.

34 Barnack JL, Chrisler, JC. (2007) The experience of chronic illness in women: a comparison between women with endometriosis and women with chronic migraine headaches. *Women and Health* **46**, 115–33.

35 Jones G, Jenkinson C, Kennedy S. (2004) The impact of endometriosis upon quality of life: a qualitative analysis. *Journal of Psychosomatic Obstetrics and Gynecology* **25**, 123–33.

36 Laumann EO, Paik A, Rosen RC. (1999) Sexual dysfunction in the United States: prevalence and predictors. *Journal of the American Medical Association* **281**, 537–44.

37 Mathias SD, Kuppermann M, Liberman RF, *et al.* (1996) Chronic pelvic pain: prevalence, health-related quality of life, and economic correlates. *Obstetrics and Gynecology* **87**, 321–27.

38 Aikens JE, Reed BD, Gorenflo DW, *et al.* (2003) Depressive symptoms among women with vulvar dysesthesia. *American Journal of Obstetrics and Gynecology* **189**, 462–66.

39 Wylie K, Hallam-Jones R, Harrington C. (2004) Psychological difficulties within a group of patients with vulvodynia. *Journal of Psychosomatic Obstetrics and Gynecology* **25**, 257–65.

40 Rabin C, O'Leary A, Neighbors C, *et al.* (2000) Pain and depression experienced by women with interstitial cystitis. *Women and Health* **31**, 67–81.

41 Granot M, Friedman M, Yarnitsky D, *et al.* (2002) Enhancement of the perception of systemic pain in women with vulvar vestibulitis. *British Journal of Obstetrics and Gynaecology* **109**, 863–66.

42 Granot M, Lavee Y. (2005) Psychological factors associated with perception of experimental pain in vulvar vestibulitis syndrome. *Journal of Sex and Marital Therapy* **31**, 285–302.

43 Nunns D, Mandal D. (1997) Psychological and psychosexual aspects of vulvar vestibulitis. *Genitourinary Medicine* **73**, 541–44.

44 Payne KA, Binik YM, Amsel R, *et al.* (2005) When sex hurts, anxiety and fear orient attention towards pain. *European Journal of Pain* **9**, 427–36.

45 Leserman J, Zolnoun D, Meltzer-Brody S, *et al.* (2006) Identification of diagnostic subtypes of chronic pelvic pain and how subtypes differ in health status and trauma history. *American Journal of Obstetrics and Gynecology* **195**, 554–61.

46 Keefe FJ, Lefebvre JC, Egert JR, *et al.* (2000) The relationship of gender to pain, pain behavior, and disability in osteoarthritis patients: the role of catastrophizing. *Pain* **87**, 325–34.

47 Meana M, Binik YM, Khalifé S, *et al.* (1999) Psychosocial correlates of pain attributions in women with dyspareunia. *Psychosomatics* **40**, 497–502.

48 Payne KA, Binik YM, Pukall CF, *et al.* (2007) Effects of sexual arousal on genital and nongenital sensation: a comparison of women with vulvar vestibulitis syndrome and healthy controls. *Archives of Sexual Behavior* **36**, 289–300.

49 Pukall CF, Binik YM, Khalifé S, *et al.* (2002) Vestibular tactile and pain thresholds in women with vulvar vestibulitis syndrome. *Pain* **96**, 163–75.

50 Reissing ED, Binik YM, Khalifé S, *et al.* (2004) Vaginal spasm, pain and behavior: an empirical investigation of the diagnosis of vaginismus. *Archives of Sexual Behavior* **33**, 5–17.

CHAPTER 32

Dyspareunia and Sexual/Physical Abuse

Barbara D. Reed

University of Michigan Health System, Ann Arbor, MI, USA

Introduction

Dyspareunia is a common complaint, affecting approximately 15% of women of all ages [1] and comprising a major symptom of women with many different genitourinary and pelvic conditions. Studies assessing women with dyspareunia in general may, in fact, include women with disparate or comorbid diagnoses [2]. For example, one study reported that 41% of chronic pelvic pain (CPP) patients reported dyspareunia [3].

Reports indicating a history of sexual abuse (SA) in women are also common; however, the prevalence varies depending on the population selection criteria, the definition of SA used, the periods of time assessed, the methods for obtaining the history selected, and the willingness of participants to report past abuse. Prevalence estimates range from 1.5% [4] to 27% [5], depending on the population studied and the methods used. A survey of over 500 women from a family practice clinic found that although 22.1% reported SA on the survey, only 2% had ever discussed this issue with a physician and 46% had told no one [6].

Although dyspareunia and SA are common, examining their link is challenging as dyspareunia may be associated with other conditions or exist in the absence of physical findings. Although one study failed to find an increased rate of SA history in women with dyspareunia complaints in general as well as in subgroups of these women compared to control women [2], studies examining SA

histories in women with CPP and other conditions have generally found such an association.

Sexual Abuse and CPP

CPP is a common condition, with one study indicating that the monthly prevalence and incidence rates of CPP to be 2.2% and 1.6%, respectively [7]. In large nonclinical populations, prevalence rates are higher (approximately 14–24%) [8, 9]. Many studies have been conducted to assess the relationship between SA and CPP. Although the characteristics and quality of the studies vary substantially (e.g., differing CPP and SA diagnoses, control group issues), most using univariate analyses report an increased risk of CPP among women with a history of SA, and those studies using multivariate analyses indicate a more complex relationship between abuse, psychological distress, and chronic pain. The assessment of the timing and severity of SA has only been recently added to the empirical literature in attempts to further clarify the characteristics of SA that may be associated with CPP.

Univariate analyses were used in most of the studies assessing the association between SA (and, in some cases, physical abuse [PA]) and CPP. Two reported on patients seeking general gynecologic care [10, 11], and although both found SA to be associated with CPP, one did not find an association between CPP and PA [10]. Several reports compared women with CPP to pain-free control women, and all except one [12] reported an increased history of SA among those with CPP compared to controls [13–17].

Patients with CPP were compared to another pain group and with pain-free control women in several studies using univariate analyses [18–23]. In five of the six studies,

Female Sexual Pain Disorders 1st edition. Edited by A. Goldstein, C. Pukall & I. Goldstein. © 2009 Blackwell Publishing, ISBN: 9781405183987.

SA was more commonly seen in the CPP group compared to the other chronic pain group and to the pain-free controls. Findings related to PA vary. Although Walling et al. [20] and Reed et al. [23] found PA to be associated with CPP compared to the other pain group and controls, no differences were found in another study [18]. Lampe et al. [21] found that PA differed between the two pain groups (which did not differ from each other) and the control group.

Despite proof of an association between SA and CPP, questions remain regarding whether this association is direct or related to confounding risk factors. Three studies used multivariate analyses to address the interrelationship of SA, PA, psychological outcomes, and CPP. Walling et al. [24] used multiple regression analysis to compare women with CPP, chronic headache, and pain-free control women. They found that SA was associated with depression, anxiety, and somatization, but this association disappeared when sociodemographic variables, chronic pain status, and childhood PA were taken into account. Alternatively, childhood PA predicted all three psychological variables (depression, anxiety, somatization) in this analysis. Poleshuck et al. [25] found that SA and PA were associated with psychological distress and anxiety among women with CPP, with PA also being associated with depression and somatization. However, in the multivariate analyses, PA, not SA, was independently associated with psychiatric outcomes.

Lampe et al. [26] modeled the relationship between SA, PA, depression, stressful life events, and chronic pain among women with CPP, low back pain, and pain-free controls. Severe childhood SA was associated with CPP (although childhood SA in general was not) and depression. Chronic pain was associated with childhood PA, stressful life events, and depression. Their model suggested that severe childhood SA was associated with chronic pain via its relationship to childhood PA, stressful life events, and depression, rather than via a direct relationship to chronic pain. These results suggest that the relationship between SA and chronic pain may be mediated by other variables (e.g., PA, depression).

Sexual Abuse and Irritable Bowel Syndrome (IBS)

IBS is a common cause of lower abdominal/pelvic pain, and due to marked symptom overlap, some suggest that

IBS and CPP are a single clinical syndrome [27]. Even when considered separately, women diagnosed with CPP often have IBS [28, 29]. In a large survey study, 30% of women with CPP reported also having been diagnosed with IBS [3].

Of patients with IBS, 40–58% report childhood or adulthood SA and PA [27]. Talley et al. [30] found that patients with IBS were more likely (43.1%) to report SA as compared with 19.4% of those without IBS, and later replicated these findings with respect to childhood SA only [31]. Further, Drossman [32] compared patients with IBS to those with inflammatory bowel disorder (IBD; a syndrome with similar symptoms, but with an organic diagnosis), and found rates of SA and/or PA of 53% among women with IBS compared to 36% of women with IBD. Similar findings were reported by Walker et al. [33].

Among patients with IBS, IBD, or other gastrointestinal (GI) disorders, those with IBS are more likely to report higher rates of childhood SA (37.9%) than those in the other two groups (9.1% and 11.6%) [34]. Creed et al. [35] found that among those with severe IBS symptoms who were undergoing psychological treatment, 12.1% reported a history of rape and 10.9% reported forced, unwanted touching. Those with a history of SA were more impaired on pain and physical functioning measures, but they were also more likely to improve with psychological treatments than those without such a history.

Some researchers have tested the belief that SA leads to increased rectal sensitivity to distention. Ringel et al. [36] assessed rectal distention pain thresholds in IBS patients and found that those with a history of severe SA had higher, rather than lower, thresholds for rectal pain and urge to defecate, disproving this theory. Guthrie et al. [37] attempted to identify subgroups of patients with severe IBS who were nonresponsive to conventional therapies based on measures of rectal sensitivity, psychological symptoms, and bowel symptoms. They found that SA history was associated with an increased number of doctor visits and psychiatric problems, interpersonal difficulties, and unemployment, but not with differences in sensitivity.

Leserman et al. [38] evaluated the severity of abuse and its relationship with outcomes among participants with GI symptoms. Of 239 women, 66.5% reported a history of SA and/or PA. Those with a history of SA had more pain, nongastrointestinal somatic symptoms, disability days, surgeries, psychiatric distress, and function disability;

similar findings were seen with PA. Age at first abuse and multiple versus single episodes were not associated with differences in outcomes.

Sexual Abuse and Urinary Symptoms

An increased prevalence of abuse has been reported among women with interstitial cystitis (IC) [39]. Peters et al. [40] surveyed 406 women diagnosed with IC and 5000 matched women and found that 49% of the clinic-based IC population reported a history of abuse (of these, 78% reported PA and 68% reported SA). Of 215 with IC, 121 with suspected IC, and 464 symptom-free controls surveyed by mail, all types of abuse (sexual, physical, and emotional) were increased in the IC groups (combined) compared to the pain-free controls (37% vs. 22%).

Sexual Abuse and Vulvodynia

Most studies examining the relationship between SA and vulvodynia have not indicated a positive association. Three studies have compared vulvodynia patients to controls and to a third group. Edwards et al. [41] found no difference in the incidence of childhood SA or PA among women with vulvodynia, other chronic vulvar diseases, and controls. Reed et al. [23] and Bodden-Heidrich et al. [22] compared patients with CPP, vulvodynia, and controls and found that women with vulvodynia were less likely to report SA than those with CPP.

Several studies compared women with and without vulvodynia, with four of the five finding no between-group difference in SA history. Three of these studies indicated no difference in either SA or PA [2, 42, 43], and one found no difference in SA (PA was not reported) [44]. The only study suggesting an association between vulvodynia and SA and PA was reported by Harlow and Stewart [45]. Results indicated that vulvodynia cases were more likely to report being sexually abused more than a few times as a child than control women (8.0% vs. 2.4%). Similarly, they were more likely to report severe PA as compared to controls (28.8% vs. 12.0%), although reports of moderate PA were similar in cases and controls (43.2% vs. 48.0%). However, SA and PA were not evaluated in a multivariate manner, and issues regarding the characteristics of the groups make conclusions regarding the contribution of each type of abuse unclear.

Sexual Abuse and Other Factors

It is important to note that a history of SA is associated with numerous medical and psychological problems. For example, a history of SA is associated with more medical problems (e.g., pelvic pain, breast disease), greater somatization, and more health risk behaviors (e.g., drug abuse) than among nonabused women, and the more severe the abuse (e.g., multiple abusers), the worse the associated problems [6]. In addition, some studies have indicated that SA is associated with other issues, including sexual problems, anxiety, depression, suicidal ideation, and sleeping disorders [46–48]. However, very few studies have addressed these associations in a multivariate or prospective manner; thus, it is difficult to determine which relationships might be causal and which are associated with other risk factors.

Theories on the Link Between Abuse and Pain

Several explanations have been offered to explain a link between a past history of SA and genitourinary/pelvic pain. Leserman et al. [38] described several potential mechanisms, including (i) a *methodological* perspective in which recall bias may amplify the relationship between abuse and disease, such that women who are more likely to remember abuse are also more likely to endorse psychological distress and illness behaviors; (ii) the *cognitive* perspective in which negative cognitions and ineffective coping styles may lead to maladaptive adjustment to illness, thereby increasing pain reporting and behaviors; and (iii) a *physiologic* perspective in which traumatic stimulation of the genitals might down-regulate the sensation thresholds of visceral nociceptors, thereby increasing sensitivity to abdominal/pelvic pain or other bowel symptoms [49].

Regarding pathophysiological explanations, an increase in noxious stimuli from the periphery can, over time, result in neuropathic changes and an upregulation of the spinal dorsal horn [50]. Fenton's hypothesis [51] builds upon recent knowledge of pain processes in the central nervous system (CNS) and of the limbic system in particular (the anterior cingulate cortex, hippocampus, and amygdala). Pain resulting from limbic dysfunction is characterized by an increased sensitivity to pain afferents from pelvic organs and abnormal efferent innervation of pelvic musculature (visceral and somatic) that creates a feedback loop between the pelvic musculature, the altered dorsal horn, and the hypervigilant limbic system. Disruption of this loop, and hence a decrease in pain, might occur by blocking afferent signals from pelvic organs via anesthesia, muscle manipulation, and/or disruption of limbic perception with psychiatric medication. Trauma from past SA might be one mechanism by which increased pain signals from the periphery, perhaps in combination with an increased susceptibility (genetic, neurologic, or other), may promote such a neuroplastic feedback loop.

Conclusions

Research on the associations between SA and dyspareunia-related disorders is fraught with methodological issues, and although the mechanisms by which SA might increase the probability of developing one or more other disorders are several, none have been identified empirically. Furthermore, despite the associations noted in some studies, it is important to keep in mind that many women with dyspareunia do not have a history of SA, and many of those abused do not develop dyspareunia-related disorders.

References

1 Laumann EO, Paik A, Rosen RC. (1999) Sexual dysfunction in the United States: prevalence and predictors. *The Journal of the American Medical Association* **281**, 537–44.

2 Meana M, Binik YM, Khalifé S, et al. (1997) Biopsychosocial profile of women with dyspareunia. *Obstetrics and Gynecology* **90**, 583–89.

3 Zondervan KT, Yudkin PL, Vessey MP, et al. (2001) Chronic pelvic pain in the community: symptoms, investigations, and diagnoses. *American Journal of Obstetrics and Gynecology* **184**, 1149–55.

4 Erickson PI, Rapkin AJ. (1991) Unwanted sexual experiences among middle and high school youth. *Journal of Adolescent Health* **12**, 319–25.

5 Finkelhor D, Hotaling G, Lewis IA, et al. (1990) Sexual abuse in a national survey of adult men and women: prevalence, characteristics, and risk factors. *Child Abuse and Neglect* **14**, 19–28.

6 Springs FE, Friedrich WN. (1992) Health risk behaviors and medical sequelae of childhood sexual abuse. *Mayo Clinic Proceedings* **67**, 527–32.

7 Zondervan KT, Yudkin PL, Vessey MP, et al. (1999) Prevalence and incidence of chronic pelvic pain in primary care: evidence from a national general practice database. *British Journal of Obstetrics and Gynaecology* **106**, 1149–55.

8 Mathias SD, Kuppermann M, Liberman RF, et al. (1996) Chronic pelvic pain: prevalence, health-related quality of life, and economic correlates. *Obstetrics and Gynecology* **87**, 321–27.

9 Zondervan KT, Yudkin PL, Vessey MP, et al. (2001) The community prevalence of chronic pelvic pain in women and associated illness behaviour. *The British Journal of General Practice* **51**, 541–47.

10 Hilden M, Schei B, Swahnberg K, et al. (2004) A history of sexual abuse and health: a Nordic multicentre study. *British Journal of Obstetrics and Gynecology* **111**, 1121–27.

11 Kirkengen AL, Schei B, Steine S. (1993) Indicators of childhood sexual abuse in gynaecological patients in a general practice. *Scandinavian Journal of Primary Health Care* **11**, 276–80.

12 Slocumb JC, Kellner R, Rosenfeld RC, et al. (1989) Anxiety and depression in patients with the abdominal pelvic pain syndrome. *General Hospital Psychiatry* **11**, 48–53.

13 Ehlert U, Heim C, Hellhammer DH. (1999) Chronic pelvic pain as a somatoform disorder. *Psychotherapy and Psychosomatics* **68**, 87–94.

14 Reiter RC. (1990) Occult somatic pathology in women with chronic pelvic pain. *Clinical Obstetrics and Gynecology* **33**, 154–60.

15 Walker EA, Katon W, Hanson J, et al. (1995) Psychiatric diagnosis and sexual victimization in women with chronic pelvic pain. *Psychosomatics* **36**, 531–40.

16 Walker E, Katon W, Harrop-Griffiths J, et al. (1988) Relationship of chronic pelvic pain to psychiatric diagnoses and childhood sexual abuse. *The American Journal of Psychiatry* **145**, 75–80.

17 Walker EA, Katon WJ, Neraas K, et al. (1992) Dissociation in women with chronic pelvic pain [see comments]. *American Journal of Psychiatry* **149**, 534–37.

18 Collett BJ, Cordle CJ, Stewart CR, et al. (1998) A comparative study of women with chronic pelvic pain, chronic nonpelvic pain, and those with no history of pain attending general practitioners. *British Journal of Obstetrics and Gynaecology* **105**, 87–92.

19 Rapkin AJ, Kames LD, Darke LL, et al. (1990) History of physical and sexual abuse in women with chronic pelvic pain. *Obstetrics and Gynecology* **76**, 92–96.

20 Walling MK, Reiter RC, O'Hara MW, et al. (1994) Abuse history and chronic pain in women: I. Prevalences of sexual abuse and physical abuse [see comments]. *Obstetrics and Gynecology* **84**, 193–99.

21 Lampe A, Solder E, Ennemoser A, et al. (2000) Chronic pelvic pain and previous sexual abuse. *Obstetrics and Gynecology* **96**, 929–33.

22 Bodden-Heidrich R, Kuppers V, Beckmann MW, et al. (1999) Chronic pelvic pain syndrome (CPPS) and chronic vulvar

pain syndrome (CVPS): evaluation of psychosomatic aspects. *Journal of Psychosomatic Obstetrics and Gynaecology* **20**, 145–51.

23 Reed BD, Haefner HK, Punch MR, *et al.* (2000) Psychosocial and sexual functioning in women with vulvodynia and chronic pelvic pain: a comparative evaluation. *The Journal of Reproductive Medicine* **45**, 624–32.

24 Walling MK, O'Hara MW, Reiter RC, *et al.* (1994) Abuse history and chronic pain in women: II. A multivariate analysis of abuse and psychological morbidity. *Obstetrics and Gynecology* **84**, 200–6.

25 Poleshuck E, Dworkin R, Howard F, *et al.* (2005) Contributions of physical and sexual abuse to women's experiences with chronic pelvic pain. *The Journal of Reproductive Medicine* **50**, 91–100.

26 Lampe A, Doering S, Rumpold G, *et al.* (2003) Chronic pain syndromes and their relation to childhood abuse and stressful life events. *Journal of Psychosomatic Research* **54**, 361–67.

27 Matheis A, Martens U, Kruse J, *et al.* (2007) Irritable bowel syndrome and chronic pelvic pain: a singular or two different clinical syndrome? *World Journal of Gastroenterology* **13**, 3446–55.

28 Williams RE, Hartmann KE, Sandler RS, *et al.* (2005) Recognition and treatment of irritable bowel syndrome among women with chronic pelvic pain. *American Journal of Obstetrics and Gynecology* **192**, 761–67.

29 Longstreth GF. (1994) Irritable bowel syndrome and chronic pelvic pain. *Obstetrical and Gynecological Survey* **49**, 505–7.

30 Talley NJ, Fett SL, Zinsmeister AR, *et al.* (1994) Gastrointestinal tract symptoms and self-reported abuse: a population-based study. *Gastroenterology* **107**, 1040–49.

31 Talley NJ, Boyce PM, Jones M. (1998) Is the association between irritable bowel syndrome and abuse explained by neuroticism? A population-based study. *Gut* **42**, 47–53.

32 Drossman DA. (1995) Sexual and physical abuse and gastrointestinal illness. *Scandinavian Journal of Gastroenterology Supplement* **208**, 90–96.

33 Walker EA, Gelfand AN, Gelfand MD, *et al.* (1995) Psychiatric diagnoses, sexual and physical victimization, and disability in patients with irritable bowel syndrome or inflammatory bowel disease. *Psychological Medicine* **25**, 1259–67.

34 Ross CA. (2005) Childhood sexual abuse and psychosomatic symptoms in irritable bowel syndrome. *Journal of Child Sex Abuse* **14**, 27–38.

35 Creed F, Guthrie E, Ratcliffe J, *et al.* (2005) Reported sexual abuse predicts impaired functioning but a good response to psychological treatments in patients with severe irritable bowel syndrome. *Psychosomatic Medicine* **67**, 490–99.

36 Ringel Y, Whitehead WE, Toner BB, *et al.* (2004) Sexual and physical abuse are not associated with rectal hypersensitivity in patients with irritable bowel syndrome. *Gut* **53**, 838–42.

37 Guthrie E, Creed F, Fernandes L, *et al.* (2003) Cluster analysis of symptoms and health seeking behaviour differentiates subgroups of patients with severe irritable bowel syndrome. *Gut* **52**, 1616–22.

38 Leserman J, Drossman DA, Li Z, *et al.* (1996) Sexual and physical abuse history in gastroenterology practice: How types of abuse impact health status. *Psychosomatic Medicine* **58**, 4–15.

39 Fenton BW, Durner C, Fanning J. (2008) Frequency and distribution of multiple diagnoses in chronic pelvic pain related to previous abuse or drug-seeking behavior. *Gynecologic and Obstetric Investigation* **65**, 247–51.

40 Peters KM, Kalinowski SE, Carrico DJ, *et al.* (2007) Fact or fiction: is abuse prevalent in patients with interstitial cystitis? Results from a community survey and clinic population. *The Journal of Urology* **178**, 891–95.

41 Edwards L, Mason M, Phillips M, *et al.* (1997) Childhood sexual and physical abuse: incidence in patients with vulvodynia. *The Journal of Reproductive Medicine* **42**, 135–39.

42 Dalton VK, Haefner HK, Reed BD, *et al.* (2002) Victimization in patients with vulvar dysesthesia/vestibulodynia: is there an increased prevalence? *The Journal of Reproductive Medicine* **47**, 829–34.

43 Plante AF, Kamm MA. (2008) Life events in patients with vulvodynia. *British Journal of Obstetrics and Gynecology* **115**, 509–14.

44 Edgardh K, Abdelnoor M. (2003) Longstanding vulval problems and entry dyspareunia among STD-clinic visitors in Oslo: results from a cross-sectional study. *International Journal of STD and AIDS* **14**, 796–99.

45 Harlow BL, Stewart EG. (2005) Adult-onset vulvodynia in relation to childhood violence victimization. *American Journal of Epidemiology* **161**, 871–80.

46 Bendixen M, Muus KM, Schei B. (1994) The impact of child sexual abuse: a study of a random sample of Norwegian students. *Child Abuse and Neglect* **18**, 837–47.

47 Randolph ME, Reddy DM. (2006) Sexual functioning in women with chronic pelvic pain: the impact of depression, support, and abuse. *The Journal of Sex Research* **43**, 38–45.

48 Bergmark K, Avall-Lundqvist E, Dickman PW, *et al.* (2005) Synergy between sexual abuse and cervical cancer in causing sexual dysfunction. *Journal of Sex and Marital Therapy* **31**, 361–83.

49 Mayer EA, Gebhart GF. (1994) Basic and clinical aspects of visceral hyperalgesia. *Gastroenterology* **107**, 271–93.

50 Butrick CW. (2003) Interstitial cystitis and chronic pelvic pain: new insights in neuropathology, diagnosis, and treatment. *Clinical Obstetrics and Gynecology* **46**, 811–23.

51 Fenton BW. (2007) Limbic-associated pelvic pain: a hypothesis to explain the diagnostic relationships and features of patients with chronic pelvic pain. *Medical Hypotheses* **69**, 282–86.

CHAPTER 33

Sexual Pain and Cancer

Don Dizon,[1] *Ann Partridge,*[2] *Alison Amsterdam,*[3]
Michael L. Krychman[4]

[1] Brown Medical School and Women and Infants, Hospital of Rhode Island, Providence, RI, USA
[2] Dana–Farber Cancer Institute, Boston, MA, USA
[3] Mount Sinai Medical Center, New York, NY, USA
[4] Hoag Hospital, Newport Beach, CA

Introduction

Sexual issues are common among female cancer survivors, and among them, pain is a frequent complaint. Such issues can result from the cancer diagnosis and/or from the multimodal treatments used in contemporary management of malignant disease. However, the detection of problems related to sexuality and intimacy must first start with a conversation. Unfortunately, this discussion is one that physicians rarely have with their patients.

In a recent study conducted at the University of Chicago, women who were long-time survivors of cervical or uterine cancer were four times as likely to have medical issues that interfered with sex compared with a healthy control group [1]. Over 60% of patients believed that their physician should initiate discussions related to sexuality, and 62% reported that they were not informed of the sexual side effects of treatment. Such research emphasizes the importance of open communication with cancer survivors.

This chapter outlines the necessary components of taking a sexual history, performing a physical examination, and conducting an objective evaluation in order to assess sexual function and dyspareunia in female cancer survivors. In addition, potential etiologies of and treatment avenues for sexual issues in female cancer patients are discussed.

Female Sexual Pain Disorders 1st edition. Edited by A. Goldstein,
C. Pukall & I. Goldstein. © 2009 Blackwell Publishing,
ISBN: 9781405183987.

How to Comprehensively Assess Sexual Function in Cancer Patients

Taking a Sexual History

The evaluation for sexual issues begins with a detailed medical history. The incorporation of several screening questions allows the patient to feel safe and protected about revealing very personal, and perhaps embarrassing, information. Open-ended questions may strategically elicit complaints related to sexual function (e.g., "Is there anything else you want to talk about?"), and more specific questions may also be helpful (e.g., "Are you having any problems with sexual arousal, desire, or orgasm?"). Inclusion of such questions on general intake forms is another way to offer patients the opportunity to discuss these topics.

Primary dyspareunia predates the diagnosis or treatment of cancer, while secondary dyspareunia occurs after cancer onset. It is important to elicit information regarding onset, duration, location, triggers, quality, characteristics, and associated symptoms of sexual pain (see Chapter 5). If symptoms existed prior to diagnosis or treatment for cancer, a search for other noncancer-related etiologies is important. For example, arthritis, uncontrolled diabetes, hyperglycemia, and underlying genital infections may all be associated with dyspareunia, and should be examined as possible explanations for pain that occurred prior to cancer diagnosis and treatment. In addition, if the history reveals prior sexual trauma such as rape or abuse, the utilization of mental or sexual health expertise may be required.

Symptoms can also develop after cancer onset; in particular, certain treatments (e.g., surgery, radiotherapy [RT], medications) can lead to dyspareunia in some patients. Specifically, for some patients, genital pain with light touch can often be encountered following radiation to the pelvis, breasts, or anogenital area. Pain with vaginal penetration can be due to prior pelvic surgery or pelvic radiation, while shortening of the vaginal vault and/or scarring can lead to a decrease in elasticity. In addition, chemotherapy and endocrine therapies, which cause ovarian failure, often lead to vaginal dryness.

A medication screen can also provide clues to the etiology of sexual dysfunction and/or pain. Most drug classes can affect the sexual response cycle and cause sexual problems; for example, antidepressants and antihypertensive medications can change sexual desire, arousal, and orgasm. In addition, decreases in arousal and desire can lead to decreased vaginal lubrication and vice versa, perhaps contributing to a vicious cycle of pain and sexual issues. Health care providers should consult sexual pharmacology resources (e.g., books, online resources) to help identify a potentially offending agent(s). Illicit drug use, alcohol consumption, and relationship functioning are also important aspects to assess, because they can impact sexual function.

With respect to assessing the sexual quality of the couple's relationship, many health care providers wrongly assume that their cancer patients are involved in heterosexual relationships. However, same-sex relationships are equally impacted by cancer. Health care providers should be sensitive to the sexual issues of all relationship types, and should be culturally aware and accepting of all individuals; as such, intake office forms should be generic and unassuming.

Physical Examination

A careful physical examination is also indicated for the evaluation of sexual complaints (see Chapter 4). For women, this includes a thorough vaginal and pelvic examination. Detailed examination of both external and internal genitalia is important. The vulva should be inspected for sores, lesions, fissures, or ulcerations. If palpation of the vestibule elicits pain, the diagnosis of provoked vestibulodynia (PVD; see Chapter 8) should be considered.

The examination should proceed with the insertion of a finger into the vaginal vault and attention to the tone of pelvic musculature. Often, penetration of the vault may

elicit involuntary contraction of the muscles, which can point toward a diagnosis of vaginismus (see Chapter 35). In addition, palpation of the urethra can be performed. If pain is elicited, urethritis should enter into the differential. A speculum exam provides direct visualization of the vaginal mucosa, cervical os, or vaginal cuff in the case of a patient with a prior hysterectomy. In addition, atrophy, dryness, and fissuring of the vaginal walls can be seen and evaluated, and areas of bleeding, nodularity or abnormal appearance should be noted. Patients with vaginismus may not tolerate a normal adult-sized speculum, which warrants the use of a pediatric speculum.

Finally, a bimanual exam is important to assess the pelvis and surrounding structures. Pain that is elicited with abdominopelvic palpation may point to an extra-vaginal etiology, such as endometriosis or adnexal lesion(s). Pain involving the rectovaginal septum may point towards adhesions or endometriosis. If the cul-de-sac appears full, fluid should be suspected and aspiration should be considered to rule out infection or malignancy. This examination, in combination with the patient's self-reported pain characteristics, can aid in determining etiology and treatment planning.

Objective Evaluation

Complete blood profile examinations should be conducted in order to rule out or confirm the involvement of other illnesses that can contribute to sexual issues. For example, a complete blood count can rule out underlying anemia as a cause of chronic fatigue. Furthermore, comprehensive tests of lipid profile, fasting glucose, prolactin levels, and thyroid function can be helpful to rule out endocrinopathies that may impact on sexual morbidity (but are less likely to cause dyspareunia).

Sexual Dysfunction in Cancer Patients

Sexual problems are common among cancer survivors. Reported rates of sexual dysfunction range widely due to the variety of cancer patient populations studied and methodologies utilized. For example, rates of sexual dysfunction among breast cancer survivors have been reported from 15% to 64% [2–8]. The etiology of sexual dysfunction in female cancer survivors is often multifactorial and can include consequences of the cancer, side effects of treatment, psychosocial issues resulting from cancer diagnosis and treatment, and/or other issues—all of which may contribute to difficulties with sexual functioning. Factors contributing to sexual dysfunction can be categorized into local and systemic issues, although there is substantial overlap among these factors.

Local Issues

Any cancer that directly affects sexual organs or the pelvis may cause sexual dysfunction. Cancers of the female reproductive tract are associated with risk of sexual dysfunction and pain, both locally and referred. Advanced cervical cancer, in particular, may invade the corpus uteri, parametrium, and/or pelvic sidewall causing bleeding and physical discomfort. Lower gastrointestinal malignancies (e.g., anorectal cancers) can also cause dyspareunia, as can local therapy for lower abdominal or pelvic region neoplasms.

Surgery can result in chronic nerve injuries and scarring in the region especially following colorectal procedures [9]. Radiation therapy to the pelvis, often utilized for cervical and anorectal cancers, is associated with decreased vaginal lubrication, scarring, and atrophy. Relative contributions of the cancer itself compared to the treatment are often not clear. For example, women undergoing radical hysterectomy for cervical cancer have significantly more problems with lubrication, sexual functioning, and decreased sexual activity compared with women undergoing hysterectomy for benign reasons [10]. This may be due to anatomic consequences from differences in surgical procedures, comorbid complications from the procedure, the psychological burden of a cancer diagnosis, or a combination of these and perhaps other factors.

Systemic Issues

Systemic therapy, including cytotoxic chemotherapy and hormonal therapy, is a substantial contributor to sexual dysfunction and pain in women with cancer. Abrupt ovarian dysfunction through chemotherapy, ovarian suppression medication, or removal/ablation of the ovaries, is associated with the greatest risk of sexual problems in young cancer survivors [11]. The resulting diminished estrogen production often causes decreased vaginal lubrication which may result in dyspareunia and, ultimately, atrophic vaginitis.

Ovarian suppression with gonadotropin-releasing hormone (GnRH) may also result in dyspareunia. An Internet-based evaluation of 371 breast cancer survivors

who had been diagnosed at age 40 or younger found that current ovarian suppression, postmenopausal status, anxiety, and receipt of chemotherapy were among the predictors associated with more bothersome menopausal symptoms [12]. Specifically, 48% of women receiving ovarian suppression experienced dyspareunia and 59% reported vaginal dryness. In addition, this study suggested that dyspareunia and vaginal dryness may be differentially associated with menopausal status and cancer-drug treatment. While dyspareunia was reported by 11% of premenopausal women not on tamoxifen and by 21% on tamoxifen, this pattern was reversed for postmenopausal women: more postmenopausal women (42%) *not* on tamoxifen reported moderate or severe dyspareunia compared to those postmenopausal women on tamoxifen (34%). A similar pattern was found for vaginal dryness.

In post menopausal women with breast cancer, aromatase inhibitors, which function by blocking the aromatization of androgens to estrogen, have been associated with near undetectable levels of estradiol and other estrogens. When GnRH analogs are used in conjunction with aromatase inhibitors, the same results are seen in premenopausal breast cancer patients. This lack of estrogen is associated with significant vaginal dryness and dyspareunia. However, tamoxifen (i.e., a selective estrogen receptor modulator) does not appear to cause vaginal dryness or dyspareunia as compared with other cancer treatment agents; instead, tamoxifen is associated with vaginal discharge, likely through its estrogen-agonist effect in the vagina and uterus. Nevertheless, tamoxifen has been associated with decreased libido.

A large randomized trial that investigated health-related quality of life among postmenopausal women with early-stage breast cancer taking either tamoxifen or anastrozole (i.e., an aromatase inhibitor) found no significant between-group differences in the Functional Assessment of Cancer Therapy for Breast Cancer measure at five years [13]. However, differences were found in patient-reported side effects. Patients receiving tamoxifen reported less vaginal dryness and dyspareunia, and higher levels of libido and vaginal discharge as compared to those taking anastrozole.

Dyspareunia related to vaginal atrophy is the most frequent sexual problem reported by young breast cancer survivors and appears to be a key factor in decreased sexual desire [11]. In a follow-up evaluation of 83 women treated by surgery or RT for cervical cancer, 40–50% reported fatigue, lack of energy, and weight gain at 97 weeks posttreatment [14]. Sixty percent had not resumed their full premorbid functional status. Mean scores for anxiety and depression were higher than those reported for the general population, and this sample scored higher for psychological distress than data quoted for disease-free cancer patients. Psychological distress scores were significantly correlated with physical complaints and functional outcomes.

For the 61 women who were sexually active, sexual function posttreatment was rated as significantly poorer than subjectively recalled premorbid sexual function. RT-treated patients were more likely to report dyspareunia and loss of sexual enjoyment than patients who received surgery, suggesting that the type of cancer treatment may influence sexual outcomes. Psychological and physical problems were highly correlated with sexual outcome. Furthermore, 44% of women reported they were unable to talk adequately with their partners about their experience. The majority of women felt that they needed more information about cervical cancer, its treatment, and how to help themselves rehabilitate, and 49% would have liked counseling. Fortunately, there is evidence that psycho-education interventions can improve sexual function in female cancer survivors [15, 16].

Treatment of Cancer-Related Sexual Pain in Women

Sexual assessment and counseling are not routinely provided in the oncology setting. Health care providers often lack experience in initiating conversations regarding sexual functioning, and patients may experience embarrassment with this sensitive subject [17]. One study indicated that almost 80% of gynecological malignancy patients wished to discuss sexual matters with their health care providers, but they avoided doing so out of fear of rejection [18]. If sexual concerns are discussed and physicians are unsure what to do, referral(s) to a sexual medicine clinic, sexual psychiatrist or psychologist, and/or other specialized professionals should be considered. A list of clinicians and ancillary staff who are sensitive to sexual issues should be readily available for cancer survivors with sexual concerns. In addition, since the etiology of sexual dysfunction is often complex and multidimensional, treatment

schemas should involve a multimodal approach, which frequently includes the patient's partner.

Multimodal Therapeutic Management

Cancer patients with sexual complaints are encouraged to make lifestyle changes. A well-balanced diet, aerobic exercise, discontinuation of tobacco and illicit drugs, and minimal alcohol consumption are all ways to improve general health and oxygenation of tissues. Good health increases metabolism, reduces body mass, and promotes central endorphin release, all of which can help alleviate some distress and symptoms.

In addition, general sex therapy techniques can be used with cancer patients who report sexual difficulties; of course, a number of special considerations must be made for fatigue and other issues that these patients face. For example, patients can be encouraged to take numerous naps and anticipate sexual contact or intimacy when well rested. An educational program should include open discussions concerning alternate forms of sexual expression (e.g., mutual massage).

Alternative sexual positions should be explained to the patient and her partner with illustrations and diagrams. The most common sexual position for heterosexual couples is the missionary position; this facilitates deep penetration but is often painful for women with a foreshortened vagina as a result of pelvic radiation, vaginal surgery, or severe atrophic vaginitis. Couples are encouraged to have sexual intercourse in other positions, including side-to-side or female superior positions. These sexual positions may minimize deep forceful pelvic thrusting, which can minimize vaginal discomfort during penetration and may enhance direct clitoral stimulation. For patients with mobility issues, pillows can be used to help facilitate a comfortable sexual situation.

Complaints of chronic discomfort or pain after cancer treatment can influence a woman's sexual response, and this discomfort will ultimately limit her desire and sexual enjoyment. Sexual health programs often incorporate techniques to help loosen tense muscles (e.g., warm soaks, genito-pelvic physical therapy programs). Other options include guided imagery, meditation, deep-muscle relaxation, and acupuncture. When appropriate, patients can be referred to local pain management specialists. Medication management may include adjusting or reducing opioid regimens, adding adjunctive or alternative analgesics, and modifying existing dosing schedules with the goal of increasing activity while maintaining satisfactory pain relief. In addition, the American Cancer Society's booklet entitled *Cancer and Sexuality* provides factual information and helpful suggestions for female cancer survivors and their partners.

Hormonal treatment, in particular local and systemic estrogen replacement, is commonly advised for female sexual complaints. Local treatments with minimally absorbed vaginal estrogen preparations, such as the 17β-estradiol tablet, have recently gained attention within the oncology community for the treatment of atrophic vaginitis, although large-scale safety studies are lacking. Patients have reported that the tablets are easier to use and less messy than cream preparations and are easier to insert than estrogen rings [19]. When vaginal (or systemic) estrogens are declined or not warranted, cancer survivors should be encouraged to use local nonmedicated, nonhormonal vaginal moisturizers or vitamin E suppositories. These agents, used two to three times weekly, can provide alternative relief for the symptoms of vaginal atrophy by maintaining the elasticity and pliability of the vaginal mucosal lining, which may decrease pain. In addition, the adjunctive use of water-based vaginal lubricants with intercourse should be encouraged. Patients should be educated regarding the irritating nature of preparations that include microbicides, perfumes, coloration, and flavors.

Unfortunately, for many cancer survivors, systemic hormonal treatment is neither warranted nor acceptable because of the increased risk of cancer. Bupropion (a dopamine agonist antidepressant medication with low sexual side effects) has been shown, in a small double blind, placebo-controlled trial, to increase sexual arousal, orgasm completion, and sexual satisfaction in women [20]. In order to manage sexual pain, graded vaginal dilators may be prescribed to help facilitate lengthening and widening of the vagina in patients with shortening, narrowing, and/or scarring. Dilators should be used on a regular basis, once daily for 10–15 min with water- or hormone-based lubricants. Clitoral stimulators can also be prescribed for patients with a history of cervical, rectal, and vaginal cancers. These sexual devices can be helpful for women who may require extra stimulation in the areas of the vagina and clitoris.

Because the approved pharmacological armamentarium is limited, many clinicians and cancer survivors have sought unconventional treatments for sexual problems. Foods such as chocolate, ginseng, oysters, and certain diet combinations have the lore of being able to facilitate improved sexual functioning. In addition, countless unregulated products on the market exist and may have detrimental side effects. Unfortunately, none have been shown in randomized clinical trials to be beneficial.

Palliative and terminal care of the female cancer patient may primarily be focused on self-image, dignity, pain, and stress management. Intimacy, sexuality, and relationship concerns remain under-researched and under-reported in the palliative care setting [21]. Providers need to reassure patients and their partners that, even at the end of life when intercourse may not be feasible, intimacy and emotional closeness are encouraged. The exchange of intimacy and sexual pleasure can be accomplished with sensual massage, oral and digital stimulation, and noncoital touching. Gentle caressing can also be very pleasurable and appropriate for use with patients at the end of their life.

Conclusions

Sexual difficulties and pain, during or following cancer therapy, are very complex and can compound an already stressful life event. The combination of anatomic, physiologic, and psychological changes following cancer treatment pose numerous challenges for health care providers. A comprehensive sexual medicine evaluation combined with sexual therapy techniques can promote healthy sexual functioning. Treatment plans should be individualized and implemented by a multidisciplinary sexual health care team, with the ultimate goal of restoring fulfilling and pleasurable sexual repertoires to cancer patients and their partners.

References

1 Lindau S, Gavrilova N, Anderson D. (2007) Sexual morbidity in very long term survivors of vaginal and cervical cancer: a comparison to national norms. *Gynecological Oncology* **106**, 413–18.

2 Kornblith AB, Ligibel J. (2003) Psychosocial and sexual functioning of survivors of breast cancer. *Seminars in Oncology* **30**, 799–813.

3 Ganz PA, Rowland JH, Desmond K, *et al.* (1998) Life after breast cancer: understanding women's health-related quality of life and sexual functioning. *Journal of Clinical Oncology* **16**, 501–14.

4 Meyerowitz BE, Desmond KA, Rowland JH, *et al.* (1999) Sexuality following breast cancer. *Journal of Sex and Marital Therapy* **25**, 237–50.

5 Friedlander M, Thewes B. (2003) Counting the costs of treatment: the reproductive and gynaecological consequences of adjuvant therapy in young women with breast cancer. *Internal Medicine Journal* **33**, 372–79.

6 Ganz PA, Kwan L, Stanton AL, *et al.* (2004) Quality of life at the end of primary treatment of breast cancer: first results from the moving beyond cancer randomized trial. *Journal of the National Cancer Institute* **96**, 376–87.

7 Stead ML. (2003) Sexual dysfunction after treatment for gynaecologic and breast malignancies. *Current Opinion in Obstetrics and Gynecology* **15**, 57–61.

8 Thors CL, Broeckel JA, Jacobsen PB. (2001) Sexual functioning in breast cancer survivors. *Cancer Control* **8**, 442–48.

9 Perera MT, Deen KI, Wijesuriya SR, *et al.* (2008) Sexual and urinary dysfunction following rectal dissection compared with segmental colectomy. *Colorectal Disease.*

10 Grumann M, Robertson R, Hacker NF, *et al.* (2001) Sexual functioning in patients following radical hysterectomy for stage IB cancer of the cervix. *International Journal of Gynecologic Cancer* **11**, 372–80.

11 Schover L. (2008) Premature ovarian failure and its consequences: vasomotor symptoms, sexuality, and fertility. *Journal of Clinical Oncology* **26**, 753–58.

12 Leining MG, Gelber S, Rosenberg R, *et al.* (2006) Menopausal-type symptoms in young breast cancer survivors. *Annals of Oncology* **17**, 1777–82.

13 Cella D, Fallowfield L, Barker P, *et al.* (2006) Quality of life of postmenopausal women in the ATAC ("Arimidex," tamoxifen, alone or in combination) trial after completion of 5 years' adjuvant treatment for early breast cancer. *Breast Cancer Research and Treatment* **100**, 273–84.

14 Cull A, Cowie VJ, Farquharson DI, *et al.* (1993) Early stage cervical cancer: psychosocial and sexual outcomes of treatment. *British Journal of Cancer* **68**, 1216–20.

15 Ganz PA, Greendale GA, Petersen L, *et al.* (2000) Managing menopausal symptoms in breast cancer survivors: results of a randomized controlled trial. *Journal of the National Cancer Institute* **92**, 1054–64.

16 Brotto L, Heiman J, Goff B, *et al.* (2008) A psychoeducational intervention for sexual dysfunction in women with gynecologic cancer. *Archives of Sexual Behavior* **37**, 317–19.

17 Auchincloss and McCartney. (1998) Gynecologic cancer. In: Holland, J. (ed.). *Psych-oncology*, pp. 359–70, Oxford University Press, New York.

18 Casey C. (1996) Psychosexual morbidity following gynecological malignancy. *Irish Medical Journal* **89**, 200–2.

19 Rioux JE, Devlin MC, Gelfand MM, *et al.* (2000) 17β-estradiol vaginal tablet versus conjugated equine estrogen vaginal cream to relieve menopausal atrophic vaginitis. *Menopause* **7**, 156–61.

20 Segraves R, Clayton A, Croft H, *et al.* (2004) Bupropion sustained release for the treatment of hypoactive desire disorder in premenopausal women. *Journal of Clinical Psychopharmacology* **24**, 339–42.

21 Stausmire JM. (2004) Sexuality at the end of life. *American Journal of Hospital Palliative Care* **21**, 33–39.

CHAPTER 34

Postpartum Dyspareunia

Colin MacNeill, Matthew F. Davies, John T. Repke

Penn State University, College of Medicine, Hershey, PA, USA

Introduction

Childbirth has a significant impact on sexual function. The number of women potentially affected is large, as approximately four million women give birth in the United States each year. The median time to resume intercourse after childbirth is 6–7 weeks; however, approximately half of the women who resume intercourse at this time experience pain, and by one year postpartum a substantial number of women continue to report pain [1].

Not all parturients carry the same risk of short-term and prolonged painful intercourse, although surprisingly, complete avoidance of vulvovaginal trauma by means of cesarean delivery does not reduce this risk completely [2]. Several routine obstetrical practices have been found to increase the risk of perineal trauma and subsequent prolonged dyspareunia, and programs instituted to systematically reduce trauma by modifying these practices have been found to be effective. Similarly, techniques aimed at preparing the perineum for childbirth have been found helpful in reducing the extent of trauma and subsequent pain [3]. Fortunately, dyspareunia resolves with time in most women, and in those with persistent pain, several interventions have been found effective in reducing pain.

In this review, we describe dyspareunia after uncomplicated, operative, and complicated vaginal deliveries, as well as cesarean deliveries. Evaluation of time course, nature, and location of postpartum dyspareunia and studies focusing on reducing recurrence are presented. We also review therapies for managing postpartum dyspareunia.

Female Sexual Pain Disorders 1st edition. Edited by A. Goldstein, C. Pukall & I. Goldstein. © 2009 Blackwell Publishing, ISBN: 9781405183987.

Postpartum Pain in Relationship to Perineal Trauma

Sexual problems, including dyspareunia and decreased libido, are reported by up to 53% of women in the immediate postpartum period, and peak at 3 months after delivery [4]. Surprisingly, Signorello et al. [1] found that 12% of first-time mothers who sustained third- or fourth-degree trauma reported improved sexual satisfaction at 6 months. These findings lead one to ask: What is the contribution of perineal trauma to sexual pain? In the past, the effect of episiotomy or laceration on dyspareunia had been open to interpretation, as most studies suffered from methodological issues related to patient selection and design (e.g., mixed degrees of perineal trauma). However, a study comparing vaginal deliveries to cesarean sections without labor reported that although women who had a cesarean birth were less likely to have urinary incontinence and perineal pain than those who delivered vaginally, there was no difference in dyspareunia rate [5].

Signorello and colleagues were among the first to provide a detailed report of the relationship between sexual function and well-defined perineal trauma in a cohort study of primiparous women at distinct postpartum time-points [1]. Patients were grouped at three trauma levels: (i) no trauma or first-degree laceration extending through the vaginal mucosa or perineal skin only; (ii) second-degree tear extending into the perineal muscles as a result of a nonextending episiotomy or laceration, and (iii) third-degree laceration involving the external anal sphincter or fourth-degree tear involving both the sphincter muscle and the anorectal mucosa as a result of either an extending episiotomy or spontaneous laceration. Results indicated that 58% of women with little or no trauma reported pain with first sexual intercourse; the percentage with pain remained relatively high at 3 and 6 months (33% and 18.6%, respectively).

As might be expected, higher degrees of trauma were associated with a greater frequency of dyspareunia. Signorello et al. found that at 3 months, 42% of those sustaining moderate trauma and 61% of those with high-degree trauma reported dyspareunia [1]. At 6 months, though, the rate of dyspareunia decreased to 24% and 27%, respectively, indicating that even dyspareunia associated with severe trauma improves with time. Given that dyspareunia persists in 18.6% of the intact group at 6 months postpartum (which could be considered the baseline rate of dyspareunia), it is reasonable to conclude that the proportion of pain attributable to high-degree perineal trauma is approximately 8%.

Regarding the mode of trauma (i.e., spontaneous tear vs. episiotomy), studies generally indicate that there is little difference in the rate of dyspareunia. Signorello et al. found no significant group differences at 3 and 6 months postpartum [1]. Similarly, Rockner and colleagues found no difference in dyspareunia between women who experienced second- or third-degree spontaneous perineal tears compared with those who underwent mediolateral episiotomy. In contrast, Larson and coworkers [6] found that 11% of women who experienced spontaneous tears reported dyspareunia, while 16% of those who underwent episiotomy reported dyspareunia at 2–3 months postpartum. More recently, Ejegard and colleagues [4] compared 110 primiparas who underwent episiotomy to 153 age-matched women who did not and found that women who underwent episiotomy reported a higher frequency of dyspareunia. In this study, women who sustained a spontaneous laceration also experienced dyspareunia at 12–18 months postpartum.

Few studies have directly compared the effect of different types of episiotomy on dyspareunia. Coats and colleagues conducted a randomized, prospective study comparing the consequences of midline and mediolateral episiotomies and found that patients' pain estimates were similar [7]. Similarly, Carolli et al. found comparable results for restrictive versus routine mediolateral versus midline episiotomy [5].

Spontaneous and assisted vaginal births have also been investigated. One study indicated that 7% of women who had a normal spontaneous vaginal birth reported a painful perineum, irrespective of episiotomy, compared with 30% of women after assisted vaginal birth [7]. Other studies have also found that after assisted vaginal birth, women have significantly more perineal pain [8]. Christianson et al. found that forceps-assisted deliveries and episiotomy also increased the rate of tears compared to noninstrumented deliveries and nonuse of episiotomy, respectively [8]. As well, this study found that nulliparous, compared to multiparous, patients were more likely to suffer a tear, suggesting that patients are less likely to suffer tears in subsequent deliveries.

Rarely, coccydynia can result from damage to the coccyx and surrounding soft tissue during childbirth [9, 10]. This pain is characterized by constant pain that is exacerbated by movement or pressure such as that brought on by sitting; it is associated with dyspareunia in 7% of cases [10].

Prevention

Conceivably, childbirth can occur without trauma, thereby preventing postpartum dyspareunia. Dyspareunia can occur, however, in the absence of observable trauma (e.g., nerve injury) or following cesarean delivery. In the latter case, the dyspareunia could be ascribed to a hypoestrogenic state as determined by vaginal pH or microscopic evaluation of a new mother who is sensitive to touch at the postpartum evaluation. Not all cases of dyspareunia can be prevented, however, as some women have dyspareunia before becoming pregnant. In the absence of other causes of vulvovaginal pain, these cases may be best conceptualized as vulvodynia [11].

Given that numerous studies indicate reduced perineal trauma with the selective use of episiotomy, it would seem that avoiding episiotomy might reduce the frequency of dyspareunia. However, when the outcome studied is dyspareunia rather than trauma, an increased rate of dyspareunia in those undergoing episiotomy has not been shown; thus, there is no evidence that avoiding episiotomy will reduce the risk of dyspareunia. Regarding methods that can aid in preventing episiotomy and, independently, dyspareunia, Beckmann's review [3] describes three studies reporting that perineal massage reduces the rate of trauma requiring suture, the use of episiotomy, and the rate of dyspareunia at 3 month follow-up. Given the low cost and safety of massage, it should be recommended as a preventative measure.

Selection of Repair Technique

Different suturing techniques have been developed in an attempt to reduce postpartum pain. Leeman et al. [12] compared nonsutured versus sutured lacerations or episiotomies, while Kettle et al. [13] and Morano et al. [14] compared interrupted to continuous running suture techniques. Nonsuturing did not reduce the incidence of dyspareunia compared to suturing [12]; in contrast, a continuous running technique led to conflicting results. Kettle et al. [13] found a decrease in postpartum dyspareunia, while Morano et al. [14] did not find changes in dyspareunia at 3 months. One study compared dyspareunia rates after one-year follow-up in which women were either repaired normally or had the deeper layers of an episiotomy or laceration repaired while the skin was left unsutured [15]. Results indicated a decrease in short-term postpartum dyspareunia with the latter technique.

Treatment

Localized Pain

Focal pain will often respond to locally applied therapies. One noninvasive measure, adapted from the vulvodynia literature, involves topical anesthetic [16]. Zolnoun and colleagues reported that overnight placement of a 5% lidocaine ointment-saturated cotton ball at the vestibule, a frequent site of dyspareunic pain, resulted in a significant decrease in pain. They found that after 7 weeks of nightly treatment, 76% of women were able to have intercourse when, prior to treatment only 36% were able to have intercourse.

Murina and colleagues [17] reported another method adapted from trigger-point injections. Working with 22 women reporting superficial dyspareunia, Murina et al. infiltrated the vestibule with a solution of methylprednisolone 40 mg/mL and lidocaine 10 mg/mL once a week for three weeks at decreasing doses (1, 0.5, 0.3 mL). Follow-up was carried out for a minimum of 9 months and in five of the subjects for 24 months. No side effects were reported at first follow-up. They found that 68% of the subjects responded favorably to the treatment, seven (32%) with absence of symptoms and eight (36%) with a marked improvement. Seven patients (32%) failed to respond in spite of a fourth dose (0.3 mL) given after 30 days. Among

responders, no relapse was observed at 9-month follow-up, while five subjects who experienced relapse at one year were given a 0.5 mL infiltration, which was followed by quick remission of symptoms. Five patients completed the 24 months' follow-up, with no need for further treatment. A substantial flaw in the study is the absence of a control group, particularly in disorders such as dyspareunia that are known to have a high spontaneous remission rate and a placebo response rate of 15–30%.

Generalized Pain

While NSAID and narcotic analgesics are often useful for vulvovaginal pain in the immediate postpartum period, these agents are generally found to be less effective in the longer term. Women in whom pain persists should undergo thorough physical evaluation, and those who are found to have microbial abnormalities or focal pain treated accordingly. Persistent postpartum dyspareunia without any identifiable cause can be treated much like generalized vulvodynia. The two most commonly used agents are the tricyclic antidepressants (e.g., amitriptyline) and gabapentin. Updike and Weisenfeld [18] surveyed vulvovaginal pain caregivers in the United States, and found the most frequently used medication for generalized vulvar pain was amitriptyline.

Physical Therapy, Ultrasound, and TENS Unit Therapy

Physical therapy is a common intervention for postpartum dyspareunia. Dyspareunia may be connected with musculoskeletal conditions such as coccydynia, sacroiliac joint dysfunction, and pubic sympholiasis. Episiotomy scarring may be treated with modalities including manual therapy and massage. Additional treatment possibilities include pelvic floor biofeedback, and manual therapy including scar friction massage and manual therapy [19]. Although transcutaneous electrical stimulation (TENS) is sometimes employed, there are currently no reported studies examining its use in postpartum pain.

In addition, deep ultrasound massage is believed to reduce pain via at least two mechanisms: (i) by decreasing the inflammatory process, and (ii) by reducing pressure on pain-sensitive tissue by aiding in local resolution of tissue edema and/or hematoma formation. Although Hay-Smith et al. performed a Cochrane Database Systematic Review of this topic [20] and found a statistically significant reduction in perineal pain, the overall consensus was that this technique does not decrease dyspareunia after vaginal delivery.

Anal Sphincter Tears

Patients may also suffer from an anal sphincter tear in their last pregnancy (partial or full third-degree tear, fourth-degree tear). Sheiner et al. [21] evaluated deliveries over 11 years and showed that forceps- and vacuum-assistance added to a statistically increased chance of anal sphincter injury. Further, Benavides et al. [22] have shown that occiput posterior versus anterior presentation further adds to this risk. Thus, a labor and delivery with spontaneous (nonassisted) vaginal delivery with the infant in an occiput anterior presentation may minimize the risk of tearing.

Conflicting data has been presented regarding the effect of mediolateral episiotomy on significant tears with involvement of the anal sphincter muscle. DeLeeuw et al. [23] documented that primiparity, occipitoposterior presentation, and increasing fetal weight are additional risk factors for anal-sphincter injury during operative vaginal delivery. In addition, they found that mediolateral episiotomy offered protection from anal sphincter injury for both vacuum- and forceps-assisted deliveries. In contrast to these findings, Hudelist et al. [24] found that only forceps with mediolateral episiotomy and high birth weight were significantly associated with anal sphincter injury.

Techniques to Minimize Trauma

Perineal massage may provide improved flexibility to contractile and noncontractile perineal structures to decrease trauma immediately and decrease dyspareunia long-term. Beckmann et al. [3] examined three studies on using massage prior to labor. They found that perineal massage for at least 4 weeks prior to delivery led to an overall reduction in the incidence of trauma requiring suturing, in the incidence of episiotomy being performed, and, for women who had already given birth, in the incidence of pain at 3 months postpartum [3]. Perineal massage has also been investigated during labor and delivery. Stamp et al. [25] randomized 1,340 women as they entered stage 2 of labor to massage versus no massage. There was no change in

incidence of intact perinea, first- or second-degree tears, or dyspareunia.

Conclusions

Postpartum dyspareunia is a common problem, with several factors influencing its risk. There appears to be little or no difference in long-term dyspareunia rates for mild or severe tears, whether they are spontaneous or from episiotomies and their extensions. Furthermore, midline (as opposed to mediolateral) episiotomies do not appear to decrease rates of postpartum dyspareunia. There is, however, evidence of heightened risk of dyspareunia from more severe versus mild tears. As much data has shown more severe tears in women undergoing episiotomy compared to restrictive use of episiotomy, minimizing the use of episiotomy when possible may help decrease postpartum dyspareunia. Data on actual clinical outcomes do not, however, corroborate this conclusion. Interventions that have negatively influenced the rate of postpartum dyspareunia include assisted delivery and delivery from an occiput posterior presentation. In contrast, practices that have decreased the short-term rate of postpartum dyspareunia include antepartum perineal massage. For those patients who present with postpartum dyspareunia or with concerns about avoiding recurrence with subsequent deliveries, the clinician must address these issues with a great deal of empathy as the impact on the existing relationship can be dramatic and the uncertainty of its course is almost certain.

References

1 Signorello LB, Harlow BL, Chekos AK, *et al.* (2001) Postpartum sexual functioning and its relationship to perineal trauma: a retrospective cohort study of primiparous women. *American Journal of Obstetrics and Gynecology* **184**, 881–90.

2 Barrett G, Peacock J, Victor CR, *et al.* (2005) Cesarean section and postnatal sexual health. *Birth* **32**, 306–11.

3 Beckmann MM, Garrett AJ. (2006) Antenatal perineal massage for reducing perineal trauma. *The Cochrane Database of Systematic Reviews* CD005123.

4 Ejegard H, Ryding EL, Sjogren B. (2008) Sexuality after delivery with episiotomy: a long-term follow-up. *Gynecologic and Obstetric Investigation* **66**, 1–7.

5 Carroli G, Belizan J. (2000) Episiotomy for vaginal birth. *The Cochrane Database of Systematic Reviews* CD000081.

6 Larsson PG, Platz-Christensen JJ, Bergman B, *et al.* (1991) Advantage or disadvantage of episiotomy compared with spontaneous perineal laceration. *Gynecologic and Obstetric Investigation* **31**, 213–16.

7 Coats PM, Chan KK, Wilkins M, *et al.* (1980) A comparison between midline and mediolateral episiotomies. *British Journal of Obstetrics and Gynaecology* **87**, 408–12.

8 Christianson LM, Bovbjerg VE, McDavitt EC, *et al.* (2003) Risk factors for perineal injury during delivery. *American Journal of Obstetrics and Gynecology* **189**, 255–60.

9 Kaushal R, Bhanot A, Luthra S, *et al.* (2005) Intrapartum coccygeal fracture, a cause for postpartum coccydynia: A case report. *Journal of Surgical Orthopaedic Advances* **14**, 136–37.

10 Peyton FW. (1988) Coccygodynia in women. *Indiana Medicine* **81**, 697–98.

11 MacNeill C. (2006) Dyspareunia. *Obstetrics and Gynecology Clinics of North America* **33**, 565–77.

12 Leeman LM, Rogers RG, Greulich B, *et al.* (2007) Do unsutured second-degree perineal lacerations affect postpartum functional outcomes? *The Journal of the American Board of Family Medicine* **20**, 451–57.

13 Kettle C, Hills RK, Ismail KM. (2007) Continuous versus interrupted sutures for repair of episiotomy or second-degree tears. *The Cochrane Database of Systematic Reviews* CD000947.

14 Morano S, Mistrangelo E, Pastorino D, *et al.* (2006) A randomized comparison of suturing techniques for episiotomy and laceration repair after spontaneous vaginal birth. *Journal of Minimally Invasive Gynecology* **13**, 457–62.

15 Grant A, Gordon B, Mackrodat C, *et al.* (2001) The Ipswich childbirth study: one-year follow up of alternative methods used in perineal repair. *British Journal of Obstetrics and Gynecology* **108**, 34–40.

16 Zolnoun DA, Hartmann KE, Steege JF. (2003) Overnight 5% lidocaine ointment for treatment of vulvar vestibulitis. *Obstetrics and Gynecology* **102**, 84–87.

17 Murina F, Tassan P, Roberti P, *et al.* (2001) Treatment of vulvar vestibulitis with submucous infiltrations of methylprednisolone and lidocaine: an alternative approach. *The Journal of Reproductive Medicine* **46**, 713–16.

18 Updike GM, Wiesenfeld HC. (2005) Insight into the treatment of vulvar pain: a survey of clinicians. *American Journal of Obstetrics and Gynecology* **193**, 1404–9.

19 Rosenbaum TY. (2007) Physiotherapy treatment of sexual pain disorders. *The Journal of Sexual Medicine* **31**, 329–40.

20 Hay-Smith EJ. (2000) Therapeutic ultrasound for postpartum perineal pain and dyspareunia. *The Cochrane Database of Systematic Reviews* CD000495.

21 Sheiner E, Levy A, Walfisch A, *et al.* (2005) Third-degree perineal tears in a university medical center where midline episiotomies are not performed. *Archives of Gynecology and Obstetrics* **271**, 307–10.

22 Benavides L, Wu JM, Hundley AF, *et al.* (2005) The impact of occiput posterior fetal head position on the risk of anal sphincter injury in forceps-assisted vaginal deliveries. *American Journal of Obstetrics and Gynecology* **192**, 1702–6.

23 de Leeuw JW, de Wit C, Kuijken JP, *et al.* (2008) Mediolateral episiotomy reduces the risk for anal sphincter injury during operative vaginal delivery. *British Journal of Obstetrics and Gynaecology* **115**, 104–8.

24 Hudelist G, Gelle'n J, Singer C, *et al.* (2005) Factors predicting severe perineal trauma during childbirth: role of forceps delivery routinely combined with mediolateral episiotomy. *American Journal of Obstetrics and Gynecology* **192**, 875–81.

25 Stamp G, Kruzins G, Crowther C. (2001) Perineal massage in labour and prevention of perineal trauma: randomised controlled trial. *British Medical Journal* **322**, 1277–80.

CHAPTER 35
Vaginismus: Evaluation and Management

Elke D. Reissing

University of Ottawa, Ottawa, Ontario, Canada

Introduction

Vaginismus is defined in the DSM IV-TR as an "*involuntary contraction of the musculature of the outer third of the vagina interfering with intercourse, causing distress and interpersonal difficulty*" [1]. This definition has received considerable criticism recently and there is no empirical basis for the vaginal spasm taxon [2]. An international consensus committee has suggested revised criteria, recommending that vaginismus be defined as "*persistent difficulties to allow vaginal entry of a penis, a finger, and/or any object, despite the woman's expressed wish to do so. There is variable involuntary pelvic muscle contraction, (phobic) avoidance and anticipation/fear/experience of pain. Structural or other physical abnormalities must be ruled out/addressed*" [3]. While more in line with the clinical presentation and available research on vaginismus, these criteria still require systematic empirical support.

· Definitional problems make it difficult to reliably estimate the prevalence of vaginismus [4], and no epidemiologically sound incidence or prevalence estimates are available [5]. Clinics and other sources [6–9] suggest referral rates ranging from 5–17%.

Vaginismus: Symptom of Dyspareunia or Diagnostic Entity?

Some researchers argue that vaginismus and dyspareunia may be impossible to differentiate because vaginal penetration problems are not specific to vaginismus but fre-

Female Sexual Pain Disorders 1st edition. Edited by A. Goldstein,
C. Pukall & I. Goldstein. © 2009 Blackwell Publishing,
ISBN: 9781405183987.

quently present as a symptom of dyspareunia [10–12]. In particular, provoked vestibulodynia (PVD) has been consistently implicated as a cause of vaginismus or complicating treatment [13–15] and, conversely, pelvic floor pathology interfering with vaginal penetration has been reported as a key symptom in virtually all women with vulvo-vaginal pain [10, 16, 17]. It is not uncommon to receive clinical referrals for a woman with vulvar pain and "some" vaginismus or "partial" vaginismus [12]. Prevalence rates may be much higher when the term *vaginismus* is used clinically to indicate pelvic floor tension.

Clinical Use of the Term *Vaginismus*

Despite a recent increase in research attention, consensus on the definition of *vaginismus* and an empirical framework for research and clinical practice are lacking. The body of literature has recently been called "virginal" [18] and is considered difficult to interpret and to generalize [4, 19]. Therefore, the current state of our knowledge of vaginismus warrants the inclusion of an explicit description of the definition [14]. The following criteria may be useful for summarizing the key symptoms.

(i) Vaginal penetration is impossible in all/the majority of attempts because of vaginal and/or pelvic muscle hypertonicity and/or muscle guarding at the entrance to the vagina.

(ii) Vaginal penetration is avoided for all/the majority of opportunities because of recurrent or chronic vulvar, vaginal, or pelvic pain.

(iii) Vaginal penetration is avoided for all/the majority of opportunities because of associated, significant anxiety and/or panic, and may be accompanied by feelings of disgust, dread, and/or fear.

Etiology

In early writings, vaginismus was conceptualized as a defense mechanism toward unresolved psychosexual conflicts in early childhood [20]. Over the past three decades, a general consensus of vaginismus as a psychophysiological problem has emerged. Various causal hypotheses exist, but none has received systematic research attention or consistent empirical support [18, 19].

Pain and fear of pain figure prominently in past and recent reports on etiology, but it has not been established whether pain is cause or consequence of vaginismus [2, 17]. Numerous organic causes for pain have been reported in the literature, for example, hymeneal abnormalities, vaginal atrophy, PVD, endometriosis, infections, vaginal lesions, and sexually transmitted diseases [21–25]. Few of these problems have received research attention. However, PVD has consistently been reported as a cause for vaginal penetration problems for many women [11, 13, 15].

A lack of or inaccurate/incomplete sex education and education biased by conservative religious beliefs have been implicated in the development of negative expectations, fears, and sexual guilt related to sexuality, vaginal intercourse, and reproductive anatomy [26]. Clinical and research reports indicate that women with vaginismus hold negative views about sexuality, in particular premarital sexual activity [22], report being brought up to believe that sex was wrong [27], and hold irrational beliefs that penetration will cause pain, injury and bleeding, and fear their vagina is too small [28].

Anxiety is increasingly considered a key factor in vaginismus [4, 17]. Negative, inaccurate, or false beliefs can result in fear and anxiety and behavioral avoidance. Display of anxiety and fear during pelvic exams and avoidance of intercourse have been noted as the only differentiating symptoms in women with vaginismus and PVD [2, 11]. It has been suggested that vaginismus may be an adaptive anticopulation defense that is "overactive" in some women who otherwise desire intercourse [29]. The development of the fear and avoidance associated with vaginismus may be similar to specific phobias that occur without negative learning events but hold evolutionary relevance [30]. In addition, women with lifelong vaginismus also report an elevated number of additional fears and phobias [26, 31, 32] and indirect evidence for the role of anxiety in vaginismus is also highlighted by the fact that nearly all published

accounts on the treatment of vaginismus include the use of anxiety reduction measures [7, 6, 31, 33, 34], and anxiolytic medication has been reported to facilitate therapy [35–37].

Sexual abuse (SA) has often been cited as a cause for vaginismus. However, in most studies with control groups, no significant differences in prevalence in SA were noted [6, 8, 22]. Only one controlled study found women with vaginismus reported a significantly higher rate of childhood SA ranging from exposure to sexual touching [38]. Although most women with SA histories do not develop vaginismus, such experiences should be assessed. Male partner or relationship factors have historically been noted as causing and/or exacerbating vaginismus; however, little research has been conducted on this topic [39]. It has been suggested that male partners may be chosen for their passive and nonthreatening personality traits or may suffer from their own sexual dysfunction. The couple thus colludes in the avoidance of intercourse and/or the maintenance of emotional balance between partners [14]. No research exists at this point supporting Masters and Johnson's [33] original report of male sexual dysfunction as the most frequent etiological factor. However, erectile dysfunction and premature ejaculation appear to be transient problems for some men following successful treatment of their female partners for vaginismus [6, 8, 9].

The current state of the literature does not point to a definite etiology for vaginismus. However, the use of the following heuristic highlighting cognitive, behavioral, and physiological factors when assessing and treating vaginal penetration problems may be helpful (see Figure 35.1). Following this model, an experience with pain, or a negative experience with or negative expectations about vaginal penetration, is associated with catastrophizing thinking. These thoughts, in turn, result in specific fears about penetration and pain associated with intercourse [40].

To cope, a woman may chose to avoid all activity related to vaginal penetration or be hypervigilant during attempts. The latter can result in an exaggerated attention to physical sensations and psychological arousal facilitating the labeling of these sensations as pain and/or fear and panic. The occasional attempt at vaginal penetration is met with a defensive pelvic floor contraction similar to flinching. Increased tonus results in painful or impossible attempts at intercourse. Not being able to "achieve"

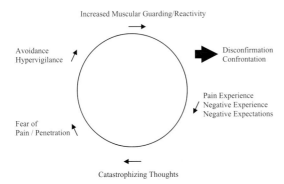

Increased Muscular Guarding/Reactivity

Avoidance
Hypervigilance

Disconfirmation
Confrontation

Pain Experience
Negative Experience
Negative Expectations

Fear of
Pain / Penetration

Catastrophizing Thoughts

Figure 35.1 The vicious cycle of vaginismus.

penetration in turn can contribute to negative experiences and confirm negative expectations. The result is maintenance and exacerbation of the "vicious cycle of vaginismus." The obvious end to this cycle is a disconfirmation and/or confrontation of fears and expectations. All elements of the vicious cycle have received some empirical support, but more research is crucial in understanding the mechanism by which these factors relate in causing a woman to develop vaginismus.

Treatment

Treatment approaches for vaginismus have primarily targeted the perceived immediate cause: the putative muscle spasm that interferes with intercourse [33, 41]. The central treatment component tends to be vaginal dilation combined with progressive desensitization and various relaxation techniques. However, a number of additional components typically make up the standard treatment protocol:

(i) Information and education intended to enhance accurate knowledge and positive beliefs about sexuality and genital anatomy.

(ii) Elimination of psychological problems, such as fear of pain and negative body or genital image via psychotherapeutic or sex therapy interventions.

(iii) Couple therapy interventions to increase communication, trust, and understanding as well as sensate focus exercises to enhance nonpenetrative sexual activities and to work gradually toward intercourse [9, 19].

A number of adjunct treatment components have also been reported in the clinical literature: educational

gynecological examinations [14], anxiolytic medication [37], hypnotherapy [42], biofeedback [8, 43], local injections of botulinum toxin [44], surgical interventions to enlarge the vaginal introitus or removal of the hymen [45], and application of topical anesthetic creams [46].

Treatment outcome for vaginismus is generally believed to be excellent [19, 23]. However, most treatment outcome reports are uncontrolled clinical studies with unspecified populations, poor design or unspecified treatment components, inadequate evaluation and outcome measures, little or no follow-up, and limited or absent statistical evaluation. At this point, the treatment of vaginismus cannot be considered "well-established" or "probably efficacious" [47], and a recent Cochrane review concluded that, despite encouraging results on the basis of uncontrolled case studies, there is very limited evidence for the effectiveness of treatments for vaginismus from controlled trials [48].

Recently, however, a well-designed, randomized controlled treatment outcome study (RCT) was conducted by Lankveld and his colleagues, and modest effectiveness of the typical combination of treatment components for vaginismus was confirmed [34]. Immediately following treatment, only 14% of women were able to experience vaginal penetration (vs. none in the control group). The researchers proceeded to examine process and prognostic factors of treatment. Successful outcome was mediated by changes in fear of intercourse and avoidance behaviors [49]. The researchers conducted a smaller treatment study to determine whether direct exposure aimed at decreasing penetration fears and avoidance behaviors would be effective in treating vaginismus. Indeed, 90% of women with lifelong vaginismus were able to experience intercourse after just two exposure sessions, and results were maintained at the 1-year follow-up [50].

Until there exists more consistent evidence for effective treatment of vaginismus from well-designed treatment outcome studies, an individualized treatment approach is necessary [14]. An educational gynecological examination is recommended to rule out or address organic factors [9]. If the client is not able to tolerate an examination, it can be postponed to a later point in therapy, for example, after learning relaxation techniques.

A thorough clinical assessment can have significant therapeutic effects. To organize the assessment and to assist the development of a treatment plan, the following steps may be helpful. First, the clinician may want to use the criteria outlined above to summarize the presenting complaint to determine what interferes with vaginal penetration (i.e., pelvic floor pathology, [fear of] pain, and/or anxiety). Second, the clinician may work with the client collaboratively to examine in detail what specific factors play a role in her "vicious cycle of vaginismus" (see Figure 35.1). In the author's experience, this exploration serves as an invaluable educational tool and provides a rationale for treatment; this, in turn, increases the credibility of and motivation for treatment.

Following the educational assessment using the "vicious cycle of vaginismus" model, the clinician may be able to prioritize therapeutic interventions. Pelvic floor pathology requires progressive desensitization to allow the woman to stay relaxed, both in mind and body, during penetration with increasingly larger sized dilators and/or more fingers. Fears and the resulting behavioral avoidance or hypervigilance are best addressed with cognitive-behavioral therapy.

Particular attention needs to be paid to absent, faulty, or incomplete sex education as the source of negative beliefs with regard to sexuality and genital anatomy. General sex education and specific education with regard to intercourse will also decrease anticipatory anxiety and prepare the woman and her partner for initial attempts at vaginal penetration. Sex therapy and couple therapy may be necessary depending on concerns about sexual response, pleasure, and couple functioning or if these factors may potentially interfere with treatment success.

Motivation to challenge and confront vaginal penetration fears is crucial for women with vaginismus because behavioral avoidance is often present for many years [2]. For some women, it is motivating to set a complete gynecological examination as her first therapy goal. This goal is considered to be more conservative, involves a medical imperative, and is an achievement "just for her." For other women, the desire for a baby can be a significant motivator. It has been suggested that artificial insemination may be an appropriate solution for women with vaginismus [51]. However, the number of pelvic examinations associated with pregnancy and labor may be sources for significant anxiety and/or pain. In addition, negative experiences and pain with pelvic examinations may potentially exacerbate vaginismus. An open discussion of the motivation for treatment and appropriate goal-setting are essential in order to assure reasonable length and success of treatment.

Summary

Vaginismus has long been a neglected woman's health problem. Currently, definitional problems complicate an examination of the research literature as well as effective assessment and management strategies. Yet, much has been gleaned from research thus far and more can undoubtedly be expected in the near future. Currently, an individualized approach at assessment and treatment are necessary to identify *what interferes* with vaginal penetration and *what maintains* the problem ("the vicious cycle of vaginismus"). Recent evidence suggests that treatment may be most effective when directly and specifically targeting fear and anxiety associated with vaginal penetration and when confronting behavioral avoidance of intercourse.

References

1 American Psychiatric Association. (2000) *Diagnostic and Statistical Manual of Mental Disorders*. 4th ed. Washington, DC.

2 Reissing ED, Binik YM, Khalifé S, *et al*. (2004) Vaginal spasm, behavior and pain: an empirical investigation of the diagnosis of vaginismus. *Archives of Sexual Behavior* **33**, 5–17.

3 Basson R, Leiblum S, Brotto L, *et al*. (2004) Revised definitions of women's sexual dysfunction. *The Journal of Sexual Medicine* **1**, 40–49.

4 Meston CM, Bradford A. (2007) Sexual dysfunctions in women. *Annual Review of Clinical Psychology* **3**, 233–56.

5 Spector IP, Carey MP. (1990) Incidence and prevalence of the sexual dysfunctions: a critical review of the empirical literature. *Archives of Sexual Behavior* **19**, 389–408.

6 Hawton K, Catalan J. (1990) Sex therapy for vaginismus: characteristics of couples and treatment outcome. *Sex and Marital Therapy* **5**, 39–48.

7 Schmidt G, Arentewicz G. (1982) Symptoms. In: Arentewicz G, Schmidt G (eds.), *The Treatment of Sexual Disorders: Concepts and Techniques of Couple Therapy*. Basic Books, New York, pp. 123–46.

8 Barnes J. (1986) Primary vaginismus (part 1): social and clinical features (part 2): aetiological features. *Irish Medical Journal* **79**, 59–65.

9 Crowley T, Richardson D, Goldmeier D. (2006) Recommendations for the management of vaginismus: BASHH Special Interest Group for Sexual Dysfunction. *International Journal of STD and AIDS* **17**, 14–18.

10 Binik YM, Bergeron S, Khalifé S. (2007) Dyspareunia and vaginismus: so-called sexual pain. In: Leiblum SR (ed.), *Principles and Practice of Sex Therapy*, 4th ed. Guilford Press, New York, pp. 124–56.

11 de Kruiff ME, ter Kuile MM, Weijenborg PT, *et al.* (2000) Vaginismus and dyspareunia: is there a difference in clinical presentation? *Journal of Psychosomatic Obstetrics and Gynecology* 21, 149–55.

12 Engman M, Lindehammar H, Wijma B. (2004) Surface electromyography diagnostics in women with partial vaginismus with or without vulvar vestibulitis and asymptomatic women. *Journal of Psychosomatic Obstetrics and Gynecology* 25, 281–94.

13 Har-Toov J, Militscher I, Lessing JB, *et al.* (2001) Combined vulvar vestibulitis syndrome with vaginismus: which to treat first? *Journal of Sex and Marital Therapy* 27, 521–23.

14 Weijmar Schultz WCM, van de Wiel HBM. (2005) Vaginismus. In: Balon R, Segraves RT (eds.), *Handbook of Sexual Dysfunction.* Taylor & Francis, New York, pp. 273–92.

15 Ter Kuile MM, Van Lankveld JJ, Vlieland CV, *et al.* (2005) Vulvar vestibulitis syndrome: An important factor in the evaluation of lifelong vaginismus? *Journal of Psychosomatic Obstetrics and Gynecology* 26, 245–49.

16 Reissing ED, Brown C, Lord MJ, *et al.* (2005) Pelvic floor function in women with vulvar vestibulitis syndrome. *Journal of Psychosomatic Obstetrics and Gynecology* 26, 107–13.

17 Weijmar Schultz W, Basson R, Binik Y, *et al.* (2005) Women's sexual pain and its management. *The Journal of Sexual Medicine* 2, 301–16.

18 Wijma B, Engman E, Wijma K. (2007) A model for critical review of literature, with vaginismus as an example. *Journal of Psychosomatic Obstetrics and Gynecology* 28, 21–36.

19 Reissing ED, Binik YM, Khalifé S. (1999) Does vaginismus exist? A critical review of the literature. *Journal of Nervous and Mental Disease* 187, 261–74.

20 Abraham HC. (1956) Therapeutic and psychological approach to cases of unconsummated marriage. *British Medical Journal* 1, 837–39.

21 Abramov L, Wolman I, Higgins MP. (1994) Vaginismus: an important factor in the evaluation and management of vulvar vestibulitis syndrome. *Gynecologic and Obstetric Investigation* 38, 194–97.

22 Basson R. (1996) Lifelong vaginismus: a clinical study of 60 consecutive cases. *Journal of the Society of Gynecologists and Obstetricians of Canada* 3, 551–61.

23 Beck JG. (1993) Vaginismus. In: O'Donohue W, Greer JH (eds.), *Handbook of Sexual Dysfunctions: Assessment and Treatment.* Allyn & Bacon, Boston, pp. 381–97.

24 Lamont JA. (1978) Vaginismus. *American Journal of Obstetrics and Gynecology* 131, 632–36.

25 Stuntz RC. (1986) Physical obstructions to coitus in women. *Medical Aspects of Human Sexuality* 20, 126–34.

26 Silverstein JL. (1989) Origins of psychogenic vaginismus. *Psychotherapy and Psychosomatics* 52, 197–204.

27 Ward E, Ogden E. (1994) Experiencing vaginismus: sufferers' beliefs about causes and effects. *Sex and Marital Therapy* 9, 33–45.

28 Reissing ED. (2008) Results of a web survey on causal hypotheses and help-seeking behavior in women with lifelong and acquired vaginismus. (Manuscript in preparation.)

29 Miller G. Vaginismus as an adaptive anticopulation defense. *HBES 2005: Human Behavior and Evolution Society Conference*, Austin, TX.

30 Poulton R, Menzies RG. (2002) Nonassociative fear acquisition: a review of the evidence from retrospective and longitudinal research. *Behavior Research and Therapy* 40, 127–49.

31 Kabakçi E, Batur S. (2003) Who benefits from cognitive-behavioral therapy for vaginismus? *Journal of Sex and Marital Therapy* 29, 277–88.

32 Reissing ED. (2006) Pain, fear, and avoidance: why a woman's body says no to sex. Paper presented at the *67th Annual Conference of the Canadian Psychological Association*, June 2006. Calgary, Canada.

33 Masters WH, Johnson VE. (1970) *Human Sexual Inadequacy.* Little, Brown and Company, Boston.

34 van Lankveld JJDM, ter Kuile MM, de Groot HE, *et al.* (2006) Cognitive-behavioral therapy for women with lifelong vaginismus: a randomized waiting-list controlled trial of efficacy. *Journal of Consulting and Clinical Psychology* 74, 168–78.

35 Kaplan HS, Fyer AJ, Novick A. (1982) The treatment of sexual phobias: the combined use of antipanic medication and sex therapy. *Journal of Sex and Marital Therapy* 8, 3–28.

36 Mikhail AR. (1976) Treatment of vaginismus by I.V. diazepam (Valium®) abreaction interviews. *Acta Psychiatrica Scandinavica* 53, 328–32.

37 Plaut SM, RachBeisel J. (1997) Use of anxiolytic medication in the treatment of vaginismus and severe aversion to penetration: case report. *Journal of Sex Education and Therapy* 22, 43–45.

38 Reissing ED, Binik YM, Khalifé S, *et al.* (2003) Etiological correlates of vaginismus: sexual and physical abuse, sexual knowledge, sexual self-schema, and relationship adjustment. *Journal of Sex and Marital Therapy* 29, 47–59.

39 Davis HJ, Reissing ED. (2007) Relationship adjustment and dyadic interaction in couples with sexual pain disorders: a critical review of the literature. *Sexual and Relationship Therapy* 2, 245–54.

40 Vlaeyen JW, Linton SJ. (2000) Fear-avoidance and its consequences in chronic musculoskeletal pain: a state of the art. *Pain* 85, 317–32.

41 Leiblum SR. (2000) Vaginismus: a most perplexing problem. In: Leiblum SR, Rosen RC (eds.), *Principles and Practice of Sex Therapy*, 3rd ed. Guilford Press, New York, pp. 181–202.

42 Araoz DL. (1982) Hypnosis and sex therapy. In: Arentewicz G, Schmidt G (eds.), *The Treatment of Sexual Disorders: Concepts and Techniques of Couple Therapy*. Basic Books: New York.

43 Seo JT, Choe JH, Lee WS, *et al.* (2005) Efficacy of functional electrical stimulation–biofeedback with sexual cognitive-behavioral therapy as treatment of vaginismus. *Urology* **66**, 77–81.

44 Brin MF, Vapnek JM. (1997) Treatment of vaginismus with botulinum toxin injections. *Lancet* **349**, 252–53.

45 Addar MH. (2004) The unconsummated marriage: causes and management. *Clinical and Experimental Obstetrics and Gynecology* **16**, 279–81.

46 Praharaj SK, Verma P, Arora M. (2006) Topical lignocaine for vaginismus: a case report. *International Journal of Impotence Research* **18**, 568–69.

47 Heiman JR, Meston CM. (1997) Empirically validated treatment for sexual dysfunction. *Annual Review of Sex Research* **8**, 148–95.

48 McGuire H, Hawton K. (2002) Interventions for vaginismus (Cochrane Review). In: *The Cochrane Library*. Oxford: Update Software.

49 ter Kuile MM, van Lankveld JJDM, de Groot E, *et al.* (2007) Cognitive-behavioral therapy for women with lifelong vaginismus: process and prognostic factors. *Behavior Research and Therapy* **45**, 359–73.

50 ter Kuile MM, Bulté I, Weijenborg PTM, *et al.* (in press) Therapist-aided exposure for women with lifelong vaginismus: a replicated single-case design. *Journal of Consulting and Clinical Psychology*.

51 Drenth JJ, Andriessen S, Heringa MP, *et al.* (1996) Connections between primary vaginismus and procreation: some observations from the clinical practice. *Journal of Psychosomatic Obstetrics and Gynecology* **17**, 195–201.

CHAPTER 36
Female Genital Cutting

Crista Johnson

Maricopa Integrated Health System, Southwest Interdisciplinary Research Center, Arizona State University, Phoenix, AZ, USA

Introduction

Female genital cutting (FGC) is an ancient tradition dating to as early as 200 B.C. in the pharaonic era of Ancient Egypt [1]. The origins are cultural rather than religious as it is practiced by Muslims, Christians, and Jews [2] and is not restricted to a particular ethnic group or religious sect. There are various customary beliefs surrounding the practice of FGC, including a rite of passage into womanhood, ensuring social acceptance and marriageability, preserving virginity, and protecting a woman's family honor. The endurance of the tradition rests in the fact that FGC defines and protects a woman's livelihood and future as a wife and mother. In these societies, circumcision is done out of love, and not circumcising one's daughter is equivalent to condemning her to a life of isolation [3]. This chapter reviews the types, epidemiology, and sequelae of FGC and offers information relevant to its surgical management, the need for culturally competent care, and rigorous research.

Types of FGC

The World Health Organization (WHO) has defined various types of FGC (Table 36.1). Type I, also known as clitoridectomy, involves partial or total removal of the clitoris and/or the prepuce. Type II (i.e., excision) consists of the partial or total removal of the clitoris and the labia minora, with or without excision of the labia majora. Type III, or infibulation, is the most extreme form of FGC. It involves the narrowing of the vaginal orifice with

Female Sexual Pain Disorders 1st edition. Edited by A. Goldstein, C. Pukall & I. Goldstein. © 2009 Blackwell Publishing, ISBN: 9781405183987.

creation of a covering seal by cutting and appositioning the labia minora and/or labia majora, with or without excision of the clitoris [4]. Type IV, which will not be further discussed, consists of all other harmful procedures (e.g., pricking) performed in the female genitalia for nonmedical purposes.

It is important to note that most studies examining FGC have relied on women's self-reports of FGC status. Studies that include clinical assessments have documented large variations in the level of agreement between self-reported descriptions and clinically observed types of FGC [5]. Furthermore, the reliability of clinical observation can be limited by natural anatomical variations and difficulty in estimating the amount of clitoral tissue under an infibulation [4].

Epidemiology

WHO estimates that 100–140 million women worldwide have undergone FGC [6]. The most recent prevalence data indicates that approximately 91.5 million females above 9 years of age in Africa are currently living with the consequences of FGC [7], with an estimated 3 million at risk of undergoing FGC every year [8]. Types I, II, and III have been documented in 28 countries in Sub-Saharan Africa, and in some countries throughout Southeast Asia and the Middle East. Some forms of FGC have also been reported in other countries, including Central and South America [4]. Eighty-five percent of all forms of FGC are type I/II, whereas 15% are type III. However, recent immigration and refugee resettlement from countries where type III FGC predominates (e.g., Somalia) have resulted in a rapid surge of females with this type throughout North America and Europe.

Table 36.1 2007 WHO Classification [8].

Type	Definition
I	Partial or total removal of the clitoris and/or the prepuce (*clitoridectomy*) *Type Ia*: removal of the clitoral hood or prepuce only *Type Ib*: removal of the clitoris with the prepuce
II	Partial or total removal of the clitoris and the labia minora, with or without excision of the labia majora (*excision*) *Type IIa*: removal of the labia minora only *Type IIb*: partial or total removal of the clitoris and the labia minora *Type IIc*: partial or total removal of the clitoris, the labia minora, and the labia majora
III	Narrowing of the vaginal orifice with creation of a covering seal by cutting and appositioning the labia minora and/or the labia majora, with or without excision of the clitoris (*infibulation*) *Type IIIa*: removal and apposition of the labia minora *Type IIIb*: removal and apposition of the labia majora
IV	Unclassified: All other harmful procedures to the female genitalia for nonmedical purposes, (i.e., pricking, piercing, incising, scraping, and cauterization)

FGC has achieved global attention due to the increasing influx of immigrants and refugees to Europe and North America, and has been the subject of increasing legislation worldwide [9]. Educational campaigns against FGC have led to a significant decline in its prevalence over the last 25 years, although support for its continuation varies widely between and within countries.

Sequelae of FGC

Medical Outcomes

Women who have undergone FGC can suffer short- and long-term complications. The range of short-term complications is rarely seen in Western countries, and may include shock, hemorrhage, infection, tetanus, urinary retention and/or oliguria, injury to adjacent structures, sepsis, and death [10–13]. The long-term complications mainly pertain to type III FGC and include epidermal inclusions cysts, keloids, dysmenorrhea, dyspareunia, apareunia (i.e., no coitus due to the inability to achieve penetration), hematometra, hematocolpos, chronic vaginal and urinary tract infections, urinary retention and voiding difficulty, urinary calculi, incontinence, fistula neuromas, and infertility [11, 14–19]. In an attempt to avoid obstetrical complications, antenatal or intrapartum defibulation may become necessary. The WHO has found that women with FGC are significantly more likely than those without to experience adverse obstetric outcomes, with the risks increasing with more extensive FGC [20].

Psychosexual Outcomes

There are cultural taboos against discussing sexual displeasure and the "pain" of circumcision; these taboos persist even among immigrant communities living in the West [21]. Admitting to interest in sex or discussing sexual pleasure and/or the genitalia may, in some settings, be regarded as inappropriate with strangers. There may also be gendered notions of proper conversation, and modesty standards in responding to private questions [22]. As such, the focus of research on FGC has paid only peripheral attention to psychosexual sequelae. It has been assumed that women with FGC experience dyspareunia, marital disharmony, and poor sexual outcomes. However, recent evidence does not support the hypothesis that FGC destroys sexual function or precludes enjoyment of sexual relations in all women [22].

There are mixed findings with regards to sexual pain associated with FGC. For example, dyspareunia was reported among 31.5% of women sampled in Egypt, the majority of whom were circumcised, and 23% of these women perceived personal distress related to sexual dysfunction [23]. In contrast, El-Defrawi et al. [24] noted that circumcised women in Egypt complained more significantly of dysmenorrhea, vaginal dryness during intercourse, lack of sexual desire, and difficulty reaching orgasm as compared to noncircumcised women, yet they did not report more dyspareunia.

When dyspareunia is present, it is most commonly reported with first intercourse, during the initial period after marriage, and with re-infibulation [25]. Male partners may also experience complications due to FGC, including difficulty with penile–vaginal entry, penile infections, and psychological sequelae [26]. However, despite these problems, sexual excitement and pleasure may be present for some women with FGC. Recent data suggests that FGC does not affect sexual function uniformly, even in societies where infibulation is performed [27].

There is concern that living in societies where FGC is not condoned may create an iatrogenic sexual dysfunction among women with FGC now living in the West; that is, women may face conflicting views and values about their bodies and sexuality [21, 28]. The messages about African women's bodies, beliefs, and cultural values that are contained in well-meaning anti-FGC campaigns [29] may also color women's views about female circumcision and sexuality. Furthermore, the concept of sexual dysfunction may not even exist in most African cultures where FGC is practiced; however, African women are beginning to associate distress concerning sexual function and their relationships with their original circumcision operation [21].

Changing viewpoints on sexuality among some women with FGC have been noted, and it appears to be related to length of time and acculturation into the host society [29]. Newly arrived older women living in Sweden conveyed a positive self-image of sexuality, with relatively few claims of a reduced ability to enjoy sex as a result of FGC. In contrast, women who lived longer in Sweden were deeply affected by the Swedish public anti-FGC discourse. This discourse has created negative expectations with regard to sexuality and the effects of FGC on sexual functioning [29].

Rigorous studies are needed to examine the influence of culture, tradition, and acculturation on women's sexuality. Unfortunately, the few published studies examining sexuality in FGC suffer from conceptual and methodological flaws and statistical inconsistencies [30–32], and often do not account for the impact of acculturation or confounding factors such as age or comorbid illness and perceived distress [24]. Furthermore, studies often generalize across various types/severity of FGC and fail to account for the unique socio-cultural beliefs, religious, and cultural attitudes toward the practice.

Neurobiological Outcomes

Recent research indicates that all types of FGC have a neuronal impact that affects genital sensation and/or function.

Depending on the type and extent of cutting, neural innervation may be damaged either directly by the cutting itself, or indirectly via injury to nerves that innervate the vulva and surrounding muscle [33]. It has been proposed that women with type III FGC may manifest similar neurological outcomes to that which occurs after radical vulvectomy [33].

Female genital cutting invariably results in wide variations in the type, depth, and extent of tissue damaged or excised, which may range from minimal to severe disfigurement. Damage to any of the neural networks associated with the vulvar and perineal areas may alter genital sensation. Clitoral neuroma formation is an underreported complication of FGC that results in chronic vulvar pain [15], and may occur up to 10 years after the original procedure. It manifests as a reactive lesion representing atypical proliferation of regenerating nerve fibers, which occurs when a nerve has been sectioned or traumatized and attempts to regenerate [15].

It is postulated that the brain and spinal cord responds to FGC as it would to any loss of neural targets or inputs by modifying neural circuits [33]. As a result, it may affect one's somatosensory response to sexual stimulation. Hence, rather than FGC resulting in an *absence* of sensation, it may cause an *altered* sensation, perhaps explaining inconsistent reports of genital feelings after FGC [33]. In fact, despite the damage to genital tissue, recent evidence suggests that women with FGC are still capable of experiencing sexual arousal and pleasure. As is similar with women with complete spinal cord injury, sexual arousal and orgasm can be achieved through stimulation of the breasts or other erogenous sites [33–35]. Similarly, women with various types of FGC have reported that their breasts and other areas such as the lips and thighs are the most sensitive part of their bodies [36, 37].

Surgical Management

It has been recommended that women with type III FGC who have experienced long-term complications and/or who are pregnant undergo surgical defibulation to release the vulvar scar tissue and alleviate the associated symptoms [14, 38–42]. The most common indications for surgical intervention include dysmenorrhea, desired vaginal birth, apareunia, dyspareunia, voiding difficulty, and engagement to be married. Defibulation may restore the

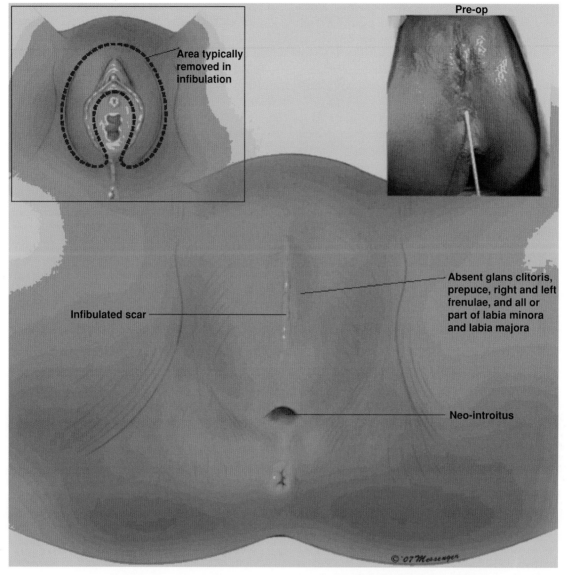

Figure 36.1 Type III female genital cutting (FGC), also known as infibulation, involves removal of part or all of the external genitalia, which generally includes the prepuce, portions of the clitoris, labia minora and/or majora. The remnant raw surfaces are sutured together (infibulated) to cover the urethra and most of the vagina. (Reprinted with permission from Johnson C, Nour NM. (2007) Surgical techniques: defibulation of type III female genital cutting. *The Journal of Sexual Medicine* **4**, 1544–47.)

external genitalia of women, with 50% of women in one study having an intact clitoris upon surgical dissection [14]. In this study, both women and their husbands noted improved sexual function, and husbands were supportive and instrumental in persuading their wives to undergo the procedure.

Defibulation is performed after counseling regarding its risks and benefits, and indications for and alternatives to the procedure. The risks include bleeding, infection, injury to adjacent structures, preterm labor (if pregnant at the time of procedure), and scar formation. The benefits include a decreased incidence

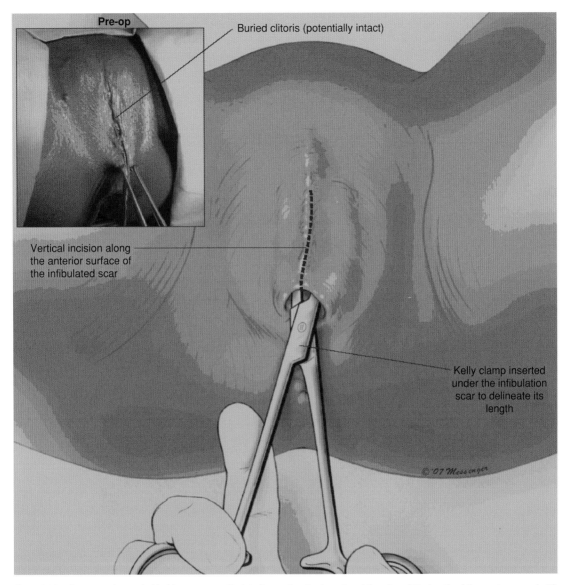

Figure 36.2 Prior to anterior vertical incision to expose the introitus and urethral meatus, delineation of the length of the scar is assessed with a Kelly clamp (Pilling, Research Triangle Park, NC) as well as palpation of the clitoral region to determine whether an intact clitoris is buried beneath the scar. (Reprinted with permission from Johnson C, Nour NM. (2007) Surgical techniques: defibulation of type III female genital cutting. *The Journal of Sexual Medicine* **4**, 1544–47.)

of chronic vaginal and urinary tract infections, voiding difficulty, dysmenorrhea, dyspareunia, and intrapartum complications. Furthermore, the procedure may help decrease obstetrical risk as well as ongoing long-term complications.

Defibulation is preferably performed as an outpatient procedure under regional or general anesthesia. Local anesthesia is not advised as the sensation of touch may trigger flashbacks of the original infibulation procedure from childhood [38]. The surgical technique of

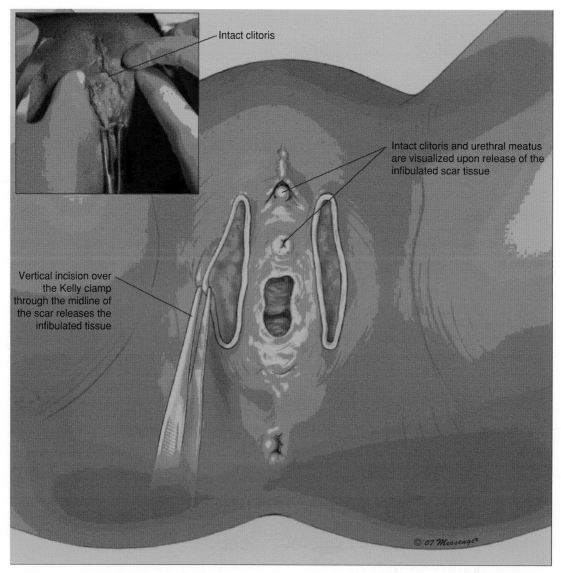

Intact clitoris

Intact clitoris and urethral meatus
are visualized upon release of the
infibulated scar tissue

Vertical incision over
the Kelly clamp
through the midline of
the scar releases the
infibulated tissue

©'07 *Messenger*

Figure 36.3 Care should be exercised to avoid injury to the clitoral tissue. (Reprinted with permission from Nour NM, Michels KB, Bryant AE. (2006) Defibulation to treat female genital cutting: effect on symptoms and sexual function. *Obstetrics & Gynecology* **108**, 55–60, and Johnson C, Nour NM. (2007) Surgical techniques: defibulation of type III female genital cutting. *The Journal of Sexual Medicine* **4**, 1544–47.)

defibulation is detailed in Figures 36.1–36.4 and summarized in Johnson and Nour's recent paper [43]. Reconstructive surgery of the clitoris may also be performed to restore both clitoral anatomy and function [44]. Excellent postoperative results have been reported with improvement in both sexual function and pain [45].

Culturally Competent Care

FGC provides a window through which we can understand the diversity in women's sexual experiences and the important role that culture plays in women's sexual health [46]. It is important to understand the specific needs of

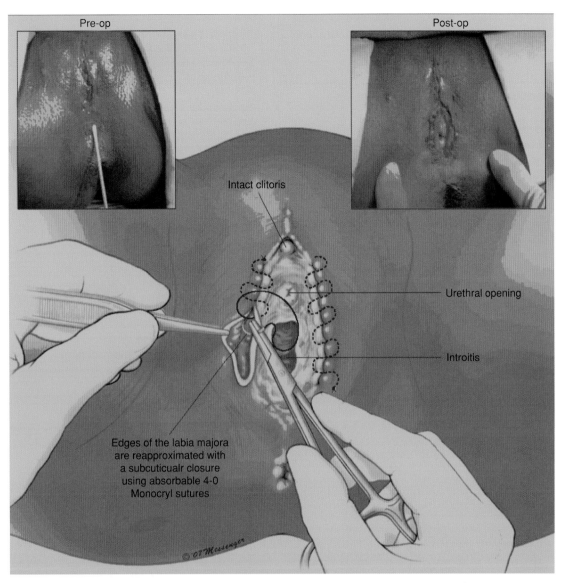

Pre-op

Post-op

Intact clitoris

Urethral opening

Introitis

Edges of the labia majora
are reapproximated with
a subcuticualr closure
using absorbable 4-0
Monocryl sutures

Figure 36.4 The raw edges of the labia majora are then reapproximated with absorbable 4.0 monocryl sutures (Ethicon, Somerville, NJ) in a subcuticular fashion. (Reprinted with permission from Johnson C, Nour NM. (2007) Surgical techniques: defibulation of type III female genital cutting. *The Journal of Sexual Medicine* **4**, 1544–47.)

women with FGC in order for health care providers to impart culturally appropriate counseling and education that will enable women to make informed decisions regarding their reproductive health care and future circumcision of their daughters.

Care should be administered in a nonjudgmental manner; engendering trust and encouraging open dialogue. Clinical evaluation should include a detailed history and physical examination documenting the type of FGC present. An exploration of the cultural significance ascribed to FGC should ensue along with elicitation of any medical sequelae experienced. An interpreter should be made available if necessary along with the woman's partner to aid in medical decision-making.

Visual aids/diagrams illustrating vulvar anatomy should also be incorporated, and sexual health counseling made available for both the woman and her partner [47].

Conclusions

Although not well studied, results concerning the sexual function of women with FGC are mixed and may depend on the type of FGC performed and other factors. To improve our knowledge of sexual outcomes among women with FGC, sexuality must be understood within a socio-cultural context, and pain/sensory function must be carefully assessed. Validated measures must be adapted, modified, and/or developed; these measures should capture the unique ideas, expectations, and experiences of women within specific sociocultural contexts of sexuality and conceptualizations of pain. Conducting rigorous scientific studies with such validated measures would aid in the development of evidence-based clinical guidelines.

References

1 Elchalal U, Ben-Ami B, Gillis R, *et al.* (1997) Ritualistic female genital mutilation: current status and future outlook. *Obstetrical and Gynecological Survey* **52**, 643–51.

2 Cohen S. (2005) *Why Aren't Jewish Women Circumcised? Gender and Covenant in Judaism.* University of California Press, Berkeley.

3 Nour N. (2000) Female circumcision and genital mutilation: a practical and sensitive approach. *Contemporary OB/GYN* **45**, 50–55.

4 WHO. (2008) *Eliminating Female Genital Mutilation: An Interagency Statement OHCHR, UNAIDS, UNDP, UNECA, UNESCO, UNFPA, UNHCR, UNICEF, UNIFEM, WHO.* World Health Organization, Geneva.

5 Elmusharaf S, Elhadi N, Almroth L. (2006) Reliability of self-reported form of female genital mutilation and WHO classification: cross-sectional study. *British Medical Journal* **333**, 124–29.

6 WHO. (2000) *Female Genital Mutilation, Fact Sheet No. 241.* World Health Organization, Geneva.

7 Yoder P, Khan S. (2007) *Numbers of Women Circumcised in Africa: The Production of a Total.* Macro International, Inc, Calverton, MD.

8 Yoder P, Abderrahim N, Zhuzhuni A. (2004)*Female Genital Cutting in the Demographic and Health Surveys: A Critical and Comparative Analysis.* ORC Macro, Calverton, MD.

9 *Female Genital Mutilation (FGM): Legal Prohibitions Worldwide.* Center for Reproductive Rights. http://www.reproductiverights.org/www_iss_fgm.html.

10 Dirie MA, Lindmark G. (1992) The risk of medical complications after female circumcision. *East African Medical Journal* **69**, 479–82.

11 Agugua NE, Egwuatu VE. (1982) Female circumcision: management of urinary complications. *Journal of Tropical Pediatrics* **28**, 248–52.

12 Aziz FA. (1980) Gynecologic and obstetric complications of female circumcision. *International Journal of Gynecology and Obstetrics* **17**, 560–63.

13 Mandara MU. (2004) Female genital mutilation in Nigeria. *International Journal of Gynecology and Obstetrics* **84**, 291–98.

14 Nour NM, Michels KB, Bryant AE. (2006) Defibulation to treat female genital cutting: effect on symptoms and sexual function. *Obstetrics and Gynecology* **108**, 55–60.

15 Fernandez-Aguilar S, Noel JC. (2003) Neuroma of the clitoris after female genital cutting. *Obstetrics and Gynecology* **101**, 1053–54.

16 Nour NM. (2003) Female genital cutting: a need for reform. *Obstetrics and Gynecology* **101**, 1051–52.

17 Nour NM. (2006) Urinary calculus associated with female genital cutting. *Obstetrics and Gynecology* **107**, 521–23.

18 Almroth L, Elmusharaf S, El-Hadi N, *et al.* (2005) Primary infertility after genital mutilation in girlhood in Sudan: a case-control study. *The Lancet* **366**, 385–91.

19 Ozumba BC. (1992) Acquired gynetresia in eastern Nigeria. *International Journal of Gynecology and Obstetrics* **37**, 105–9.

20 WHO Study Group on Female Genital Mutilation and Obstetric Outcome. (2006) Female genital mutilation and obstetric outcome: WHO collaborative prospective study in six African countries. *The Lancet* **367**, 1835–41.

21 Ahmadu F. (2007) Ain't I a Woman Too? In: Hernlund Y, Shell-Duncan B (eds.), *Transcultural Bodies: Female Genital Cutting in Global Context.* Rutgers University Press, New Brunswick, NJ, pp. 278–310.

22 Obermeyer CM. (2005) The consequences of female circumcision for health and sexuality: an update on the evidence. *Culture, Health and Sexuality* **7**, 443–61.

23 Elnashar AM, El-Dien Ibrahim M, El-Desoky MM, *et al.* (2007) Female sexual dysfunction in lower Egypt. *British Journal of Obstetrics and Gynecology* **114**, 201–6.

24 El-Defrawi MH, Lotfy G, Dandash KF, *et al.* (2001) Female genital mutilation and its psychosexual impact. *Journal of Sex and Marital Therapy* **27**, 465–73.

25 Elnashar A, Abelhady R. (2007) The impact of female genital cutting on health of newly married women. *International Journal of Gynecology and Obstetrics* **97**, 238–44.

26 Almroth L, Almroth-Berggren V, Hassanein OM, *et al.* (2001) Male complications of female genital mutilation. *Social Science and Medicine* **53**, 1455.

27 Gruenbaum E. (2001) *The Female Circumcision Controversy: An Anthropological Perspective.* University of Pennsylvania Press, Philadelphia.

28 Catania L, Abdulcadir O, Puppo V, *et al.* (2007) Pleasure and orgasm in women with female genital mutilation/cutting (FGM/C). *The Journal of Sexual Medicine* **4**, 1666–78.

29 Johnsdotter S, Essen B. (2004) Sexual health among young Somali women in Sweden: living with conflicting culturally determined sexual ideologies. *Conference on Advancing Knowledge on Psycho-Sexual Effects of FGM/C: Assessing the Evidence.* Alexandria, Egypt.

30 Odoi A, Brody SP, Elkins TE. (1997) Female genital mutilation in rural Ghana, West Africa. *International Journal of Gynecology and Obstetrics* **56**, 179–80.

31 Adinma JI. (1997) Current status of female circumcision among Nigerian Igbos. *West African Journal of Medicine* **16**, 227–31.

32 Knight R, Hotchin A, Bayly C, *et al.* (1999) Female genital mutilation: experience of The Royal Women's Hospital, Melbourne. *The Australian and New Zealand Journal of Obstetrics and Gynaecology* **39**, 50–54.

33 Einstein G. (2008) From body to brain: considering the neurobiological effects of female genital cutting. *Perspectives in Biology and Medicine* **51**, 84–97.

34 Whipple B, Komisaruk BR. (2002) Brain (PET) responses to vaginal–cervical self-stimulation in women with complete spinal cord injury: preliminary findings. *Journal of Sex and Marital Therapy* **28**, 79–86.

35 Tepper MS, Whipple B, Richards E, *et al.* (2001) Women with complete spinal cord injury: a phenomenological study of sexual experiences. *Journal of Sex and Marital Therapy* **27**, 615–23.

36 Okonofua FE, Larsen U, Oronsaye F, *et al.* (2002) The association between female genital cutting and correlates of sexual and gynaecological morbidity in Edo State, Nigeria. *British Journal of Obstetrics and Gynecology* **109**, 1089.

37 Lightfoot-Klein H. (1989) The sexual experience and marital adjustment of genitally circumcised and infibulated females in the Sudan. *Journal of Sex Research* **26**, 375–92.

38 McCaffrey M. (1995) Management of female genital mutilation: the Northwick Park Hospital experience. *British Journal of Obstetrics and Gynecology* **102**, 787–90.

39 McCaffrey M. (1995) Female genital mutilation: consequences for reproductive and sexual health. *Journal of Sex and Marital Therapy* **10**, 189–200.

40 Toubia N. (1994) Female genital mutilation and the responsibility of reproductive health professionals. *International Journal of Gynecology and Obstetrics* **46**, 127–35.

41 Nour NM. (2004) Female genital cutting: clinical and cultural guidelines. *Obstetrical and Gynecological Survey* **59**, 272–79.

42 Toubia N. (1994) Female circumcision as a public health issue. *The New England Journal of Medicine* **331**, 712–16.

43 Johnson C, Nour NM. (2007) Surgical techniques: defibulation of type III female genital cutting. *The Journal of Sexual Medicine* **4**, 1544–47.

44 Foldes P. (2006) Reconstructive surgery of the clitoris after ritual excision. *The Journal of Sexual Medicine* **3**, 1091–94.

45 Foldes P. (2004) Reconstructive plastic surgery of the clitoris after sexual mutilation. *Progres en Urologie* **14**, 47–50.

46 Fourcroy JL. (2006) Customs, culture, and tradition: what role do they play in a woman's sexuality? *The Journal of Sexual Medicine* **3**, 954–59.

47 Goodman M, Bachmann G, Johnson C, *et al.* (2007) Is elective vulvar plastic surgery ever warranted, and what screening should be conducted preoperatively? *The Journal of Sexual Medicine* **4**, 269–76.

CHAPTER 37

Practical Aspects of Establishing a Sexual Pain Center

Susan Kellogg Spadt, Kristene E. Whitmore
Drexel University College of Medicine, Philadelphia, PA, USA

Introduction

Female sexual pain is a complex perceptive biologic phenomenon, which can have physical and psychosexual implications for the individual experiencing the pain as well as for the relationship(s) that is/are affected by the sexual pain condition [1]. The purpose of this chapter is to suggest a practical multidisciplinary care-based approach for establishing a center that focuses on the treatment of sexual pain in women. The specific approaches employed by our established pelvic and sexual health institute will be given, and alternative approaches will also be discussed.

Developing an Approach, Philosophy, and Mission Statement

Prior to incorporating sexual pain management into an existing practice or opening a new practice, it is important for the health care team to be clear about their philosophical stance regarding pain, sexuality, and wellness. It should be determined if the approach to treating sexual pain will be from a predominantly clinical, traditional medical "illness-based" model (or from a wellness perspective) and whether a patient will be managed entirely by one health care provider or by a team of providers. Philosophies about treating each woman with sexual pain on an individual basis or within a partner/family systems framework should be clarified. It is important for health care providers to be clear about their philosophies on chronic pain, including the use of narcotics and other controlled substances to manage pain. Decisions about the use of alternative therapies including massage, stress management, homeopathy, herbology, acupuncture, hypnosis, etc., are also important. Goals or endpoints for care, limitations of clinical services (medical, surgical, psychological) and triage routes should be established. Lastly, a statement(s) regarding beliefs about sexual pain and goals of the care team should be agreed upon and compiled in the form of a mission statement [2].

Categories of Sexual Pain Etiologies: A Framework to Guide Center Development

When designing a center that can address the complexity of sexual pain, the potential etiologies of sexual pain can serve as a framework from which to identify members of the health care team, collaborating professionals, modes of assessment, diagnostic testing, and treatment options. Although a wide range of disorders can be associated with chronic pain, most sexual concerns arise from one or more of six basic categories: neurological, dermatologic, musculoskeletal, inflammatory, infectious, and psychological [1–7].

Identifying Goals, Care Providers, and Support Services

Sexual pain disorders are multifaceted and, as such, best results are obtained when sexual pain is addressed by a

Female Sexual Pain Disorders 1st edition. Edited by A. Goldstein,
C. Pukall & I. Goldstein. © 2009 Blackwell Publishing,
ISBN: 9781405183987.

multidisciplinary team. Identification of the members of the team is based on the specific skill set of each member of the team. As an aggregate, the team must possess the skills needed to accomplish the specific goals of sexual pain management. These goals include [1, 3, 5–7]

1 Identification of the specific disease process (e.g., lichen sclerosus, endometriosis, etc.) or disorder (e.g., pelvic floor dysfunction, irritable bowel syndrome, etc.) causing the sexual pain;

2 Initiate proper treatment of the specific disease or disorder;

3 Reduction in inflammation, vulvar hypersensitivity, and hyperreactivity;

4 Restoration of tissue elasticity, moisture, integrity, and removal of chemical allergens, dietary, and lifestyle irritants;

5 Identification, treatment, and suppression of recurrent infection according to specific species type;

6 Restoration of adequate strength and tonus to the pelvic core, and superficial and deep pelvic floor muscles;

7 Comprehensive management of individual and couple/family psycho-behavioral issues to facilitate sexual and psychological wellness.

The Integrated Approach

An integrated approach to treating the sexual pain patient has as its goal an understanding of how various illness states, physical sensations, and psychological processes have interacted to cause suffering in a woman who presents for care. In addition, it is imperative to understand the issues surrounding the initiation of pain problem, its chronology, and the progression of the pain to its present state (e.g., vestibular pain, hypertonus of the pelvic floor, depression, etc.) so that appropriate interventions can be designed. Integrated does not always mean interdisciplinary. Theoretically, an integrated approach could be carried out by one (very busy) provider or it can be carried out by a number of collaborating subspecialists, depending on the complexity and severity of the problem. In most cases, sexual pain is treated by several members of an integrated team who view the patient as a functional unit of mind and body, and who work together so that healing occurs in an integrated fashion [1, 2].

The sexual pain care team can involve several key professionals. In our center, these include:

Sexual Pain Team (within the center):
Team Leaders:
Urologist or gynecologist/surgeon (MD) and medical sexologist (PhD, NP)

Team Members:
OB/GYN nurse practitioners
Manual physical therapist: specialization in pelvic floor disorders
Massage/craniosacral/yoga therapist: specialization in neuromuscular re-education
Compounding pharmacist
Hypnotherapist: specialization in pain/stress management
Nutritionist
Homeopathist
Sexual relationship therapists: specialization in pain, sexual trauma, and eye movement desensitization and retraining (EMDR)
Marriage and family therapists
Research coordinator

Support Services (outside the center):
Consulting dermatologist
Consulting dermatopathologist
Consulting infectious disease specialist
Consulting acupuncturist/herbalist
Consulting anesthesiologist/pain management specialist
Consulting colorectal surgeon
Consulting gynecologic surgeon
Consulting internist or family practitioner

The structure of our team, and the individual duties within the group, have been established with a thorough understanding of the specific skills of each individual team member. As such, other sexual pain teams might have a gynecologist, dermatologist, infectious disease specialist, or pain management specialist as a team leader.

In some treatment centers, members of the entire sexual pain team have offices "under one roof." In such a clinical setting, a patient can be provided with the full variety of services that she requires, and can see many team members during serial appointments with specialists who are located within the same physical space. This type of clinical program requires a very significant investment in time, space, financial resources, and organizational support. This can be accomplished in the setting of an academic medical center if administrators are aware of the large scope of sexual pain clinic. Alternatively, the sexual pain care team may be located in a free standing "center" but this often requires significant financial investment of the team leaders.

In other settings, "virtual" multidisciplinary centers are created, where a woman visits her primary sexual pain specialist and subsequently is triaged to specialty support services in outside centers. Careful, prioritized communication patterns (e.g., email, fax, priority phone lines) as well as regular "team meetings" are essential in order for the team to coordinate patient care and work as a unified whole.

Setting Is Key

The physical setting of a sexual pain center should portray a calming, caring, nonrushed professional attitude. Staff should be educated regarding the sensitive nature of the disorders and be careful to maintain patient privacy at all times. In our center, there are comfortable upholstered chairs, fresh flowers, plants, soothing music, and an office-sized waterfall to greet women and partners as they arrive.

In centers where sexual pain is integrated into a busy gynecologic, primary care, or urologic practice, providers can separate privacy needs of sexual pain patients by seeing them on certain days of the week or by designating the quieter "corner" examination rooms for sexual medicine.

To facilitate patient comfort, many centers have an office area where patients are initially interviewed before they are moved to an examination room. In other centers, such as ours, there is a comfortable "conversation area" within each examination room that is used for interviewing a woman and her partner. After a clothed sexual history interview, which generally takes 20–30 min, the woman undresses and moves to another side of the room where there are traditional examination tables with stirrups, brighter examination lighting, instruments, measurement devices, and laboratory supplies. The woman may choose to have her partner stay or leave during her examination. After the examination, the woman dresses and joins her provider in the conversation area again, allowing time for questions and home care program instructions. Most new patient visits take 60–90 min.

Assessment and Diagnostic Testing

Ot is imperative that methods of data collection and medical record keeping facilitate communication between members of the sexual pain team. The keeping of electronic medical records (EMR) is one method that facilitates effective communication between members of the sexual pain team. In addition, it assists in gathering data for retrospective studies or for the identification of patients who might benefit from new treatment modalities.

The diagnostic work-up of a woman with sexual pain is explained in great detail in other portions of this book. In our clinic, assessment is systematic (summarized below) and focuses on each of the possible etiologic origins for sexual pain [1, 3–10]:

1 *Psycho-behavioral assessment:* Women are asked to complete several validated inventories including Female Sexual Function Inventory, Beck Depression Inventory, O'Leary Sant Symptom Index, and Visual Analog Pain Scale. These are useful in face-to-face interviews by the psychological counselor. Inventories also aid in the development of specific psycho-behavioral, sex, and relationship interventions and can help to monitor progress.

2 *Dermatologic assessment:* We perform a thorough colposcopic evaluation of the vulva and perianal regions using 3% acetic acid. Any lesions, pigment variations, or topographic changes are biopsied and sent for histopathologic evaluation by a dermatopathologist.

3 *Muscle assessment:* As discussed more thoroughly in other chapters in this textbook, evaluation of the musculoskeletal system of the pelvis is an essential component of the evaluation of sexual pain. A perineometer can be used to gather objective data regarding the tone of a woman's pelvic floor muscles. This tampon-shaped electronic device is inserted into a woman's vagina and digitally records the relative resting tone and voluntary contraction tone of the pelvic floor muscles (PFMs). Precision perineometry, in concert with the patient's response to PFM palpation, can serve as a basis for initiating physical therapy and aides in evaluation of the success of programs such as biofeedback and graduated dilator use. Additional pelvic floor muscle testing may include internal or external electromyography, PFM real-time ultrasound with maneuvers, urodynamic testing, pudendal nerve motor latency, or anal manometry.

4 *Infection assessment:* Urine and vaginal cultures are routinely performed, evaluated microscopically, then sent to

a microbiology laboratory for fungal/bacterial speciation (with sensitivities, if indicated). "Test of cure cultures" may be performed after treatment. At subsequent visits, interim cultures can assure the provider and patient that an infection has not recurred.

5 *Neurological assessment:* Pain mapping during the physical examination is used to define the extent of vulvar, urologic, rectal, and upper pelvic pain and clarifies precise anatomical locations associated with the patient's symptoms. Pain mapping is performed with a saline moistened cotton swab, placed at specific points on the outer vulva and within the vulvar vestibule. Patients rate their discomfort on an escalating scale (either 1–10 or 1–5 depending on clinic preference). A biothesiometer adds additional sensory data by assessing several points (both tender and nontender) within the vulva. This device measures vibratory thresholds (expressed in volts) and is a general indicator of peripheral nerve competency in the genital region. Gross deviation from the sensory threshold norms for areas within pudendal nerve distribution may indicate alterations in sexual response and infer the need for a more extensive neurological evaluation.

Coordinating Treatment

Specific medical and surgical treatment regimens for sexual pain are detailed in other chapters of this book. Implementing a comprehensive treatment program requires coordination, and it is important to have procedures in place that optimize the communication between team members (particularly if they are not in one physical space) [2].

In our clinic, care is managed by the primary MD or NP provider, who is in charge of communicating with other team members (verbally and in writing) and documenting their involvement, progress, and basic care plan in the patient's medical chart. Due to the fact that we are in one practice setting, there is ample opportunity for team members to informally update one another on patient progress and for various members of the team to have access to diagnostic testing results and the medical plan of care. In addition, monthly team meetings are held, during which there are presentations of challenging sexual pain case studies and time for clinicians to privately discuss progress being made with individual cases. Most clinics exchange phone calls, secure e-mails, faxes, or letters that document their multidisciplinary treatment.

Reimbursement and Coding

The clinical practice guidelines and references to coding discussed here reflect the experiences of the authors in caring for sexual pain patients, which, because of many local and regional trends, is a tertiary referral practice. Most patients referred to our practice have been previously evaluated by several other providers and are physician-referred. Additionally, many patients have been referred by patient advocacy organizations such as the National Vulvodynia Association and the Interstitial Cystitis Association. Lastly, patients are increasingly using the Internet to find providers knowledgeable in the evaluation and treatment of sexual pain disorders.

In order for any sexual pain program to continue to serve patients, it must have a means of insuring revenue. In countries where health care is funded by the government, it may be necessary to convince authorities responsible for funding of the prevalence and importance of the treatment of sexual pain disorders. In the United States, revenue can be generated in several ways discussed below.

In the *cash payment model*, patients are required to pay for services at the time of their clinic services. They are provided with a coded superbill, which they may choose to submit to their insurance provider after the time of service. As many patients have out-of-network benefits, they are often able to recuperate a moderate percentage of their "out-of-pocket" expenditures. Most sexual pain centers have a sliding scale fee schedule so that women unable to pay the full amount are still able to obtain care.

In the *insurance model*, most medical care, procedures, diagnostic testing, surgeries, and physical therapy are billed directly to insurance from the primary sexual medicine provider's office or PT office. In this model, the patient is responsible for any deductible, copay, or partial payment percentage that their individual insurance requires. In addition, providers of psychological services, compounded medications, massage, nutrition, and other alternative therapies are paid in cash (often on a sliding scale basis) directly by the patient. In the case of our clinic, most medical insurance plans are accepted. Because most patients have been physician-referred, new sexual pain patients are often coded as an initial consultation, Level 4 or 5 (99244, 99245). If patients self-refer, we use either 99204 (Level 4) or 99205 (Level 5). The exact coding depends upon the complexity of their problems and time invested both directly interacting with the patient,

Table 37.1 Common Diagnostic Codes and Procedure Codes in Sexual Pain Management [11, 12].

ICD-9 Codes	CPT Codes
Vulvodynia/genital pain 625.8	Vaginal wet mount Q0111
Female pelvic pain 625.9	Urinalysis 81000
Dyspareunia 302.76	Colposcopy of vulva (no biopsy)
Vaginismus 306.51	56820
Pelvic floor dysfunction 739.5	Colposcopy of vulva with biopsy
Unspecified cystitis 595.3	56821
Interstitial cystitis 595.1	Injection of anesthetic agent
Painful menstruation 625.3	64450
Atrophic vulvitis 627.3	Perineometry 95999 or 90911
Vaginitis and vulvovagintis 616.10	Biothesiometry 95999 or 0107T
Herpes, genital vulvovaginitis	Anal manometry/PFM
054.11	biofeedback 90911
Streptococcus, group B 041.02	
Candidiasis, vulva and vagina	
112.1	
Other vaginal bacterial infection	
041.84	
Unspecified inflammatory disease	
of female pelvic organs/tissues	
(lichenoid dermatoses, contact	
irritant dermatitis) 614.9	
Perimenopausal sexual	
dysfunction 302.70	
Sexual arousal disorder 302.72	
Sexual aversion disorder 302.79	
Depression 296.2	
Anxiety 300.01	
Urgency 788	
Hematuria 599.7	
Urethral syndrome 597.81	
Trigonitis 595.4	

and indirectly during review of previous medical records. For follow-up visits, which usually take 20–50 min, levels 3, 4, and 5 (99213, 99214, and 99215) are used. Specific diagnostic or procedural codes that are frequently used in our center are listed on Table 37.1.

Another type of business plan is the *"all-inclusive" model*. In this situation, patients pay an initial "flat fee" for care, which is inclusive of all their medical evaluation, diagnostic testing, physical therapy, sex therapy, compounded medications, and other team services. This may or may not be formatted into a superbill for submission to insurance companies for reimbursement. This model is often adopted by practices that see patients from outside of their geographic region for a limited number of consultative visits, rather than for ongoing care.

Patient Convenience Items

As a courtesy service to patients, many sexual pain practices stock and sell a variety of "support" items that facilitate sexual rehabilitation and comfort. These may include hypoallergenic water–based or silicone lubricants, graduated sizes of flexible or rigid vaginal dilators, curved dilators to assist in PFM rehabilitation, home biofeedback units, home clitoral therapy devices, selected erotic reading, magnifying mirrors, and educational pamphlets and books.

Conclusion

Sexual pain often represents the complex interplay of several physiologic and psychosocial etiologies. Coincident pelvic floor muscle dysfunction is extremely common as are concomitant pain conditions that affect the adjacent urinary, reproductive, or gastrointestinal systems. Depression, anxiety, as well as a myriad of relationship issues require active intervention throughout each phase of medical management and therapy. Establishing a sexual pain center is a challenging clinical endeavor, as well as a truly rewarding one. It perpetuates academic, clinical, and personal growth for the health care providers who care for this deserving patient population.

References

1 Graziottin A, Dennerstein L, Alexander JL, *et al.* (2006) Classification, etiology, and key issues in female sexual disorders. In: Porst H, Buvat J (eds.), *Standards of Practice in Sexual Medicine.* Blackwell Publishing, Malden, MA, pp. 305–14.

2 Steege JF. (1998) Basic philosophy of the integrated approach: overcoming the mind–body split. In: Steege JF, Metzger DA, Levy BS (eds.), *Chronic Pelvic Pain: An Integrated Approach.* WB Saunders, Philadelphia, pp. 5–12.

3 Lucas M, Pickersgill A, Smith ARB. (2006) Chronic pelvic pain: diagnosis and management. In: Chapple CR, Zimmern PE, Brubaker L, Smith ARB, Bo K (eds.), *Multidisciplinary Management of Female Pelvic Floor Disorders.* Churchill Livingstone Elsevier, Philadelphia, pp. 319–34.

4 Basson R, Leiblum S, Brotto L. (2004) Revised definitions of women's sexual dysfunction. *The Journal of Sexual Medicine* **1**, 40–48.

5 Binik YM, Reissing E, Pukall C, *et al.* (2002) The female sexual pain disorders: genital pain or sexual dysfunction? *Archives of Sexual Behavior* **31**, 425–29.

6   Grazziotin A, Brotto LA. (2004) Vulvar vestibulitis syndrome: a clinical approach. *Journal of Sexual Marital Therapy* **30**, 125–39.

7   Goldstein A, Burrows L. (2008) Vulvodynia. *Journal of Sexual Medicine* **5**, 5–15.

8   Whitmore K, Siegel JF, Kellogg-Spadt S. (2007) Interstitial cystitis/painful bladder syndrome as a cause of sexual pain in women: a diagnosis to consider. *The Journal of Sexual Medicine* **4**. 720–27.

9   Hundley AF, Wu JM, Visco AG. (2005) A comparison of perineometer to brink scores for assessment of pelvic floor muscle strength. *American Journal of Obstetrics and Gynecololgy* May, **192**, 1583–91.

10 Connell K, Guess MK, Bluestein CB, *et al.* (2005) Effects of age, menopause, and comorbidities on neurological function of the female genitalia. *International Journal of Impotence Research.* **17**, 3–70.

11 *Physicians' Professional ICD-9-CM International Classification of Diseases: Vols. 1 & 2.* (2008) Medical Management Institute, Salt Lake City, UT.

12 Beebe M, Dalton JA, Espronceda M, *et al. Current Procedural Terminology 2008 (Professional Edition.* American Medical Association, Chicago, IL.

CHAPTER 38
The Power of Patient Advocacy

Phyllis Mate, Christin Veasley

National Vulvodynia Association, Silver Spring, MD, USA

Introduction

In 1994, after being brought together by their mutual physician, five vulvodynia patients from Washington, DC, came to the conclusion that they couldn't possibly be the only women in the world suffering from vulvodynia. This realization was momentous, as they had all been suffering in isolation for many years without receiving a diagnosis. In some cases, physicians who questioned the legitimacy of their condition had referred them to psychiatrists with the idea that the pain was entirely "in their heads."

These five women exchanged contact information and started a local support group for women suffering from chronic vulvar pain and related disorders. Later that year, they made a long-term commitment to become patient advocates and the National Vulvodynia Association (NVA) was founded. What began as a small, local support group grew into an international organization serving tens of thousands of women with vulvodynia, as well as health care providers committed to treating this disorder. The NVA founders' intuition that they were not the only ones suffering from vulvodynia was confirmed by prevalence studies indicating that there are actually *millions of women* suffering from the disorder in the United States alone!

Educational Information

When the NVA started, there was virtually no public information on vulvodynia. Fittingly, the organization's first priority was to develop educational materials for both the patient and medical communities. The NVA drafted an informative brochure and began distributing it to health care providers and patients who contacted the organization. The NVA also created the *NVA News*, its highly praised informative newsletter published three times yearly. With nearly 40 issues in print to date, the newsletter contains articles written by experts in the field who provide a wealth of information on the diagnosis and treatment of vulvodynia. It also features news articles summarizing the latest research findings, as well as events on Capitol Hill aimed at increasing federal funds for research.

The NVA firmly believes that the more patients know about the diagnosis and treatment of the condition, the better equipped they will be to discuss their options with their health care providers. In addition, because the etiology of the condition is poorly understood and likely multifactorial, the organization's philosophy is to present information on *all* types of medically responsible treatment and encourage women to work as a team with their providers in order to decide which treatment options are most appropriate for them.

Support Network and Online Support

The NVA's next priority was to establish a national support network modeled upon the Washington, DC, area support group. Many women find that mutual support is both a good source of information and the best way to overcome the emotional isolation that often results from having vulvodynia. Today, the NVA has nearly 100 support leaders in place throughout the United States, Canada, and a handful of other countries, including Israel and Australia. The role

Female Sexual Pain Disorders 1st edition. Edited by A. Goldstein, C. Pukall & I. Goldstein. © 2009 Blackwell Publishing, ISBN: 9781405183987.

of the NVA support leaders is to accept phone calls and emails from affected women in their geographic area. In some cities, leaders organize regular support group meetings or communicate online with their group members. The purpose of the groups is to provide emotional support, host speakers from different medical specialties, and raise public awareness by hosting local events and reaching out to media professionals. In addition, the NVA refers interested women to online e-groups and bulletin boards that can provide support to those who are incapacitated, prefer online communication, or need support in between their local group meetings.

Health Care Provider Referrals

When the NVA started receiving calls, the first question women tended to ask was, "Can you give me the name of a health care provider in my area?" Although the NVA initially did not plan on offering this service, it was apparent that providing this information was essential for most patients. Therefore, the NVA began to gather names and contact information of doctors, nurse practitioners, physical therapists, and other health care providers across the country familiar with vulvodynia. The NVA now maintains the most comprehensive database of health care professionals interested in treating vulvar pain disorders in the United States and Canada; the list also contains information for health care providers in several other countries. In an effort to assist women in making more informed choices about their health care, the NVA has recently expanded the database to include information on specialty, type of practice, average number of vulvodynia patients seen monthly, percentage of the practice devoted to vulvar disorders and chronic pain, and degree of involvement in vulvodynia research.

Lobbying for Research Funding

Within a year of its incorporation, NVA headed to Capitol Hill to educate members of Congress about vulvodynia and promote the urgent need for federal research funding. As a result of numerous Congressional meetings and briefings that have taken place over the years, substantial progress has been made. Senator Tom Harkin (D-IA), a well-known women's health advocate, has been the most prominent champion, ensuring that language on vulvodynia has been included in the National Institutes of Health (NIH) appropriations report every year since 1998. The FY2008 NIH appropriations report contained the following language:

> In the last decade, the NIH has supported three important research conferences on vulvodynia, as well as the first prevalence study and clinical trial on the disorder. These efforts have both clearly demonstrated the need for substantial additional research and served to heighten the research community's level of interest in studying vulvodynia. The Committee calls upon the Director to build upon these initial successes by coordinating through the Office of Research on Women's Health (ORWH) an expanded, collaborative extramural and intramural research effort into the causes of, and treatments for, vulvodynia. This effort should involve the National Institute of Child Health and Human Development, the National Institute of Neurological Disorders and Stroke and other relevant NIH Institutes and Centers (ICs), as well as the NIH Pain Consortium. The Committee also commends ORWH for working with patient groups, other relevant ICs and women's health offices in other governmental agencies to plan an educational outreach campaign on vulvodynia, as previously requested by the Committee. Finally, the Committee encourages the Director to work with the Center for Scientific Review and ICs to ensure that experts in vulvodynia, and related chronic pain and female reproductive system conditions, are adequately represented on peer-review panels.

In early 2001, the NIH allocated $5 million for vulvodynia research and funded its first four studies on the disorder. One of the first grants awarded was to fund a prevalence study by Bernard Harlow (University of Minnesota) and Elizabeth Stewart (Harvard University). Their study was the first to substantiate that vulvodynia is a highly prevalent condition, affecting up to 16% of women of all ages and ethnic/racial backgrounds. In 2002, the NIH awarded funding to David Foster (University of Rochester) to conduct the first randomized, placebo-controlled, double-blinded clinical trial on the efficacy of four medical regimens for provoked vestibulodynia (PVD), also referred to as vulvar vestibulitis syndrome, a major subtype of vulvodynia. This study was completed in 2007, and Foster and his colleagues are currently analyzing the data and preparing a manuscript for publication. The NIH has funded nine other studies at institutions including the University of Michigan, Yale University, the University of Medicine and Dentistry of New Jersey, and the University of North Carolina. For summaries of these studies, see http://www.nva.org/for_medical_professionals/nih_funding.html.

In 2006, Congress directed the NIH Office of Research on Women's Health (ORWH) to plan the first Vulvodynia Awareness Campaign to disseminate information on vulvodynia's symptoms, diagnosis and treatment to patients, health care providers, and the public. In October 2007, the campaign was launched at the National Press Club in Washington, DC. Over 30 government agencies and health organizations (e.g., American College of Obstetricians and Gynecologists, American Medical Women's Association, Society for Women's Health Research) have partnered with the NIH in this campaign. The NVA, ORWH, and the National Women's Health Resource Center have led the publicity charge by contacting editors and writers at popular magazines, newspapers, and Web sites. Since the launch of the campaign, several publications have included articles on vulvodynia, such as the *New York Times* article by respected health columnist Jane Brody (January 2008).

The NVA continues to work cooperatively with NIH representatives on public awareness and federal research funding efforts. In addition, the organization continues its Congressional outreach efforts through its annual grassroots advocacy campaign. During this week-long campaign, vulvodynia sufferers, along with their family members and health care providers, meet with or write to their Congressional representatives. Through this effort, nearly every senator and representative in the U.S. Congress has been contacted by a constituent about vulvodynia!

Medical Research Fund

In response to scientists' growing need for funding to gather preliminary data for their grant applications, the NVA created its Medical Research Fund. In 1997, NVA awarded its first grant to an investigator at Johns Hopkins School of Medicine. Since then, the organization has awarded more than $300,000, supporting a total of 21 studies. Several of the NVA's grant recipients have used

data gathered with this funding to obtain large grants from the NIH. For a summary of NVA-funded studies, see http://www.nva.org/for_medical_professionals/research_fund.html.

Career Development Award

In 2006, the NVA created the Dr. Stanley C. Marinoff Vulvodynia Career Development Award to encourage interested faculty to pursue a clinical or academic interest in the field. The award provides seed money to conduct research, write a publication, or develop/expand a vulvar pain clinic. As a result of this funding mechanism, two new vulvodynia clinics opened in New Jersey and Michigan in 2006. The NVA is hopeful that the continuation of this program will increase the number of qualified, knowledgeable clinicians and scientists in the field. A summary of award recipients' projects can be viewed at: http://www.nva.org/for_medical_professionals/career_development_award.html.

Professional Education

Although the NVA's primary focus has been serving the patient community, the organization also develops educational programs for the medical community. For years, members of the NVA's medical/scientific advisory board have given presentations at national and international conferences. The NVA also exhibits at several medical conferences each year, where staff members and volunteers disseminate complimentary educational materials to medical professionals in different specialties, including gynecology, pain management and family medicine.

In addition, to promote research interest and establish future directives for vulvodynia research, the NVA collaborated with the NIH in 1997, 2003, and 2004 to organize conferences on the disorder. Specialists from all over the world have come to these conferences to exchange treatment information and discuss recent research findings.

The NVA also publishes a quarterly electronic newsletter, *NVA Research Update*, providing abstracts on vulvodynia from journals and conference presentations. In addition, the NVA, in consultation with its medical advisory board members, developed the first online vulvodynia tutorial to offer continuing medical education credits, *Vulvodynia: Integrating Current Knowledge into Clinical Practice.* This complementary program (http://learn.nva.org) provides a self-guided presentation on etiology/risk factors, differential diagnosis, and treatment of vulvodynia.

Public Awareness

When the NVA was founded in 1994, the media expressed little interest in covering vulvodynia. Since then, the NVA has reached out to interested media professionals and interest has steadily grown. Vulvodynia first received major publicity in 1999 when one of the NVA's support leaders was featured on a CBS primetime special, *The Body Human.* Two years later, on the Oprah Winfrey show, Drs. Laura and Jennifer Berman answered a question from an audience member about painful intercourse and vulvodynia. The NVA's Web site was visited by more than 10,000 people in the next 24 hours!

Later that year, millions of television viewers learned about vulvodynia on HBO's award-wining show *Sex and the City.* In the episode, Charlotte, played by Kristen Davis, is examined by her gynecologist and told that she may have vulvodynia. She is perplexed when her gynecologist recommends an antidepressant and tells her to keep a daily pain journal. Consistent with the series' lighthearted tone, Charlotte's friends joke that her "vagina is depressed." The NVA received hundreds of phone calls from vulvodynia sufferers who were indignant about the show's unsympathetic portrayal of the painful condition. In response, NVA issued a press release praising HBO for tackling the subject, but criticizing its insensitive portrayal. In the weeks following, eight major newspapers, including the *Chicago Sun-Times*, the *New York Daily News*, and the *Chicago Tribune* responded to the release and published articles on the reality of living with vulvodynia.

In October 2001, Susanna Kaysen, author of *Girl Interrupted*, released her second memoir, *The Camera My Mother Gave Me.* In this autobiographical account of her desperate search to find treatment for chronic vulvar pain, she writes, "It isn't cancer. It isn't diabetes. It isn't life threatening. It's just horrible." The memoir details both Kaysen's interactions with numerous medical professionals and the wide array of treatments that she tried. Vulvodynia sufferers around the world identified with

Ms. Kaysen's experiences and praised her for her candor in revealing the details of this private condition.

In the summer of 2002, two ground-breaking books on vulvodynia and vulvovaginal health, authored by NVA medical/scientific advisory board members, Howard Glazer and Elizabeth Stewart, were released. Glazer and co-author, Gae Rodke, wrote *The Vulvodynia Survival Guide* to give women with vulvodynia guidance on how to alleviate their pain and reclaim their lives. *The V Book,* written by Elizabeth Stewart and Paula Spencer, was the first comprehensive guide to vulvovaginal health. In this book, questions about common vulvovaginal ailments that are often embarrassing to discuss with others are answered. Together, these books have sold over 50,000 copies and continue to provide women with valuable information, guidance and most importantly, hope.

English novelist, Fay Weldon, once said that, "Nothing happens, and nothing happens, and then everything happens." For the NVA, October 2007 was one of those months when *everything happened.* In addition to the launch of the first NIH Vulvodynia Awareness Campaign (see Lobbying for Research Funding), ABC's hit show, *Private Practice,* featured a woman who was unable to have sex with her new husband. During her gynecological exam, she screams in pain and is diagnosed with vulvar vestibulitis and vaginismus. In addition to the show's 12.2 million viewers, the episode was made available online at abc.com and was viewed by thousands more. Also in October, NVA approached *New York Times* health columnist, Jane Brody, to write an article on vulvodynia. Continuing conversations over the following months led to an article that appeared in the January 29, 2008, edition. In addition to the paper's daily circulation of 1.1 million, Ms. Brody's column is syndicated and appears in nearly 100 other newspapers across the country and abroad. In the following weeks, the NVA and Ms. Brody were flooded with letters and e-mails from grateful readers. One reader wrote, "Having chronic pain is terrible, but not being believed is unbearable. Thanks for sending me this wonderful reminder that I am not alone, and I am not imagining this condition."

Hundreds of other reporters, freelance writers, and radio and television personalities who have covered vulvodynia over the years. The condition has been featured in many popular women's magazines, such as *Redbook*, on Web sites such as WebMD and health.com, and on several television and radio shows. Cumulatively, these features have reached tens of millions of people across the world, greatly raising the public's awareness of vulvodynia.

NVA Partners

The NVA has worked cooperatively with several other advocacy groups over the years, including the Society for Women's Health Research, the American Pain Foundation, and the Interstitial Cystitis Association (ICA). Through their efforts, these organizations have significantly advanced awareness of, and research on, women's health and chronic pain conditions. Because many women suffer from both vulvodynia and interstitial cystitis (IC), the NVA has worked most closely with the ICA in the past decade. This patient advocacy group was founded in 1984 by Vicki Ratner, a physician who developed IC during medical school. Among its many accomplishments, the ICA has secured over $100 million of research funding from the NIH, worked with the Centers for Disease Control on the first IC national awareness campaign, and obtained recognition of IC from the Social Security Administration.

Moving Forward: The Power of Advocates

The NVA's accomplishments demonstrate how great a difference a small group of committed volunteers can make. The NVA did not start with a multimillion dollar seed grant and a team of executives. It began with a modest $5,000 donation from a private donor, to whom the NVA and millions of women worldwide are forever grateful,

and a few vulvodynia patients who cared deeply about their cause. Marian Wright Edelman, children's advocate and president of the Children's Defense Fund, once said, "We must not, in trying to think about how we can make a big difference, ignore the small daily differences we can make which, over time, add up to big differences that we often cannot foresee." In addition to two committed staff members, hundreds of NVA volunteers have worked tirelessly over the past 14 years on behalf of women suffering from vulvodynia. These efforts are making a difference in the lives of millions of women!

Even though the organization has accomplished a great deal since its inception, work remains to be done. Everything NVA does is with one goal in mind: We want *every* woman to be able to seek medical care without embarrassment, be accurately diagnosed by the *first* health care provider she consults, and then immediately receive effective treatment. The movement for change has begun; however, in order to reach this goal more quickly, people who have a vested interest in the condition—patients, their family members and friends, and health care providers who treat vulvar pain disorders—must become advocates themselves. There is power in numbers. Media attention and Congressional allocation of research dollars to a medical condition are largely influenced by public outcry. Please join the NVA in our effort to end the unnecessary suffering of vulvodynia by writing to, or meeting with, your Congressional representatives, contacting your local media and/or educating your colleagues unfamiliar with the condition. For additional information on Congressional and media outreach, which includes a vulvodynia fact sheet and talking points, visit: http://www.nva.org/about_nva/awareness.html.

CHAPTER 39
The Future of Vulvodynia Research

David C. Foster
University of Rochester School of Medicine and Dentistry Rochester, NY, USA

Introduction

A chapter charged with predicting future vulvodynia research necessarily reflects personal opinion rather than fact, in contrast to the other scholarly efforts of this book. The perspective reflected in this chapter is based on my many years of attempting to understand and treat vulvodynia. The chapter is divided into two major sections: first, research avenues to help strengthen the foundation of vulvodynia research are described, and second, specific research ideas are proposed.

Avenues of Research

The Need for Improved Diagnostic Categories

Recognizing the need for an updated vulvodynia classification, the 1999 World Congress of the International Society for the Study of Vulvovaginal Disease (ISSVD) convened a discussion group to update the classification of chronic vulvar pain, resulting in the publication of a new classification system [1] (Table 39.1). *Chronic vulvar pain* refers to vulvar pain lasting more than three months; this category is subdivided into *vulvar pain related to a specific disorder* (e.g., infectious conditions) and *vulvodynia*, chronic vulvar pain that exists in the absence of a specific, clinically identifiable disorder.

The category of vulvodynia, in turn, is subdivided according to the pain location (*generalized* vs. *localized*) and temporal characteristics (*provoked* vs. *unprovoked* vs.

Female Sexual Pain Disorders 1st edition. Edited by A. Goldstein, C. Pukall & I. Goldstein. © 2009 Blackwell Publishing, ISBN: 9781405183987.

mixed) [1]. The ISSVD specifically recommended replacing the term *vestibulitis* with *vestibulodynia*, as the former, implying inflammation, was deemed misleading because of the poor demonstrated correlation between vestibular pain and inflammatory indicators. This classification system and associated terminology has met with slow approval. For example, many clinicians continue to use the term vestibulitis and some have questioned whether the divisions truly reflect distinct conditions.

What could explain the slow acceptance of this classification? A useful system should meet at least one of the following goals: (i) it should reflect an understanding of the pathophysiology involved; (ii) it should provide insight into the choice of therapy; or (iii) it should predict prognosis of defined disease subsets. However, the pathophysiology of vulvodynia remains obscure, and therapeutic options have not been well studied for efficacy and prognosis. In addition, a diverse group of providers (e.g., gynecologists, dermatologists, neurologists, etc.), each with their own professional language, manage vulvodynia differently, thereby contributing to various perspectives related to the understanding of the condition and the focus of treatment.

The long-term goal in the treatment of vulvodynia will be the development of a mechanism-based classification system and the practice of making treatment decisions based upon the most effective option against the identified mechanism. Presently, an understanding of the pathophysiology of vulvodynia is uncertain, and such doubt leads to indecision when faced with treatment options. However, in spite of the large number of randomized clinical trials (RCTs) for neuropathic pain, an adequate understanding of *any* chronic pain condition that might permit a rational selection of treatment based on mechanism has yet to be achieved [2].

Table 39.1 ISSVD classification of chronic vulvar pain (vulvodynia)

ISSVD Terminology and Classification of Vulvar Pain

Vulvar pain related to a specific disorder

Infectious, Inflammatory, Neoplastic, Neurologic

Vulvodynia (vulvar dysesthesia)

Generalized (provoked, unprovoked, mixed)

Localized (provoked, unprovoked, mixed)

The Necessity for More Epidemiological Research

An estimated 7% of women will meet the diagnostic criteria for vulvodynia at some time in their lives, and many will report significant psychosocial problems, including sexual dysfunction, anxiety, depression, and relationship distress [3–6]. Fortunately, the National Institutes of Health (NIH) has been involved in research funding for vulvodynia. However, obtaining increased NIH support is unlikely because of limited budgets and competition for other medical priorities; thus, a significant amount of future research funding may arise from the private pharmaceutical sector.

Before such funding can be obtained, however, epidemiologists will need to clearly answer the questions of prevalence, population proportions of vulvodynia subsets, long-term morbidity of chronic vulvar pain, the financial impact of vulvodynia, and, ultimately, the cost/benefit ratio of various treatment options. Although the work of Harlow and Stewart [7, 8] has provided an excellent epidemiologic foundation, far more still needs to be done. For example, information on whether vulvodynia is an *orphan disease* or *just the tip of the iceberg* needs to be clarified [8].

Molecular epidemiology, as a unique discipline within epidemiology, may help in mapping future directions in vulvodynia research. The power of this approach is based upon the identification of molecular markers at the sub-

cellular, cellular, tissue, and organism levels [9], which are followed through a mechanistic continuum from exposure to manifestation of clinical disease. An excellent example is illustrated by the exposure to human papillomavirus (HPV) and subsequent development of cervical neoplasia.

Figure 39.1 demonstrates the steps of molecular epidemiology as might be applied to vulvodynia. As is evident, the contemporary understanding of vulvodynia is the equivalent of a "black box": we have yet to identify agents of exposure and we have yet to fully appreciate the tissue alterations in the presence of disease.

Refining RCT Methods

In the future, RCTs for vulvodynia will require clear and widely accepted definitions of disease, inclusion/exclusion criteria, and outcome measures [10]. Expert panels such as the *Initiative on Methods, Measurements, and Pain Assessment in Clinical Trials* (IMMPACT) group have convened to define what is "success" (i.e., a core outcome domain) [11] and how to measure it (i.e., patient-reported outcome measure) in pain RCTs [12, 13]. The IMMPACT group has focused much of their effort on widely studied chronic pain conditions, such as postherpetic neuralgia (PHN) and diabetic neuropathy, but the principles apply to vulvodynia as well.

In vulvodynia outcome studies to date, selected primary outcome variables have fallen into three major categories,

Sequential events of molecular epidemiology as applied to vulvodynia*

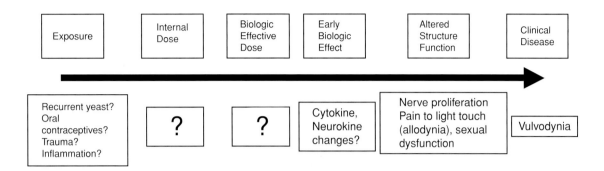

*Adapted from Schulte PA, A conceptual and historical framework for molecular epidemiology. in Molecular Epidemiology Schulte PA, Perera FP eds. Academic press Inc. San Diego CA, 1993, pp 3-44.

Figure 39.1 Research methods of molecular epidemiology applied to the question of vulvodynia etiopathogenesis.

each one with strengths and weaknesses: (i) composite pain scores [14, 15]; (ii) individually designed patient- or clinician-reported assessments [16, 17]; and (iii) quantitative sensory testing (QST) [18, 19]. Composite pain score measures consist of one or several psychometric tests combined with other measures of patient- and clinician-reported outcomes. Although the use of reliable and well-validated tools adds important dimensions for analyses, many psychometric measures lack specificity with regards to vulvodynia. Further, scores can potentially be influenced by coexisting pain conditions (e.g., interstitial cystitis, irritable bowel syndrome, etc.). The complexity of composite scores may increase the difficulty of study replication, and subtle variations of method (e.g., order of administration) may influence the outcome. Although individually designed patient- or clinician-reported measures are specific to the condition under investigation, they hold variable degrees of reliability and validity. RCTs using such measures commonly fail to report their associated reliability and validity, thereby weakening the impact of RCT findings.

QST provides concrete and reliable measures, often specifically designed for vulvar pain assessment. Several researchers have developed QST instruments for vulvar pain testing [18–20]. Unfortunately, QST may be dimensionally limited as a primary outcome variable, and may overlook particular psycho-affective aspects of pain

experience. In addition, the techniques are instrument-dependent, making replication difficult, and data generated by QST may be difficult to extrapolate to real-world pain experiences. At the present time, it appears as if there is no single ideal outcome measure for vulvodynia.

More RCTs Are Required

Although vulvodynia is common, evidence-based treatment options are few. Research efforts to identify effective treatments for vulvodynia via RCTs have been limited to date. To compare treatment options, the gold standard is the back-to-back RCT of one treatment versus another. Practically speaking, however, large-scale RCTs will necessitate a collaborative, multisite design, and it will be physically impossible to involve back-to-back comparisons of all potential treatments. Unfortunately, RCTs are expensive and time-consuming, and they require an adequate number of dedicated patients who are willing to potentially receive placebo. Due to limited resources, an alternative comparison of RCT results have begun to emerge, which involves pooling RCT data through meta-analysis and cross-comparing therapeutic options using two statistically-defined measures: "number needed to treat" (NNT; how many patients are treated before a first success) and "number needed to harm" (NNH; how many patients are treated before a first serious side effect) [21].

Such measures are intuitively attractive because of the impression of a common denominator on which various treatments can be compared. Such meta-analyses necessitate similarly conducted RCTs, with standard protocols that include definitions of disease, inclusion/exclusion criteria, outcome measures, and side effect profiles. The scientific merit of such analyses is subject to question due to the potentially false assumption of similar or equivalent research techniques that may ultimately weaken the conclusion from pooled data. Presently, we lack adequate RCTs in vulvodynia to be capable of generating NNTs and NNHs when comparing various options. As an expanding number of smaller vulvodynia clinical trials are reported, such meta-analyses may be undertaken with caution.

Basic Science Research

Vulvodynia pain mechanisms will undoubtedly be heterogeneous with respect to predominance of peripheral and central neural activity, nerve type/density, neurotransmitters, neurokines, and cytokines. QST profiling is a developing area of research where a more precise somatosensory phenotype is determined by various measurements of sensation (e.g., allodynia, pain with heat, cold, touch) [22]. Imaging peripheral and central nerves should be facilitated by imunohistochemical markers used in tissue and tissue cultures [23] and by vital imaging such as functional magnetic resonance imaging (fMRI) [24]. The role of genetics and epigenetics in vulvodynia will be further strengthened by the development of specific genetic and proteinomic arrays and the development of an animal model for vulvodynia. Ideally, the mouse model should be of central interest because of the potential of developing "vulvodynia knock-outs."

Address the Comorbidity Between Vulvodynia and Other Pain Conditions

Vulvodynia frequently coexists with other chronic somatic and visceral pain conditions, such as irritable bowel syndrome (IBS), interstitial cystitis (IC), and fibromyalgia (FM). Research has only recently tackled this issue and suggests that one or several factors may be involved, including, but not limited to central centralization, viscerosomatic convergence, somatic muscle hypertonicity/instability, and autonomic dysfunction.

Similar to IBS, IC, and FM patients, vulvodynia patients report lowered pain thresholds to pressure and pinprick stimuli and to pain-producing substances such as capsaicin [25–28]. Vulvodynia has also been associated with chronic systolic hypotension similar to that seen in other chronic pain conditions, suggesting a common autonomic dysregulation [27, 29, 30]. The pathophysiologic interrelationships between vulvodynia, IC, IBS, and FM are intriguing but yet unexplained.

Sexual Dysfunction and Relationships Should Be Examined

Population-wide, 43% of women aged 18–59 report sexual problems, with sexual pain being a common complaint [31] and many affected women suffering from significant psychosocial problems [3–6]. Although the interpersonal impact of vulvodynia is believed to lead to unique psychosexual stresses in both members of the couple, most studies have focused solely on the affected woman [32]. However, it can be expected that partner reactions and emotional dynamics can result in significant struggles for some couples and may even affect therapy motivation and adherence. Research should examine these factors.

Specific Research Avenues to Pursue

Diagnostic

QST Profiling: Somatosensory phenotypes have been shown to be heterogeneous within chronic pain conditions (e.g., PHN) and can vary across age and gender categories [22]. Standardized QST protocols have been developed to rapidly provide a profile of 13 parameters, including thermal detection threshold for perception of cold, warm, and paradoxical heat sensations, thermal pain to cold and hot stimuli, and mechanical detection for touch and vibration. QST may permit a vulvodynia classification based upon neurophysiology and, potentially, pathogenesis.

Laser-Evoked Potentials: Neurophysiological function of small fibers (C-fiber and A-delta) can be assessed with CO_2 laser evoked potentials (LEPs). The response to CO_2 laser stimuli within specific dermatomes is measured through cortical activity (scalp potentials). This technique has not yet been used in vulvodynia, but is being used to characterize the varied presentations of PHN [33].

Fibroblast Cell Culture Research: A mechanistic connection has been proposed between pro-inflammatory stimulants (e.g., candida antigen), anatomically specific fibroblasts, enhanced regional IL-1β, IL-6, and IL-8 syntheses, and vestibulodynia [34]. Future fibroblast cell culture research may evolve into the equivalent of a "culture and sensitivity" test for determining effective medical treatments.

Modulation of Schwann Cell Activation: In the peripheral nerve microenvironment, the Schwann cell provides myelin encapsulation of axons, and, following neural injury, it undergoes phenotype changes, leading to proliferation, migration, and the secretion of various neurotropic factors [35]. Given the central role that Schwann cells provide in response to injury, a focus on the modulation of Schwann cell activity may be another research avenue in understanding the pathophysiology of vulvodynia.

Treatment

Cone Snail Research: Carnivorous sea snails (genus: *Conus*) have been found to produce over 500 venoms with 50–200 different peptides, which have a wide range of targets and possible blocking effects on neural fiber activity, producing analgesic properties. One such conotoxin (Ziconodine) is of interest because of its selective blockade of N-type voltage-sensitive calcium channels found in the dorsal root ganglion. The drug has been approved for intrathecal use [34].

Systemically Acting Agents (Cannabinoids): The CB2 cannabinoid has been shown to inhibit acute pain, inflammatory hyperalgesia, and peripheral neuralgia [37]. This antinociceptive effect appears to be independent of a narcotic (endorphin) effect and could provide another novel and effective therapy for vulvodynia.

siRNA Targeting: RNA interference is an evolutionally conserved process where small, interfering double-stranded RNA leads to degradation of homologous messenger RNAs, ultimately leading to reduced protein product. The logical end result with respect to therapy would be to develop antisense strategies to lower various pain-producing proteins, such as the vanilloid receptor, TRPV1 [38].

fMRI: Patients can be trained to modify cortical activity in specific brain areas (e.g., anterior cingulate cortex), leading to threshold changes in pain perception [39]. Such training may provide a feedback tool to facilitate the training of pain modulation in vulvodynia.

References

1 Moyal-Barracco M, Lynch PJ. (2004) ISSVD terminology and classification of vulvodynia: a historical perspective. *The Journal of Reproductive Medicine* **49**, 772–77.

2 Woolf CJ, American C, American P. (2004) Pain: moving from symptom control toward mechanism-specific pharmacologic management. *Annals of Internal Medicine* **140**, 441–51.

3 Goetsch MF. (1991) Vulvar vestibulitis: prevalence and historic features in a general gynecologic practice population. *American Journal of Obstetrics and Gynecology* **164**, 1609–14.

4 Stewart DE, Reicher AE, Gerulath AH, *et al.* (1994) Vulvodynia and psychological distress. *Obstetrics and Gynecology* **84**, 587–90.

5 Nunns D, Mandal D. (1997) Psychological and psychosexual aspects of vulvar vestibulitis. *Genitourinary Medicine* **73**, 541–44.

6 Meana M, Binik YM, Khalifé S, *et al.* (1999) Psychosocial correlates of pain attributions in women with dyspareunia. *Psychosomatics* **40**, 497–502.

7 Harlow BL, Wise LA, Stewart EG. (2001) Prevalence and predictors of chronic lower genital tract discomfort. *American Journal of Obstetrics and Gynecology* **185**, 545–50.

8 Harlow BL, Stewart EG. (2003) A population-based assessment of chronic unexplained vulvar pain: have we underestimated the prevalence of vulvodynia? *Journal of the American Medical Women's Association* **58**, 82–88.

9 Schulte PA. (1993) A conceptual and historical framework for molecular epidemiology. In: Schulte PA, Perera FP (eds.), *Molecular Epidemiology*, 3rd ed. Academic Press, San Diego, pp. 3–44.

10 Landry T, Bergeron S, Dupuis MJ, *et al.* (2008) The treatment of provoked vestibulodynia: a critical review. *Clinical Journal of Pain* **24**, 155–71.

11 Turk DC, Dworkin RH, Allen RR, *et al.* (2003) Core outcome domains for chronic pain clinical trials: IMMPACT recommendations. *Pain* **106**, 337–45.

12 Turk DC, Dworkin RH, Burke LB, *et al.* (2005) Developing patient-reported outcome measures for pain clinical trials: IMMPACT recommendations. *Pain* **125**, 208–15.

13 Dworkin RH, Turk DC, Farrar JT, *et al.* (2005) Core outcome measures for chronic pain clinical trials: IMMPACT recommendations. *Pain* **113**, 9–19.

14 Bergeron S, Binik YM, Khalifé S, *et al.* (2001) A randomized comparison of group cognitive-behavioral therapy, surface electromyographic biofeedback, and vestibulectomy in the treatment of dyspareunia resulting from vulvar vestibulitis. *Pain* **91**, 297–306.

15 Danielsson I, Torstensson T, Brodda-Jansen G, *et al.* (2006) EMG biofeedback versus topical lidocaine gel: a randomized

study for the treatment of women with vulvar vestibulitis. *Acta Obstetricia et Gynecologica Scandinavica* **85**, 1360–67.

16 Bornstein J, Livnat G, Stolar Z, *et al.* (2000) Pure versus complicated vulvar vestibulitis: a randomized trial of fluconazole treatment. *Gynecologic and Obstetric Investigation* **50**, 194–97.

17 Nyirjesy P, Sobel JD, Weitz MV, *et al.* (2001) Cromolyn cream for recalcitrant idiopathic vulvar vestibulitis: results of a placebo-controlled study. *Sexually Transmitted Infections* **77**, 53–57.

18 Eva LJ, Reid WM, MacLean AB, *et al.* (1999) Assessment of response to treatment in vulvar vestibulitis syndrome by means of the vulvar algesiometer. *American Journal of Obstetrics and Gynecology* **181**, 99–102.

19 Pukall CF, Young RA, Roberts MJ, *et al.* (2007) The vulvalgesiometer as a device to measure genital pressure–pain threshold. *Physiological Measurement* **28**, 1543–50.

20 Curnow JS, Barron L, Morrison G, *et al.* (1996) Vulval algesiometer. *Medical and Biological Engineering and Computing* **34**, 266–69.

21 Finnerup NB, Otto M, McQuay HJ, *et al.* (2005) Algorithm for neuropathic pain treatment: an evidence-based proposal. *Pain* **118**, 289–305.

22 Rolke R, Baron R, Maier C, *et al.* (2006) Quantitative sensory testing in the German Research Network on Neuropathic Pain (DFNS): standardized protocol and reference values. *Pain* **123**, 231–43.

23 Tympanidis P, Casula MA, Yiangou Y, *et al.* (2004) Increased vanilloid receptor VR1 innervation in vulvodynia. *European Journal of Pain* **8**, 129–33.

24 Schweinhardt P, Glynn C, Brooks J, *et al.* (2001) An fMRI study of cerebral processing of brush-evoked allodynia in neuropathic pain patients. *Neuroimage* **32**, 256–65.

25 Verne GN, Robinson ME, Price DD. (2001) Hypersensitivity to visceral and cutaneous pain in the irritable bowel syndrome. *Pain* **93**, 7–14.

26 Giesecke J, Reed BD, Haefner HK, *et al.* (2004) Quantitative sensory testing in vulvodynia patients and increased peripheral pressure pain sensitivity. *Obstetrics and Gynecology* **104**, 126–33.

27 Foster DC, Dworkin RH, Wood RW. (2005) Effects of intradermal foot and forearm capsaicin injections in normal and vulvodynia-afflicted women. *Pain* **117**, 128–36.

28 Moshiree B, Price DD, Robinson ME, *et al.* (2007) Thermal and visceral hypersensitivity in irritable bowel syndrome patients with and without fibromyalgia. *Clinical Journal of Pain* **23**, 323–30.

29 Bou-Holaigah I, Calkins H, Flynn JA, *et al.* (1997) Provocation of hypotension and pain during upright tilt table testing in adults with fibromyalgia. *Clinical and Experimental Rheumatology* **15**, 239–46.

30 Gupta V, Sheffield D, Verne GN. (2002) Evidence for autonomic dysregulation in the irritable bowel syndrome. *Digestive Diseases and Sciences* **47**, 1716–22.

31 Laumann EO, Paik A, Rosen RC. (1999) Sexual dysfunction in the United States: prevalence and predictors. *The Journal of the American Medical Association* **281**, 537–44.

32 Foster D, Kotok M. (2007) Vulvodynia's psychological impact on the partner. *NVA News* **12**, 1–5

33 Truini A, Haanpaa M, Zucchi R, *et al.* (2003) Laser-evoked potentials in post-herpetic neuralgia. *Clinical Neurophysiology* **114**, 702–09.

34 Foster DC, Piekarz KH, Murant TI, *et al.* (2006) Enhanced synthesis of proinflammatory cytokines by vulvar vestibular fibroblasts: implications for vulvar vestibulitis. *American Journal of Obstetrics and Gynecology* **196**, 346.

35 Campana WM. (2007) Schwann cells: activated peripheral glia and their role in neuropathic pain. *Brain, Behavior, and Immunity* **21**, 522–27.

36 Sharp D. (2006) Novel pain relief via marine snails. *Lancet* **366**, 439–40.

37 Ibrahim MM, Rude ML, Stagg NJ, *et al.* (2006) CB2 cannabinoid receptor mediation of antinociception. *Pain* **122**, 36–42.

38 Rohl T, Kurreck J. (2006) RNA interference in pain research. *Journal of Neurochemistry* **99**, 371–80.

39 deCharms RC, Maeda F, Glover GH, *et al.* (2005) Control over brain activation and pain learned by using real-time functional MRI. *Proceedings of the National Academy of Sciences of the United States of America* **102**, 18626–31.

Conclusion

The cardinal rule in medicine is *primum non nocere*—above all do no harm. Unfortunately, too many women suffering from sexual pain disorders have not been helped by their health care providers—through being ignored, being told the pain was purely psychologic without a biologic evaluation, being told it was purely biologic without a psychologic assessment, being prescribed medications for other purposes without full disclosure regarding potential side effects, being treated with ineffective therapies, or simply not being referred to a specialist when the problem warranted. This book should serve as a resource for health care providers, so that ultimately women receive appropriate multidisciplinary attention and care for their sexual pain disorders.

The field of sexual medicine has grown significantly over the last decade with regard to women's sexual health. Models of the sexual response cycle have moved from Masters and Johnson straight-line model engaging arousal, to Helen Singer Kaplan's linear concept engaging desire, to Rosemary Basson's circular model. Michael Sand and Bill Fisher have shown that each of these models may be correct depending upon the sexual function or dysfunction of the particular women. None of these models mentions sexual pain. Is it a sexual disorder or a pain disorder? Perhaps this is why we have not seen any one specialty focused on providing care in this area: gynecology, psychology, sexual medicine, urology, dermatology, physical therapy, despite the focus by basic scientists to learn more about sexual physiology.

Physiology implies normal function. While there has been research in the physiology of desire, arousal, and orgasm, there has been limited study into the absence of pain, although by definition, the absence of pain is normal function. Pathophysiology of desire, arousal, and orgasm problems has also been studied, and validated outcome scales exist to help assess these issues.

It is only recently that behavioral models of pain have been developed, but biologic pathophysiologic models are still lacking, and a specific outcome scale targeting sexual pain is yet to be validated. It is difficult to envision an easy fix to pain problems when no one claims it as their turf. There are too many groups looking at small pieces of the puzzle without integrating those pieces into a finished picture.

It is our sincerest hope that this book will offer the tools required by both generalists and specialists to begin to address women's sexual pain problems. For them, whether or not this is a sexual disorder or a pain disorder has no bearing. For women suffering, all they ask is that you, the provider, help them stop hurting.

Index

Note: Italicised f and t refer to figures and tables.

mast cells, 176–8
  clinical significance of, 178
  functional role of, 177–8
    inflammatory response, 177
    neovascularization, 177–8
    neurogenic inflammation, 177
    neurogenic response, 177
    re-epithelialization, 177–8
    scarring, 178
    vascular response, 177
  importance of, 176
  morphology of, 176–7
  overview of, 176
Mayer Roikitansky Kuster Hauser
    (MRKH) syndrome, 121
McCoy Female Sexuality
    Questionnaire (MFSQ), 23
McGill Pain Questionnaire, 11
McGill Melzack Pain Questionnaire
    (MPQ), 22
medical history, 14–15, 28
Medical Research Fund, 252
medications, and dyspareunia, 15–17
Medoc Thermal Genital Sensory
    Analyzer, 24
Medoc Vibratory Sensory Analyzer,
    24
meperidine, 173
methadone, 173
methylprednisolone, 159
metronidazole, 71*t*, 99
miconazole, 102*t*
mifepristone, 197
Mirena IUD, 197
Mittleshmertz, 196
modified vestibulectomy, 162
morphine, 173
mucous membrane pemphigoid,
    54–5
Müllerian duct, 119
muscle assessment, 246
musculoskeletal exam, 29
myofascial trigger point release, 83

National Institutes of Health (NIH),
    251–2, 256
National Vulvodynia Association
    (NVA), 250–54
  advocates, 254
  career development award, 252
  educational information, 250

healthcare provider referrals,
    251
  lobbying for research funding,
    251–2
  medical research fund, 252
  online support, 250–51
  partners, 254
  professional education, 252–3
  public awareness campaign,
    253–4
  support network, 250–51
Neisseria gonorrhea, 69, 72
neovascularization, 177–8
neural mobilization, 83–4
neuralgia, pudendal, 112–6
  anatomy of, 112–4
  clinical features of, 112–6
  diagnosis of, 114–5
  etiology of, 114
  modification of activities in, 115
  neurophysiologic testing, 114
  overview, 112
  pharmacological measures, 115
  physical therapy treatment of,
    115–6
  pudendal nerve block, 114–6
  pudendal nerve decompression,
    116
neurogenic inflammation, 177
neurological assessment, 247
Neurontin, 79
nitroglycerin, 158
nitroimidazole, 99
noninfectious vaginitis, 105–10
  atrophic, 105–7
    diagnosis of, 106–7
    etiology of, 105
    sexual dysfunction in, 105–6
    treatment of, 107
  desquamative inflammatory,
    107–10
    diagnosis of, 109
    epidemiology, 108
    etiology of, 108–9
    microscopic findings in, 109*f*
    overview of, 108–9
    treatment of, 109–10
  treatment of, 102–3
Norpramin, 78
nortriptyline, 78, 90, 172
nysatin, 102*t*

Office of Research on Women's
    Health (ORWH), 252
OLeary Sant Symptom and Problem
    Index (OSSOI), 89–90
opioids, 173
oral contraceptives, 15, 69, 197
ovarian masses, 195–6
ovarian suppression, 220
ovulatory pain, 196
oxycodone, 173

pain, 199–200. *See also* dyspareunia
  animal models of, 199–205
    colitis, 203–4
    common pain behaviors, 201*t*
    endometriosis, 202–3
    evaluation of, 199–200
    interstitial cystitis, 203
    parturition, 203–4
    uretheral calculosis, 200
    uterine distension, 202
    uterine inflammation, 200–202
    vaginal distension, 202
    validity of, 204–5
    yeast-induced sensitization to
      touch, 204
  behaviors, 201*t*, 205*t*
  injectable therapy, 158–60
    anesthetics, 159
    benefit of, 156
    botulinum toxin, 159–60
    corticosteroids, 158–9
    interferon, 159
    side effects and limitations, 157
  interference and comorbid
      problems, 21–2
  mediators, 21
  in pelvic floor dysfunction, 160
  properties, 21
  self-administered measures, 22–3
  topical therapy, 156–9
    anesthetics, 157
    benefit of, 156
    capsaicin, 157–8
    drug trials, 157
    estrogen, 158
    gabapentin, 158
    nitroglycerin, 158
    side effects and limitations, 157
    testosterone, 158
    tricyclic antidepressants, 158